Virtual Medical Office

for

Beik:
Health Insurance Today: A Practical Approach
Fifth Edition

Virtual Medical Office

for

Beik:
Health Insurance Today: A Practical Approach
Fifth Edition

Textbook by

Janet Beik, AA, MA, MEd
Southeastern Community College (Retired)
Administrative Instructor
Medical Assistant Program
West Burlington, Iowa

Software developed by

Wolfsong Informatics, LLC
Tucson, Arizona

Study Guide prepared by

JRC Press
Honey Brook, Pennsylvania

ELSEVIER

ELSEVIER

3251 Riverport Lane
St. Louis, Missouri 63043

VIRTUAL MEDICAL OFFICE FOR
BEIK: HEALTH INSURANCE TODAY: A PRACTICAL APPROACH
FIFTH EDITION

ISBN: 978-0-323-22119-1

Notices

Knowledge and best practice in this field are constantly changing. As new research and experience broaden our understanding, changes in research methods, professional practices, or medical treatment may become necessary.

Practitioners and researchers must always rely on their own experience and knowledge in evaluating and using any information, methods, compounds, or experiments described herein. In using such information or methods they should be mindful of their own safety and the safety of others, including parties for whom they have a professional responsibility.

With respect to any drug or pharmaceutical products identified, readers are advised to check the most current information provided (i) on procedures featured or (ii) by the manufacturer of each product to be administered, to verify the recommended dose or formula, the method and duration of administration, and contraindications. It is the responsibility of practitioners, relying on their own experience and knowledge of their patients, to make diagnoses, to determine dosages and the best treatment for each individual patient, and to take all appropriate safety precautions.

To the fullest extent of the law, neither the Publisher nor the authors, contributors, or editors, assume any liability for any injury and/or damage to persons or property as a matter of products liability, negligence or otherwise, or from any use or operation of any methods, products, instructions, or ideas contained in the material herein.

International Standard Book Number: 978-0-323-22119-1

Executive Content Strategist: Jennifer Janson
Content Development Manager: Luke Held
Senior Content Development Specialist: Jennifer Bertucci
Publishing Services Manager: Debbie Vogel
Project Manager: Pat Costigan

Printed in the United States of America

Last digit is the print number: 9 8 7 6 5 4 3 2

Table of Contents

GETTING STARTED

The product you have purchased is part of the Evolve Learning System. Please read the following information thoroughly to get started.

HOW TO ACCESS YOUR VMO RESOURCES ON EVOLVE

There are two ways to access your VMO Resources on Evolve:

1. If your instructor has enrolled you in your VMO Evolve Resources, you will receive an email with your registration details.

2. If your instructor has asked you to self-enroll in your VMO Evolve Resources, he or she will provide you with your Course ID (for example, 1479_jdoe73_0001). You will then need to follow the instructions at https://evolve.elsevier.com/cs/studentEnroll.html.

HOW TO ACCESS THE ONLINE VIRTUAL MEDICAL OFFICE

The Virtual Medical Office simulation is available through the Evolve VMO Resources. There is no software to download or install: the Virtual Medical Office simulation runs within your Internet browser, directly linked from the Evolve site.

HOW TO ACCESS THE WORKBOOK

There are two ways to access the workbook portion of *Virtual Medical Office:*

1. Print workbook
2. An electronic version of the workbook, available within the VMO Evolve Resources

TECHNICAL SUPPORT

Technical support for *Virtual Medical Office* is available by visiting the Technical Support Center at http://evolvesupport.elsevier.com or by calling 1-800-222-9570 inside the United States and Canada.

Virtual Medical Office Quick Tour

Welcome to *Virtual Medical Office* (VMO), a virtual office setting in which you can work with multiple patient simulations and also learn to access and evaluate the information resources that are essential for providing high-quality medical assistance.

VMO's medical office is called Mountain View Clinic. Once you have signed in to Mountain View Clinic, you can access the Reception area, Exam Room, Laboratory, Office Manager area, and Check Out area, as well as a separate room for Billing and Coding.

BEFORE YOU START

Make sure you have your textbook nearby when you use VMO. You will want to consult topic areas in your textbook frequently while working online and using this Study Guide.

HOW TO SIGN IN

- Access the simulation on the Evolve resource page for your textbook. See the **Getting Started** instructions on page 1 of the Study Guide for information on accessing your Evolve resources.
- Enter your name on the medical assistant identification badge. The name entered here will print out on your performance summary reports.
- Click **Start Simulation**.

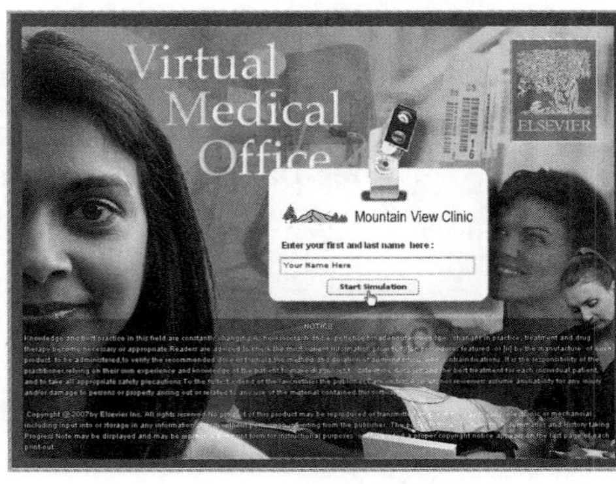

- This takes you to the office map screen. Across the top of this screen are photos of patients available for you to follow throughout their office visit.

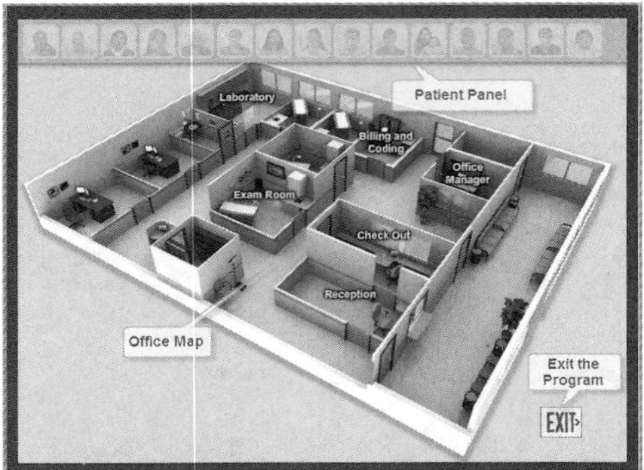

PATIENT LIST

1. **Janet Jones (age 50)**—Ms. Jones has sustained an on-the-job injury. She is in pain and impatient. By working with Ms. Jones, students will learn about managing difficult patients, as well as the requirements involved in workers' compensation cases.

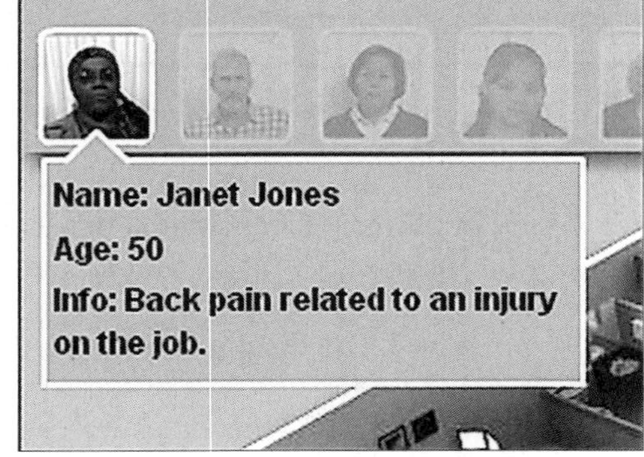

2. **Wilson Metcalf (age 65)**—A Medicare patient, Mr. Metcalf is being seen for multiple symptoms of abdominal pain, nausea, vomiting, and fever. He is seriously ill and might need more specialized care in a hospital setting.

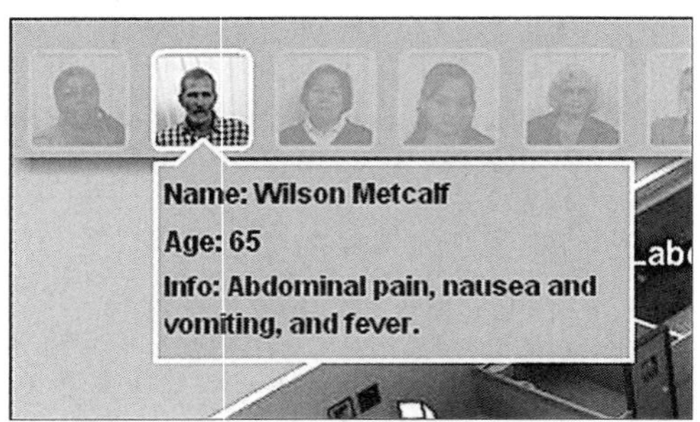

3. **Rhea Davison (age 53)**—An established patient with chronic and multiple symptoms, Ms. Davison does not have medical insurance.

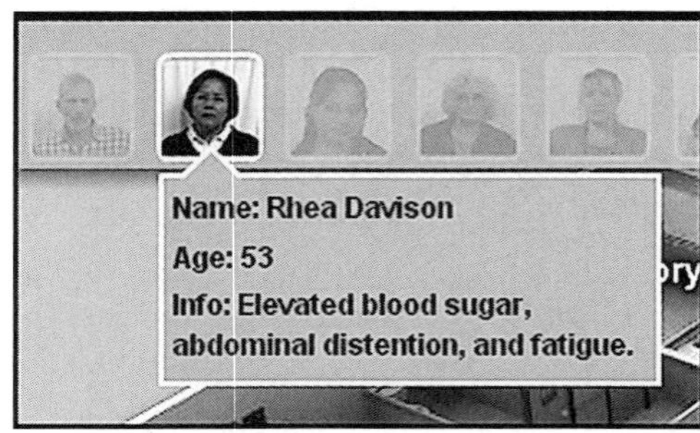

4. **Shaunti Begay (age 15)**—A new patient, Shaunti Begay is a minor who has an appointment for a sports physical. Upon arrival, Shaunti and her family learn that Mountain View Clinic does not participate in their health insurance.

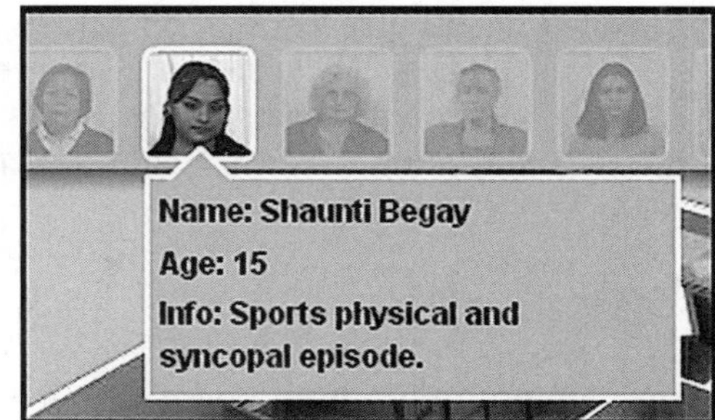

5. **Jean Deere (age 83)**—Accompanied by her son, Ms. Deere is an established Medicare patient being evaluated for memory loss and hearing loss.

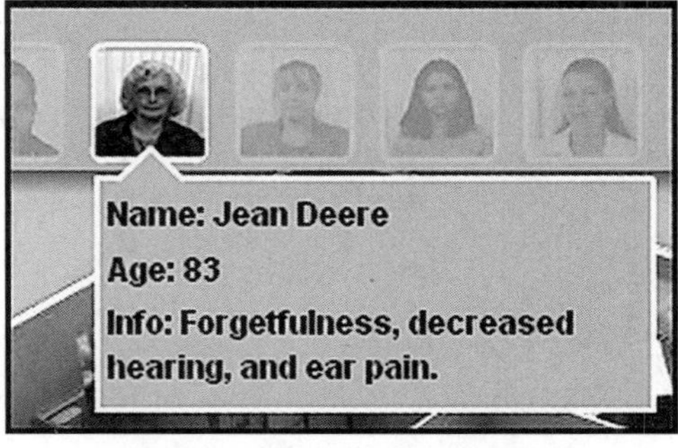

6. **Renee Anderson (age 43)**—Ms. Anderson scheduled her appointment for a routine gynecologic exam but exhibits symptoms that suggest she is a victim of domestic violence.

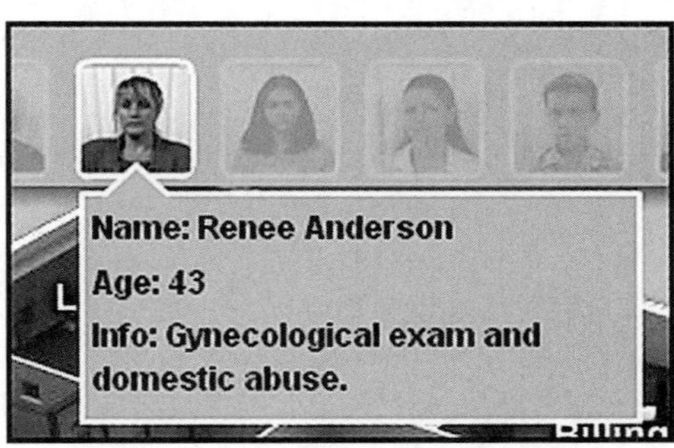

7. **Teresa Hernandez (age 16)**—Teresa is a minor patient who is unaccompanied by a parent for her appointment. She is seeking contraceptive counseling and STD testing.

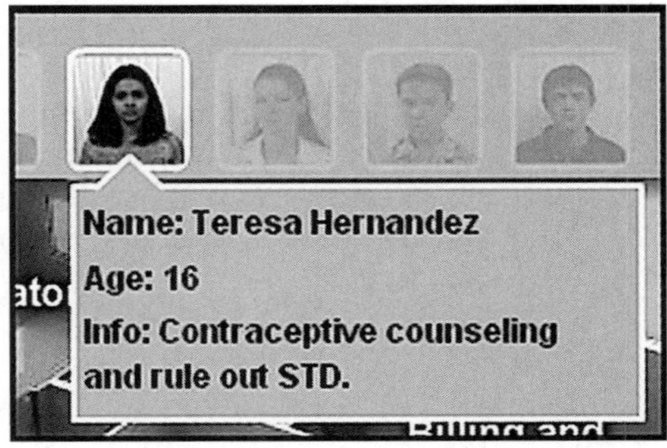

8. **Louise Parlet (age 24)**—Ms. Parlet is an established patient being seen for a pregnancy test and examination. She will also need to be referred to an OB/GYN specialist.

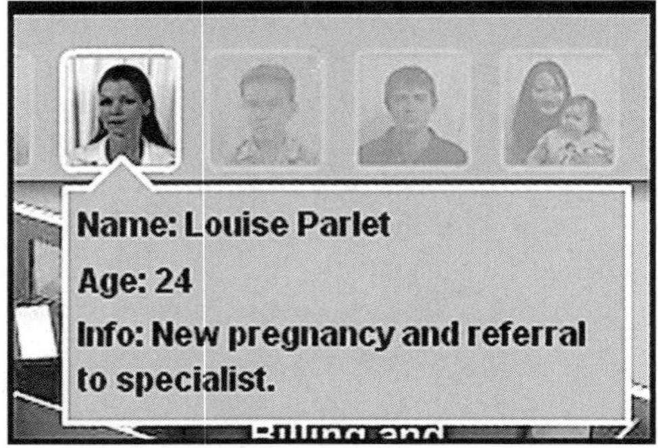

9. **Tristan Tsosie (age 8)**—A minor patient accompanied by his older sister and younger brother, Tristan is having a splint and sutures removed from his injured right arm.

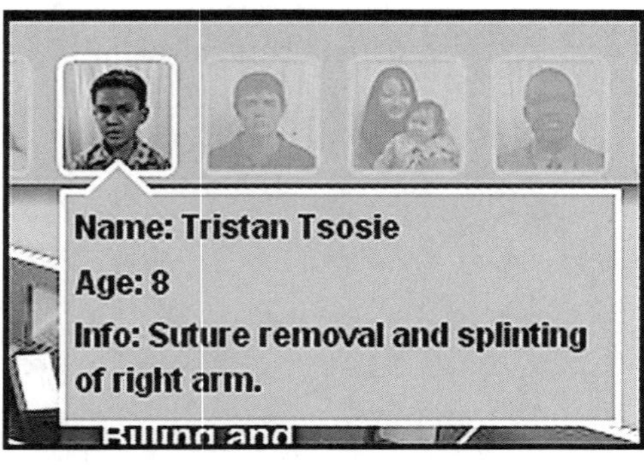

10. **Jose Imero (age 16)**—Jose is a minor patient who is scheduled for an emergency appointment to have the laceration on his foot sutured.

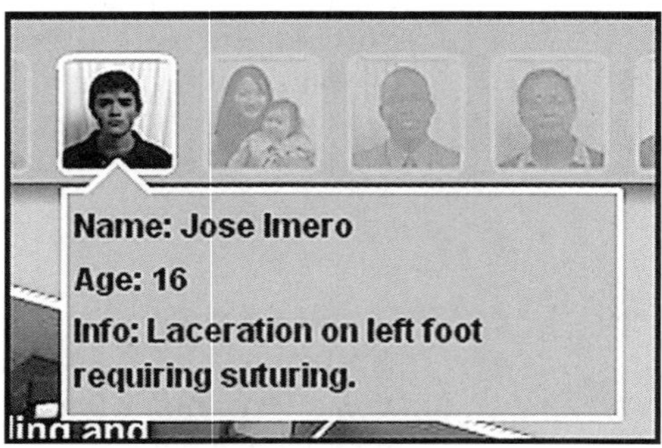

11. **Jade Wong (age 7 months)**—Jade and her parents are new patients to Mountain View Clinic. Jade needs a checkup and updates to her immunizations. Her mother does not speak English.

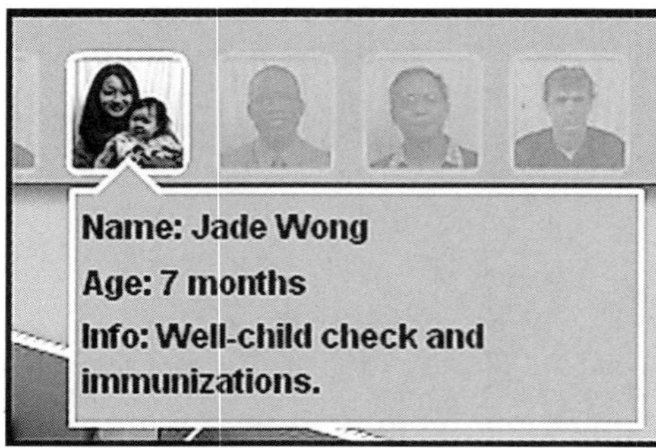

12. **John R. Simmons (age 43)**—Dr. Simmons is a new patient with a history of high blood pressure and recent episodes of blood in his urine.

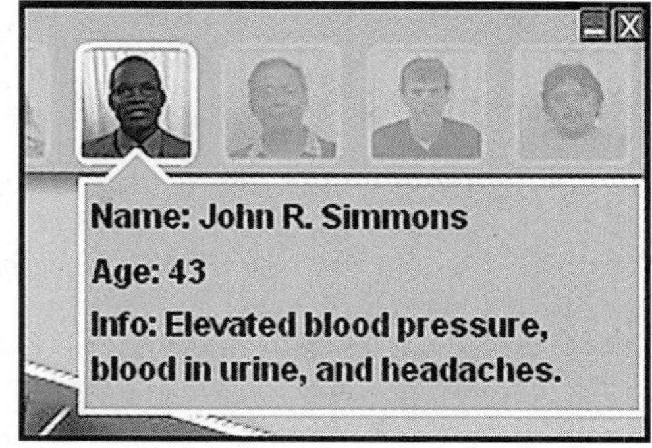

13. **Hu Huang (age 67)**—Mr. Huang developed a severe cough and fever after returning from a recent trip to Asia.

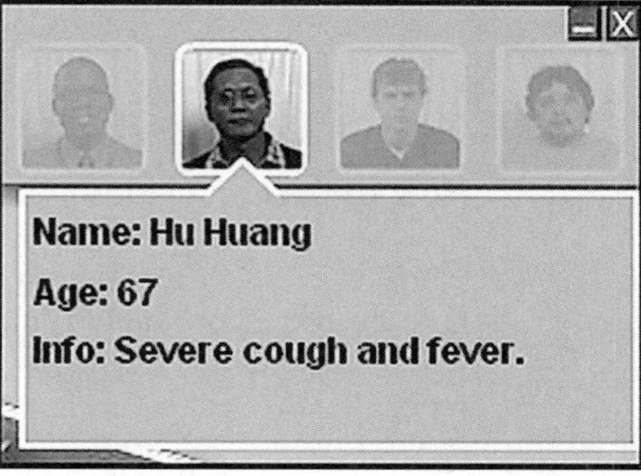

14. **Kevin McKinzie (age 18)**—Mr. McKinzie has made an appointment because of his nausea and vomiting. He is insured through the restaurant where he works.

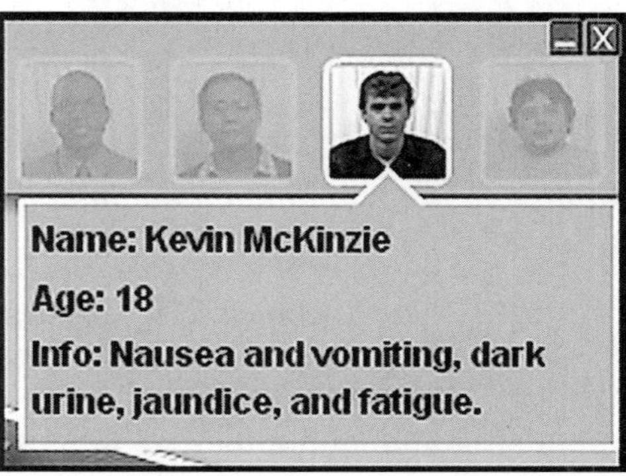

15. **Jesus Santo (age 32)**—Mr. Santo has been brought to the office as a walk-in appointment by his employer for leg pain and a fever. He has no insurance or identification, but his employer has offered to pay for the visit.

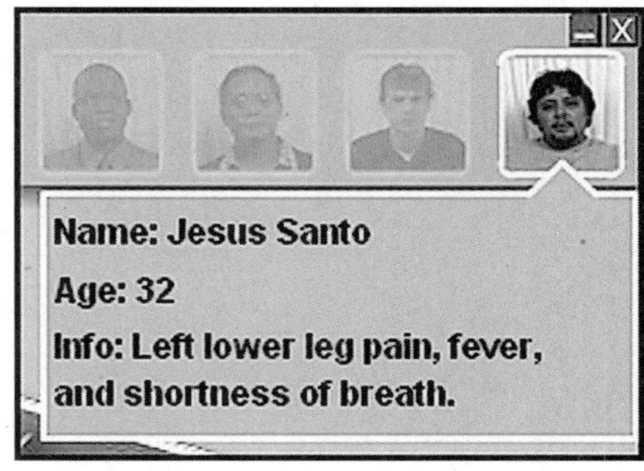

■ BASIC NAVIGATION

HOW TO SELECT A PATIENT

The list of patients is located across the top of the office map screen. Pointing your cursor at the various patients will highlight their photo and reveal their name, age, and medical problem (see examples in the illustrations on the previous pages). When you click on the patient you wish to review, a larger photo and description will appear in the lower left corner of the screen.

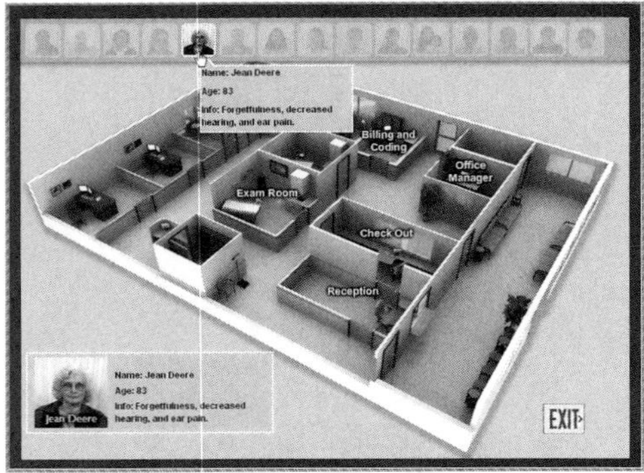

HOW TO SELECT A ROOM

After selecting a patient, use your cursor to highlight the room you want to enter. The active room will be shaded blue on the map. Click to enter the room.

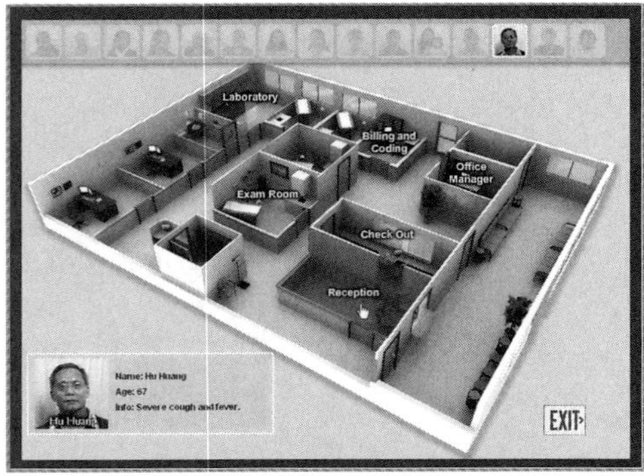

Note: You ***must*** select a patient before you are allowed access to any room, except for the Office Manager's area.

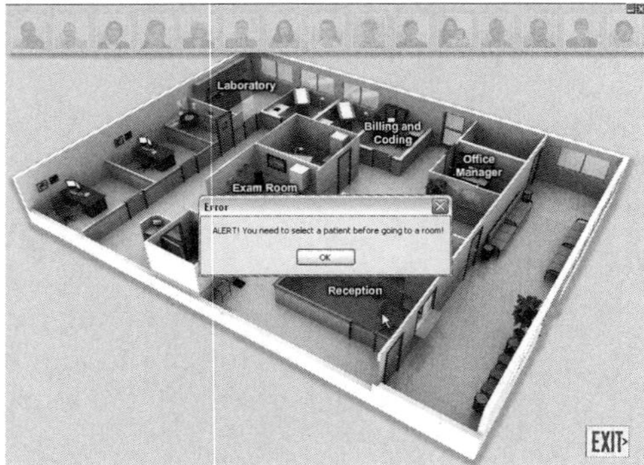

HOW TO LEAVE A ROOM

When you are finished working in a room, you can leave by clicking the exit arrow found at the bottom right corner of the screen.

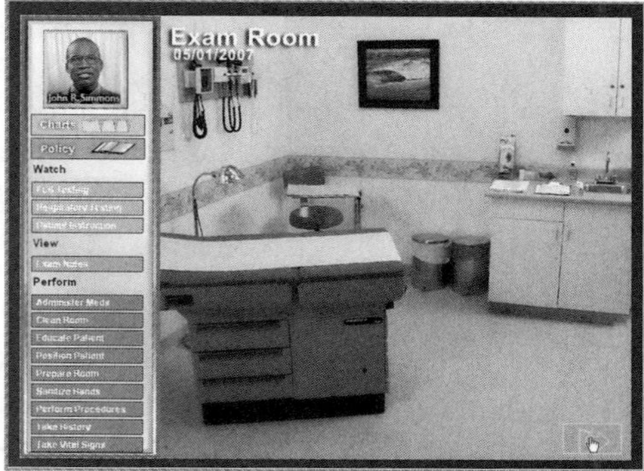

Leaving a room will automatically take you to the Summary Menu.

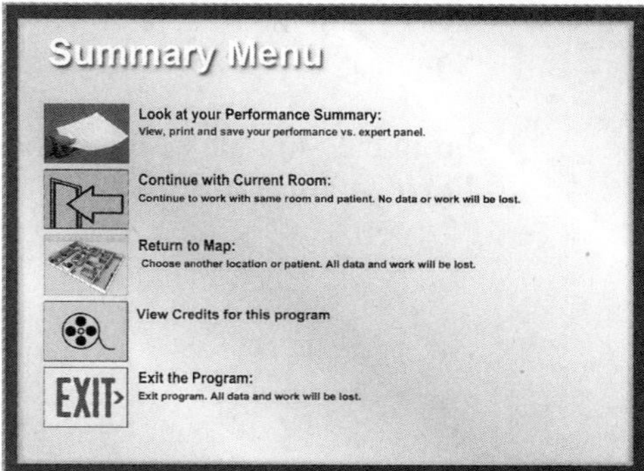

From the Summary Menu, you can choose to:

- **Look at Your Performance Summary**
  In each room there are interactive wizards or tasks that can be completed. The Performance Summary lets you compare your answers with those of the experts.
- **Continue with Current Room**
  This takes you back to the last room in which you worked. This option is not available if you have already reviewed your Performance Summary.
- **Return to Map**
  This reopens the office map for you to select another room and/or another patient.
- **View Credits for This Program**
  This provides a complete listing of software developers, publisher, and authors.
- **Exit the Program**
  This closes the *Virtual Medical Office* software. You will need to sign in again before you can use the program.

Note: If you choose to return to the office map, VMO alerts you that all unsaved room data will be lost. This means that any tasks completed in that room will be reset. Choose **Yes** to continue to the office map or **No** to return to the Summary Menu, where you can choose to continue working in the room or look at your Performance Summary.

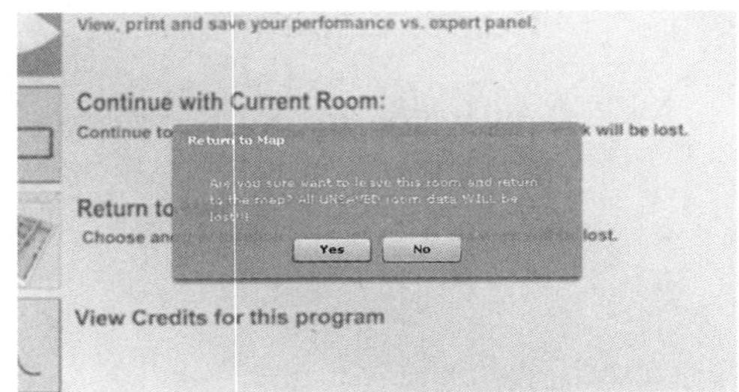

HOW TO USE THE PERFORMANCE SUMMARY

If you completed any of the interactive wizards in a room, you can compare your answers with those of the experts by accessing your Performance Summary. This feature can be accessed after working in the Reception area, Exam Room, Laboratory, and Check Out area. The Performance Summary is not a grading tool, although it is valuable for self-assessment and review.

From the Summary Menu, click on **Look at Your Performance Summary**.

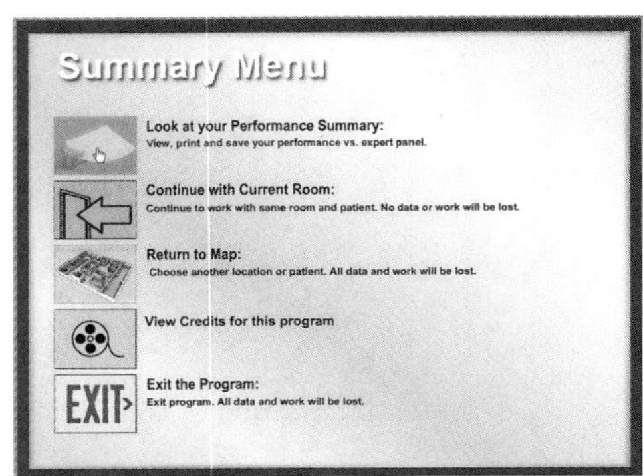

The complete list of tasks associated with the active room will appear with two columns showing the results of your choices. Your answers will appear in the column labeled **Your Performance**, and the answers chosen by the expert will appear in the **Expert's Performance** column. A check mark in both columns for a given task indicates that your answer matched the expert's answer. The Performance Summary can be saved to your computer or disk by clicking on the disk icon at the upper right side of the screen. The saved file can be printed or e-mailed to your instructor. A hard copy can also be printed without saving by clicking on the printer icon at the upper right corner of the screen.

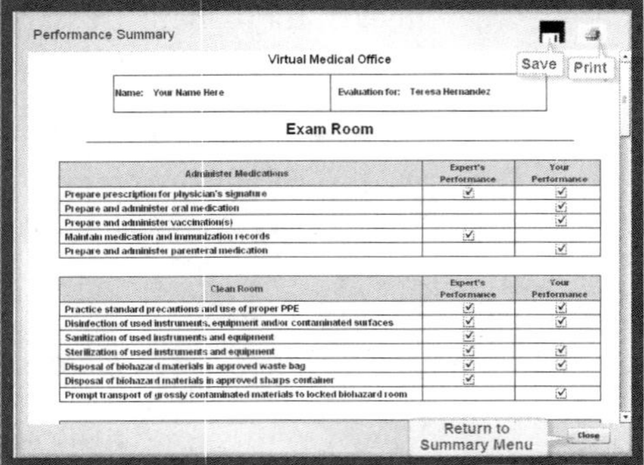

ROOM DESCRIPTIONS

All rooms can be entered at any time and in any order. You can follow a patient's visit from Reception to Check Out, or you can choose to observe patients at any point in their care. Below is a description of the information and activities that can be found in various rooms.

ALL ROOMS

- You can access the patient's medical record (Charts) and the office Policy Manual in all rooms.
- Each room has a sidebar Room Menu, from which you can choose to view documents, perform tasks, and watch videos.

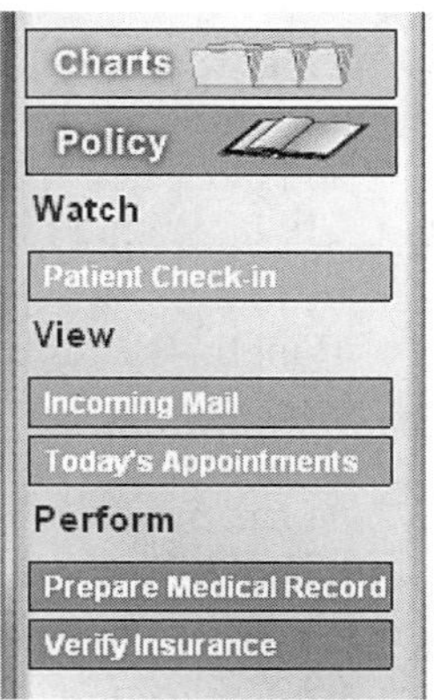

- The Reception area, Exam Room, and Check Out areas all feature videos in which you can watch the medical assistant interact with other Mountain View Clinic personnel and patients. Within the video screen you have a variety of options for navigating. Hover your cursor over the controls and status bar along the bottom of the video screen to reveal how each functions. By clicking various controls, you can play the video, pause it, forward or rewind using the scroll bar, and adjust the volume. Pressing the square stop button will stop the video and return the scroll bar to the beginning. Close the video screen by clicking on the **X** in the upper right corner of the screen.

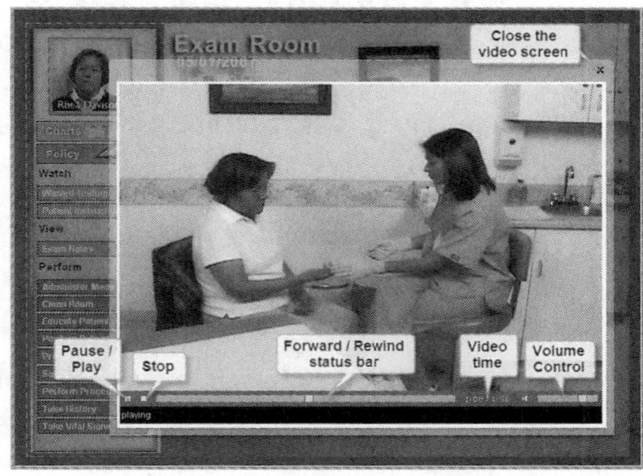

- Almost all rooms have **View** and **Perform** options on the Room Menu (***Note:*** The Billing and Coding area does not have any Perform functions). These tasks can be completed either by clicking on the task description in the Room Menu or by clicking on the corresponding object in the room area. (For example, during an exercise, if you are required to perform the task of sanitizing your hands, the instructions may be worded as "Click on **Sanitize Hands** under Perform on the Room Menu," or you may simply be asked to "Click on the **Sink**." Both routes take you to the same task.) As you move your cursor over each item connected to one of the tasks on the View or Perform menu, both the object and the corresponding task in the Room Menu will highlight and become active. (***Note:*** All corresponding pairs of instruction cues are listed in the individual room descriptions on the following pages.)

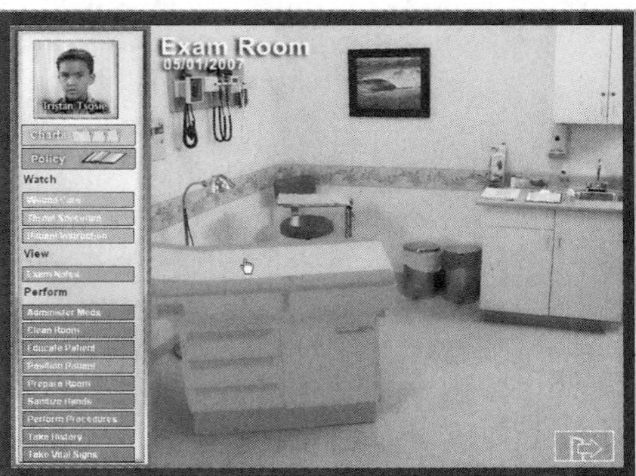

RECEPTION

In the Reception area, you can choose:

- **Charts**—Look at the patient's chart. ***Note:*** For new patients, there will be no information available in the chart at this time, although you do have the option of assembling a new medical record.
- **Policy**—Open the office Policy Manual and review the established administrative, clinical, and laboratory policies for Mountain View Clinic. Within the Policy Manual you will also find the Coding and Billing Manual.
- **Watch**—Watch a video of the patient's arrival. Each patient is shown checking in at the front desk so that you can observe the procedures typically performed by the receptionist and consider some of the various problems that might arise.
- **View**—Look at the Incoming Mail for the day by clicking on the stack of letters located on the **Stackable Trays** on the Reception desk. Review Today's Appointments by clicking on the **Computer** on the Reception desk to open up the day's schedule.
- **Perform**—Perform tasks at the Reception desk that are part of an administrative medical assistant's duties. Practice how to Prepare a Medical Record for a patient by clicking on the **Medical Record** file folder on the Reception desk. Verify Insurance for a patient by clicking on the **Insurance Card** on the counter at the Reception desk window.

EXAM ROOM

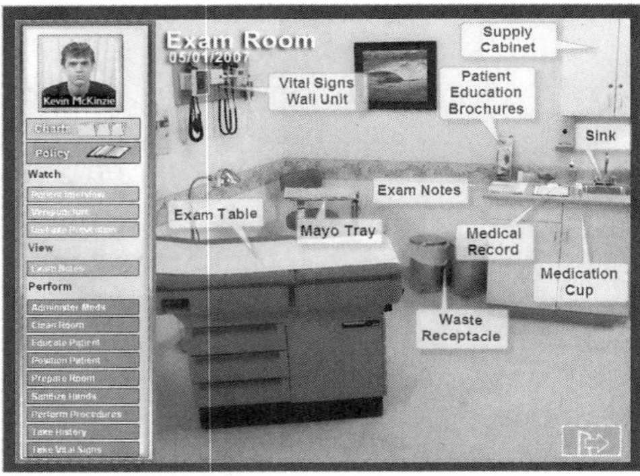

- **Charts** and **Policy**—Access the patient's chart and the office Policy Manual.
- **Watch**—View videos of different parts of the patient's exam. Observe the actions of the medical assistants in the videos and critique the competencies demonstrated.
- **View**—Review the physician's documented findings for the current visit in the Exam Notes. These notes are added to the full Progress Notes in the patient's chart as the patient continues on to Check Out. This can be accessed by clicking on the **Exam Notes** on the Exam Room counter.
- **Perform**—Perform multiple tasks that are required of a clinical medical assistant, such as preparing the room for the exam, taking vital signs and patient history, and properly positioning the patient for an exam. For each task listed under Perform on the Room Menu (cues on the left below), a corresponding object in the room area (cues on the right below) can also be clicked to access and perform the task:
  - **Administer Meds = Medication Cup**
  - **Clean Room = Waste Receptacles**
  - **Educate Patient = Patient Education Brochures**
  - **Position Patient = Exam Table**
  - **Prepare Room = Supply Cabinet**
  - **Sanitize Hands = Sink**
  - **Perform Procedures = Mayo Tray**
  - **Take History = Medical Record**
  - **Take Vital Signs = Vital Signs Wall Unit**

LABORATORY

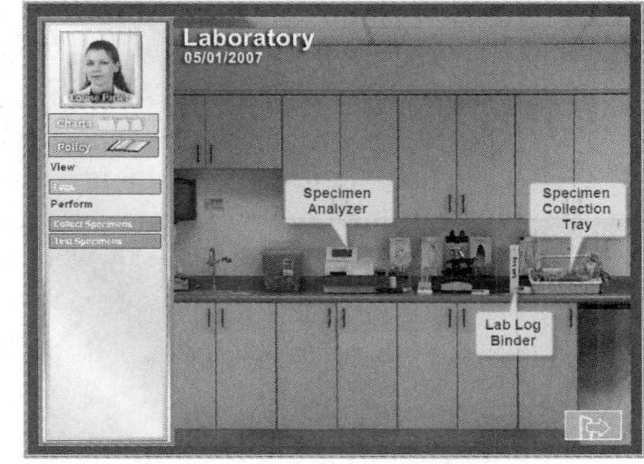

- **Charts** and **Policy**—Access the patient's chart and the office Policy Manual.
- **View**—View the laboratory's log of specimens sent out for testing. Opportunities to practice filling out laboratory logs are included in the Study Guide exercises. This can be accessed by clicking on the **Lab Log Binder** on the Laboratory counter.
- **Perform**—Perform specific tasks as needed in the laboratory, such as collecting and testing specimens. These interactive wizards walk you through the steps for collecting and testing specimens ordered by the physician as part of the patient's exam. Access the Collect Specimens function by clicking on the **Specimen Collection Tray** on the counter. Complete the Test Specimens task by clicking on the **Specimen Analyzer**, also on the laboratory counter.

CHECK OUT

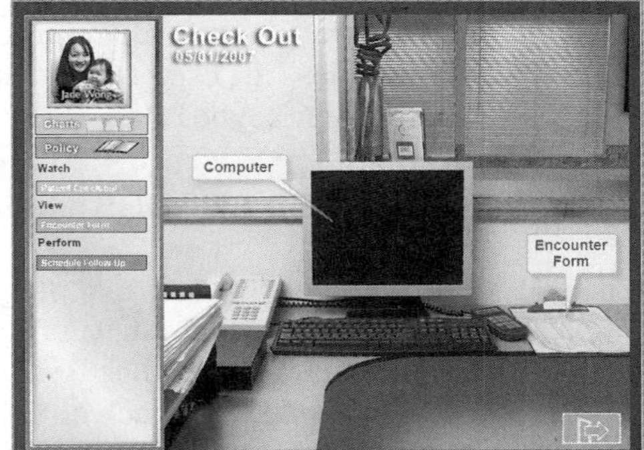

- **Charts** and **Policy**—Access the patient's chart and the office Policy Manual.
- **Watch**—Watch a video of the patient checking out of the office at the end of the visit. Observe the administrative medical assistants as they schedule follow-up appointments, accept payments, and manage the various duties and problems that may arise.
- **View**—The Encounter Form for each patient's visit can be accessed by clicking on the **Encounter Form** on the clipboard on the Check Out desk.
- **Perform**—Certain patients will require a return visit to the office. Schedule their follow-up appointments as needed by clicking on the **Computer** on the Check Out desk.

BILLING AND CODING

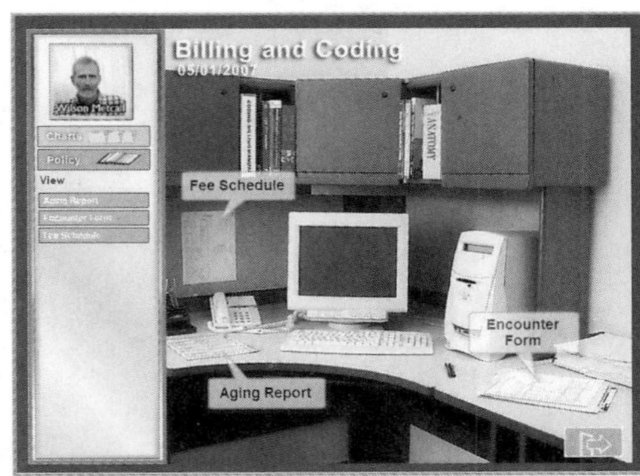

- **Charts** and **Policy**—Access the patient's chart and the office Policy Manual.
- **View**—Review the outstanding balances on various patient accounts and assess when to implement different collection techniques by clicking on the **Aging Report** on the left side of the Billing and Coding desk. Use the patient's **Encounter Form** on the right side of the desk to determine whether the proper procedures were followed to ensure accurate billing and coding. The office's **Fee Schedule** (on the wall to the left of the computer) is used to calculate the proper charges for the patient's visit.

OFFICE MANAGER

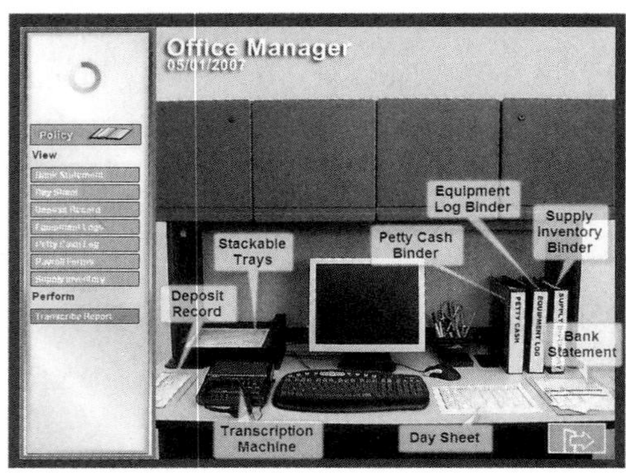

- **Policy**—View the office Policy Manual. Note that patient charts are not available from the Office Manager area.
- **View**—A variety of financial and administrative documents are available for viewing in the Office Manager area to practice managing office finances. Corresponding clues are listed below (menu terms on left; object cues on right):
  - **Bank Statement** = **Bank Statement** green file folder
  - **Day Sheet** = **Day Sheet** to the right of the computer keyboard
  - **Deposit Record** = **Deposit Record** to the left of the **Transcription Machine**
  - **Equipment Logs** = **Equipment Log Binder**
  - **Petty Cash Log** = **Petty Cash Binder**
  - **Payroll Forms** = located in the **Stackable Trays**
  - **Supply Inventory** = **Supply Inventory Binder**
- **Perform**—A recorded medical report is included for transcription practice with full player controls. This can be accessed by clicking on the Transcription Machine to the left of the computer keyboard.

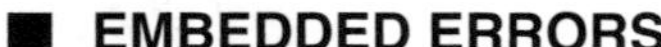

■ EMBEDDED ERRORS

The individual lessons and patient scenarios associated with the *Virtual Medical Office* program were designed to stimulate critical thinking and analytical skills and to help develop the competencies you will be tested on as part of your course work. Thus deliberate errors have been embedded into each of the 15 patient scenarios and in the Billing and Coding and Office Manager activities. Many of the exercises in the Study Guide draw attention to these errors so that you can learn to recognize when and why a correction needs to be made, as well as how to correct it. Other errors have not been specifically addressed, and you may discover them as you work through the various rooms and tasks. These errors, when found, provide great learning opportunities to further develop the essential critical thinking and decision-making skills needed for professional work in the clinical office.

The following icons are used throughout the Study Guide to help you quickly identify particular activities and assignments:

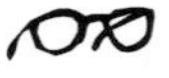 Reading Assignment—tells you which textbook chapter(s) you should read before starting each lesson

 Writing Activity—certain activities focus on written responses such as filling out forms or completing documentation

 Online Activity—marks the beginning of an activity that uses the *Virtual Medical Office* simulation software

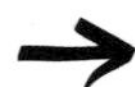 Online Instructions—indicates the steps to follow as you navigate through the software

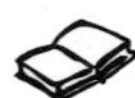 Reference—indicates questions and activities that require you to consult your textbook

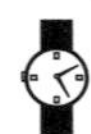 Time—indicates the approximate amount of time needed to complete the exercise

Virtual Medical Office Detailed Tour

If you wish to understand the capabilities of *Virtual Medical Office* more thoroughly, take a detailed tour by completing the following exercises. During this tour, we will work with a specific patient to introduce you to all the different components and learning opportunities available within the VMO software for the Medical Insurance/Billing & Coding student.

Exercise 1

Online Activity—Role of an Insurance Billing Specialist

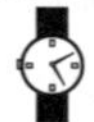

45 minutes

- Sign in to Mountain View Clinic and select **Shaunti Begay** from the patient list. Highlight the **Reception** area and click to enter. Remember, except for the Office Manager's area, you cannot enter any of the rooms on the map until a patient is selected.

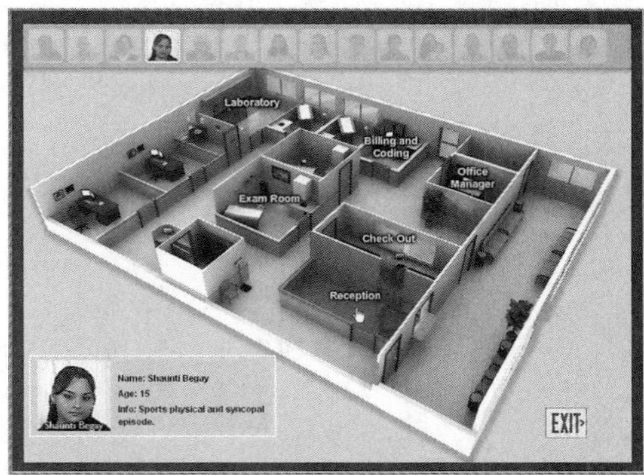

- You are now at the **Reception** desk, where Shaunti Begay will check in for her appointments. In this room you can watch the Check-In video for important information about her visit and review her insurance information.

- From the Room Menu under the Watch heading, select **Patient Check-In** and watch the video of Shaunti checking in for her appointment. You can use the video controls to pause, rewind, fast-forward, and adjust the volume as you watch.

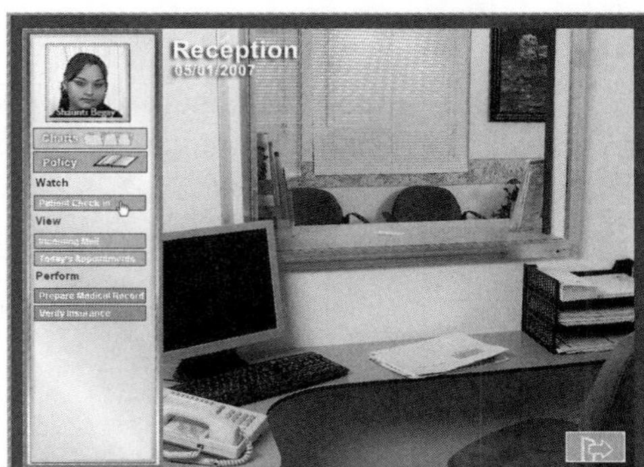

1. What information about Shaunti Begay and her visit were you able to gather from the video? Select all that apply from the list below.

   _____ Shaunti is a new patient at the practice.

   _____ Shaunti is an established patient at the practice.

   _____ Shaunti has an appointment with Dr. Hayler.

   _____ Shaunti is being seen for a sports physical examination.

   _____ Shaunti's father works on Fifth Avenue.

→ • When you are finished, click on the **X** at the top right of the video screen to close the video and return to the Reception desk.

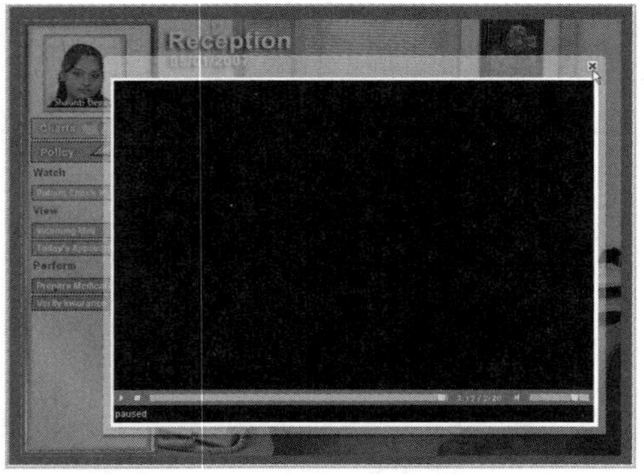

• To confirm Shaunti's appointment, click on the **Computer** to view Today's Appointments. This will open Mountain View Clinic's appointment schedule for the day's visits. ***Note:*** The virtual date for simulations in Mountain View Clinic is May 1, 2007. Use the scroll bar to view both morning and afternoon appointments.

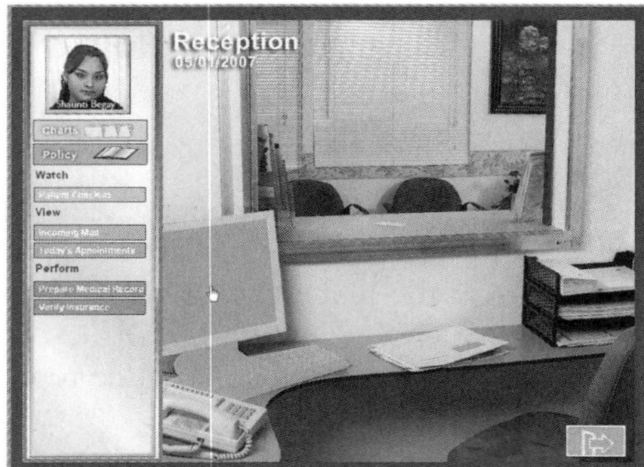

2. Which provider is Shaunti scheduled to see?
   a. Dr. Hayler
   b. Dr. Meyer

3. What time is Shaunti's appointment scheduled for?

4. Take a moment to skim over the rest of today's appointments. Of the other patients being seen today, which one has SMO insurance?

- Click **Finish** to return to the Reception desk. According to the video you watched, a problem has developed with Shaunti's insurance. Click on the **Insurance Card** on the counter to verify her insurance.

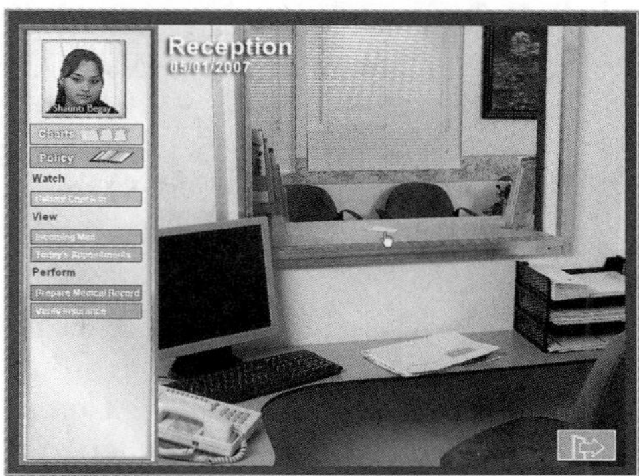

- You are instructed to choose an appropriate question to ask Shaunti. Selecting the correct question depends on whether she is a new or an established patient. Because this is Shaunti's first visit to the office, she is a new patient. Thus the second question choice does not apply because no records are currently on file that need to be changed or updated. Click the **Ask** button next to "Do you have insurance?"

- Next, you will be asked to follow through on the information provided by the patient to complete her insurance verification. If you need more information about the patient's insurance, you can use the buttons at the bottom left of the screen to view her insurance card or her completed Patient Information Form. Click on **Insurance Card(s)** to view the back and front of Shaunti's insurance card.

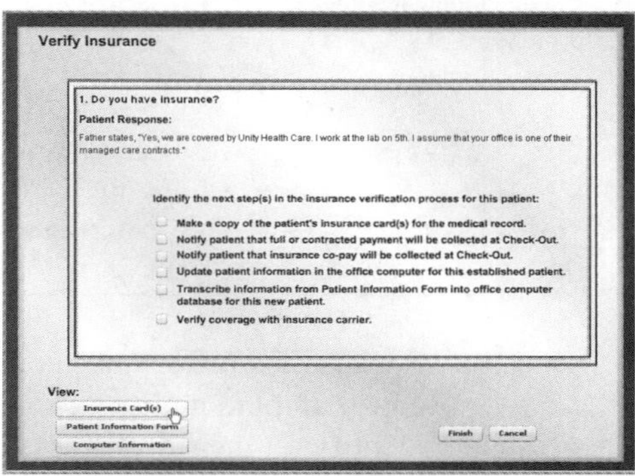

5. Shaunti's insurance card was issued by:
   a. Blue Cross/Blue Shield.
   b. Medicaid.
   c. Unity Health Care.

6. The Group Number indicated on Shaunti's insurance card is:
   a. 4B22.
   b. 6144.
   c. M238458888.
   d. 86756.

7. The issue date on Shaunti's insurance card is:
   a. May 1, 2007.
   b. April 1, 2001.

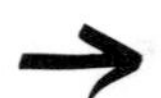

- Click the **Back** button to return to the Verify Insurance screen. (***Note:*** If you select Finish, you will be taken back to the Reception desk and you will not be able to return to the Verify Insurance task unless you exit to the office map and reenter the Reception desk.)

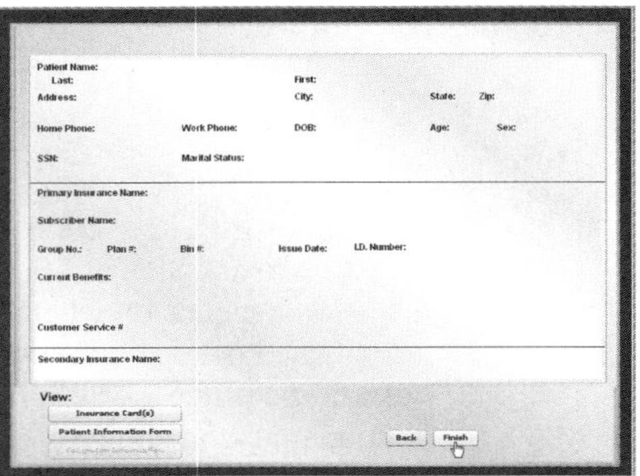

- Many physicians' offices now use computers to track their patients' personal and medical information. Click on the **Computer Information** button on the lower left of the screen to see a typical screen used for entering this information.

8. Below, practice filling in Shaunti's information for the first section of the screen. You can locate all the data you need to complete this screen by clicking to view the **Insurance Card(s)** and **Patient information Form** at the lower left side of your screen.

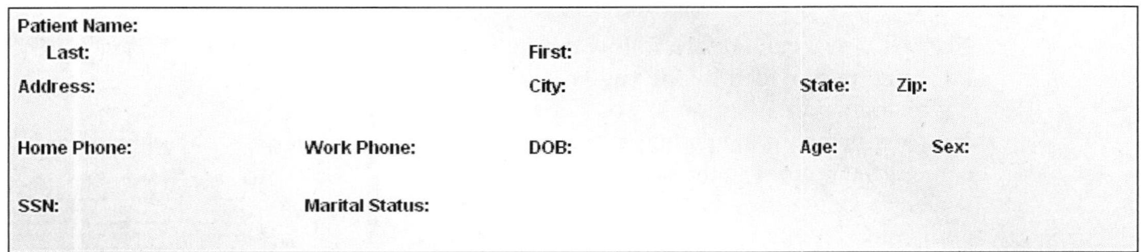

Patient Name:
Last: First:
Address: City: State: Zip:
Home Phone: Work Phone: DOB: Age: Sex:
SSN: Marital Status:

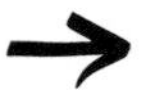

- Because the office does not accept the Begays' insurance plan, the staff cannot accept the copay amount and must collect the full amount due when Shaunti checks out. Make sure you identify all the steps necessary to finish verifying her insurance. The next steps are to:
  - Make a copy of the insurance cards for the medical record.
  - Notify Shaunti's parents that full payment will be expected at the end of the visit.
  - Enter the new patient information in the computer.
  - Verify coverage with the insurance carrier.

- Click on **Finish** to return to the Reception desk.

- Before we continue, look at the Verify Insurance button on the Room Menu. Has anything changed? Note that each time you complete a task under the Perform menu in any room, the corresponding menu selection bar lightens and a check mark appears next to the task. Because you have completed this task (Verify Insurance), you will not be able to access the task again unless you exit the room, return to the office map, and select this room again. (***Note:*** The tasks on the Room Menu do not necessarily appear in the order in which they should be completed.)

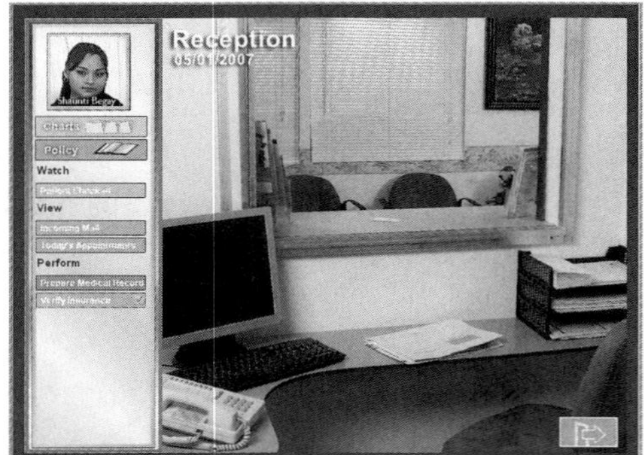

- In the video, Kristin, the receptionist, offered the Begays a copy of the office's policies. Click on the **Policy** button to review Mountain View Clinic's policies.

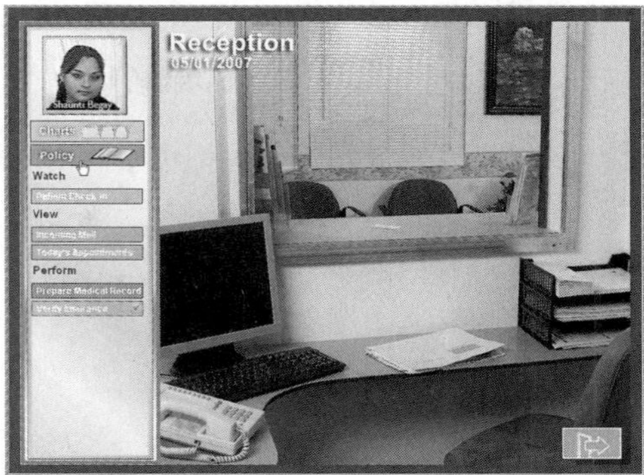

- You have several options for searching and navigating the Policy Manual. You can type specific keywords in the search bar, use the Table of Contents menu on the left to browse through particular sections, use the scroll bar and arrows on the right side of the screen, or jump to a specific page by using the page number box or the page-turn arrows.

- The policy on accepted insurance carriers is located on page 33 of the Policy Manual. Using any of the methods described above will take you to the correct location. Try all four routes for practice:
  - Type the word *insurance* in the search bar and click on the magnifying glass or press Enter on your keyboard. This will search the Policy Manual for that specific term. You will need to continue to click on the magnifying glass until you locate the section of the Policy Manual you need. (***Remember:*** The magnifying glass is for finding, not for zooming in. To enlarge text for easier reading, use the zoom bar to the right of the magnifying glass.)

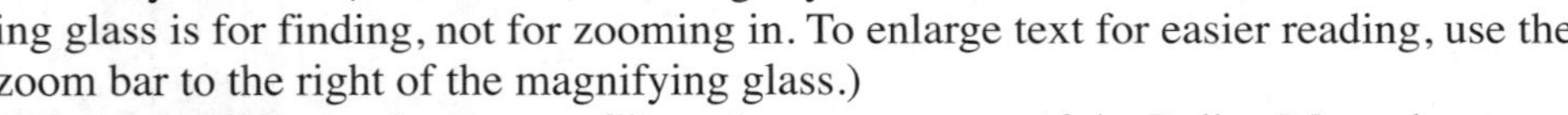

  - Use the scroll bar and arrows to flip to the correct page of the Policy Manual.
  - Type *33* in the page number box and press Enter on your keyboard.
  - Expand the Table of Contents until you find the correct area. Click on the relevant heading to go there. (***Note:*** Mountain View Clinic's policy on accepted insurance carriers is located in the Billing and Coding Manual under the Financial Policy section.)

9. Which of the following are accepted insurance carriers at Mountain View Clinic? Select all that apply.

_____ State Health Insurance

_____ Unity Health Care

_____ Oasis Health

_____ Star Insurance

_____ Local Supplement Health Group

_____ Medicaid

_____ Mutual Health Insurance Company

_____ Midwestern HMO

_____ Workers' Compensation

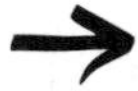

- Click **Close Manual** at the bottom of the screen to return to the Reception desk.
- Click on **Charts** button at the top of the Room Menu. Because Shaunti is a new patient, there are no records yet in her chart. As Shaunti progresses through her visit, forms and charts will be added to her medical record.

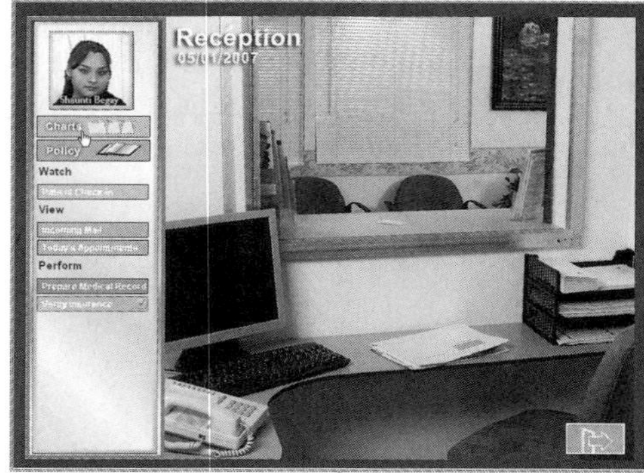

- Click on **Close Chart** to return to the Reception desk.

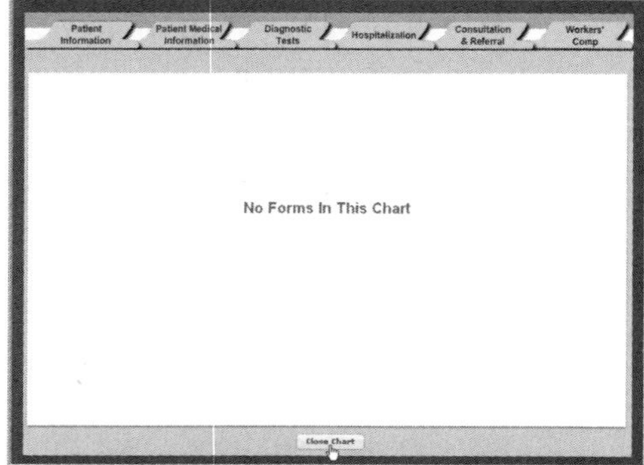

- Take a moment to look through the day's mail. Click on the pile of letters in the **Stackable Trays** on the right side of the Reception desk. The screen opens to reveal a letter to Dr. Meyer from Dr. William Neurg.

- To see the rest of the day's mail, use the directional arrows at the top of the screen or click on the number of the piece of mail you want to review. Click to view each piece of the **Incoming Mail**.

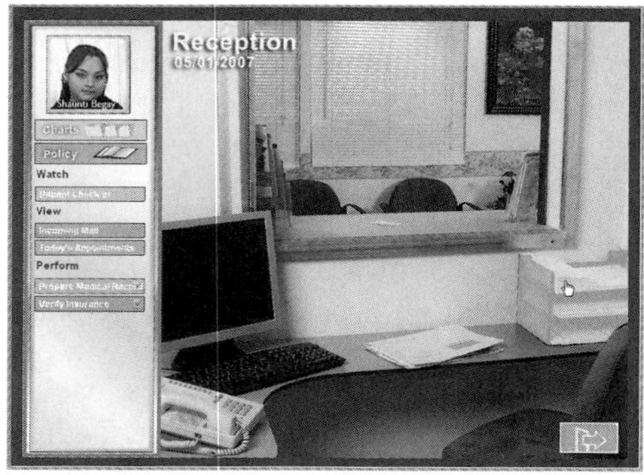

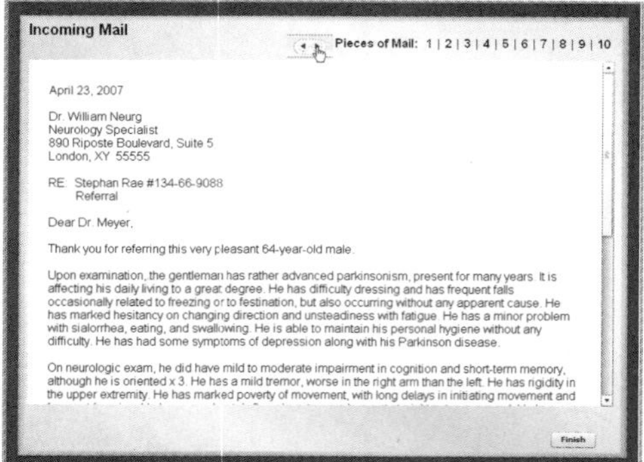

April 23, 2007

Dr. William Neurg
Neurology Specialist
890 Riposte Boulevard, Suite 5
London, XY 55555

RE: Stephan Rae #134-66-9088
Referral

Dear Dr. Meyer,

Thank you for referring this very pleasant 64-year-old male.

Upon examination, the gentleman has rather advanced parkinsonism, present for many years. It is affecting his daily living to a great degree. He has difficulty dressing and has frequent falls occasionally related to freezing or to festination, but also occurring without any apparent cause. He has marked hesitancy on changing direction and unsteadiness with fatigue. He has a minor problem with sialorrhea, eating, and swallowing. He is able to maintain his personal hygiene without any difficulty. He has had some symptoms of depression along with his Parkinson disease.

On neurologic exam, he did have mild to moderate impairment in cognition and short-term memory, although he is oriented x 3. He has a mild tremor, worse in the right arm than the left. He has rigidity in the upper extremity. He has marked poverty of movement, with long delays in initiating movement and

10. How many total pieces of mail are there to be reviewed?

11. How many checks were received in the mail?

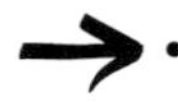

- Click on **Finish** to return to Reception. It is time to leave the room and follow Shaunti to the Exam Room. Click on the exit arrow in the lower right corner of the screen to leave the Reception desk.

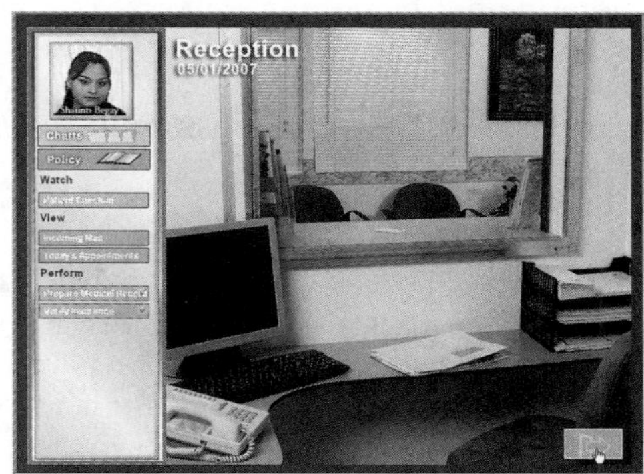

- At the Summary Menu screen, click on **Return to Map** to follow Shaunti's progress in the Exam Room.

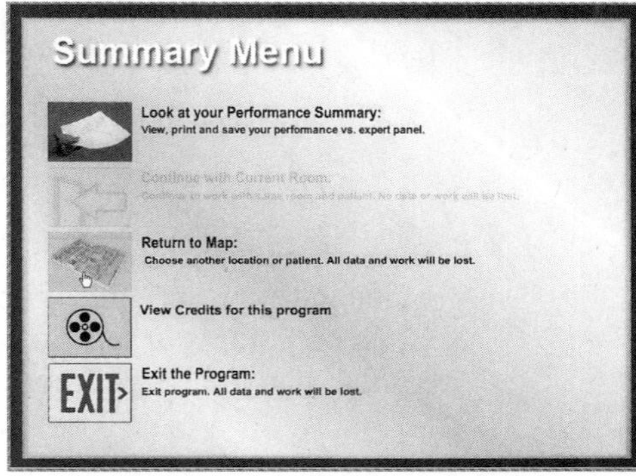

- Each time you return to the Office Map, *Virtual Medical Office* alerts you that all unsaved room data will be lost. This means any tasks completed, such as verifying insurance, will be reset. If you choose No, you will be returned to the Summary Menu, where you can continue working in the current room, review your Performance Summary, or exit the program. For your current assignment, click **Yes** to return to the Office Map.
- You are now ready to follow Shaunti to the Exam Room.

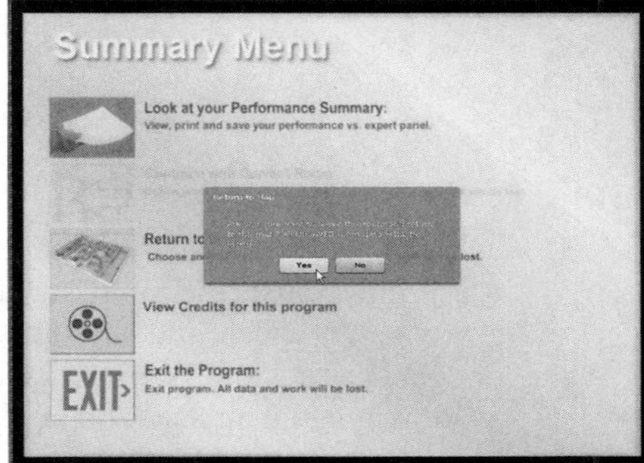

Exercise 2

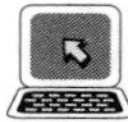

Online Activity—Exam Room

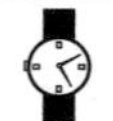

10 minutes

- Shaunti Begay will remain as your patient unless you exit the VMO software or select another patient. Keep Shaunti as your patient for this exercise. It is time for her to see the physician in the Exam Room. To go there, click on the **Exam Room** on the office map.

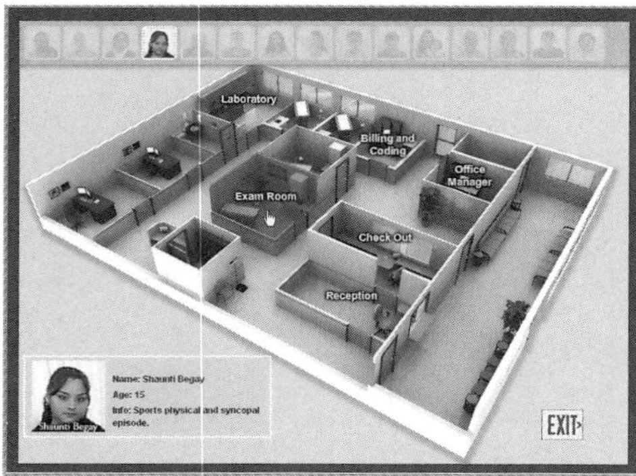

- Both Shaunti's chart and the office Policy Manual can be accessed within the room. Click on **Charts** to see what information is available in the Exam Room.

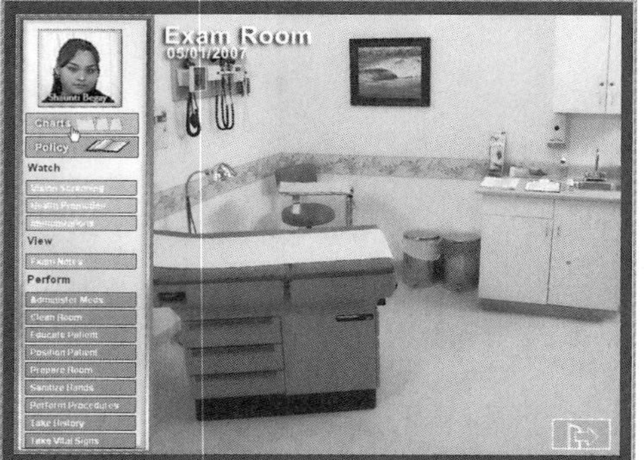

- The chart opens to Shaunti's Patient Information Form. Across the top of the chart are tabs under which you can find additional information about Shaunti's visit. As you click on each tab, a drop-down menu appears, listing all the available information under that tab.

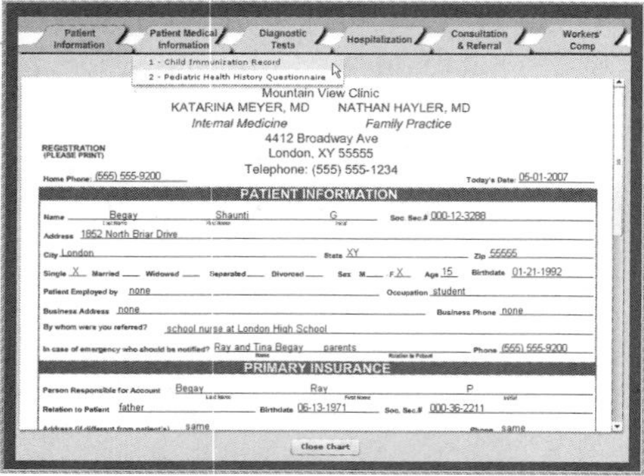

1. Click on the **Patient Information** tab. What documentation is included under this tab?

   (1)

   (2)

   (3)

   (4)

   (5)

2. Which of the following tabs do not currently have any forms? Select all that apply.

_____ Patient Information

_____ Patient Medical Information

_____ Diagnostic Tests

_____ Hospitalizations

_____ Consultation & Referral

_____ Workers' Comp

→ • Click **Close Chart** at the bottom of the screen to return to the Exam Room.

• Click on the **Exam Notes** clipboard to view Shaunti's Exam Notes as summarized from her Progress Notes by the physician.

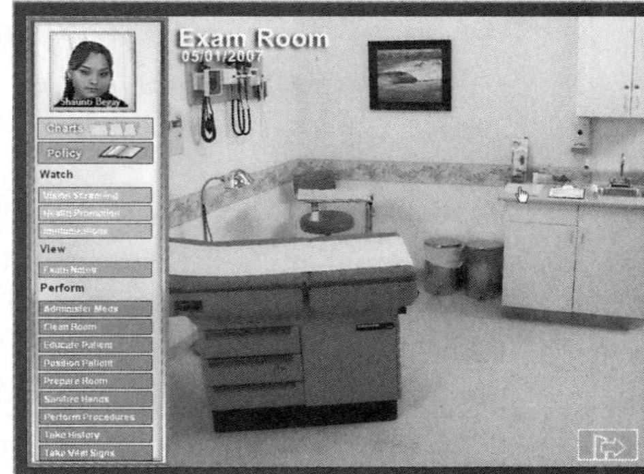

3. Where will the ECG testing for Shaunti be performed?
   a. At Shaunti's home
   b. At Mountain View Clinic
   c. At the hospital

4. Indicate whether the following statement is true or false.

_____ The Health Assessment for Teens (HEADSS) finds Shaunti to be an underactive teenager.

→ • Click the **Finish** button to return to the Exam Room. Click on the exit arrow at the bottom right of the screen to exit the room. On the Summary Menu, click **Return to Map**. Again, a pop-up message will inform you that all data will be lost. Click **Yes** to return to the office map and continue with Shaunti to the Check Out area.

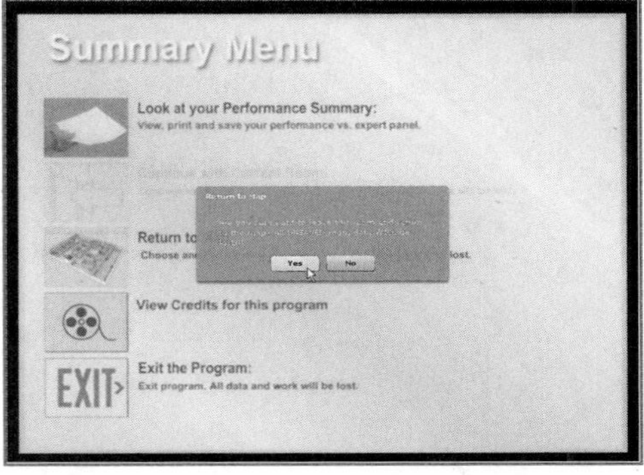

Exercise 3

Online Activity—Check Out Area

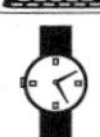

30 minutes

- Shaunti and her family are ready to proceed to Mountain View Clinic's Check Out area, where they will pay for Shaunti's visit and collect any information they might need for after they leave.
- On the office map, click on **Check Out**.

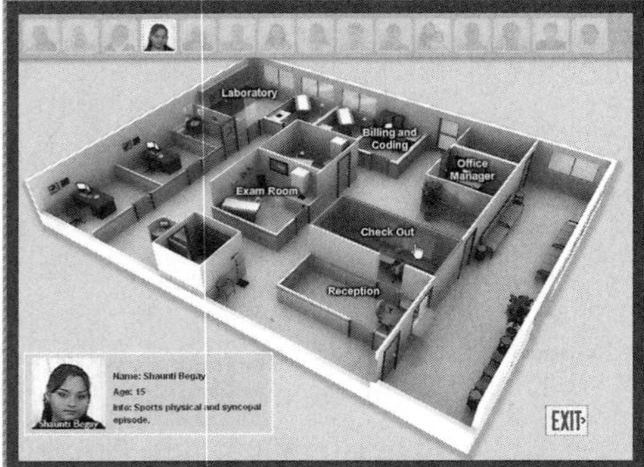

- Once again, Shaunti's chart and the office Policy Manual are both accessible. Click on **Charts** to review the documents added to Shaunti's medical record since she left the Exam Room.

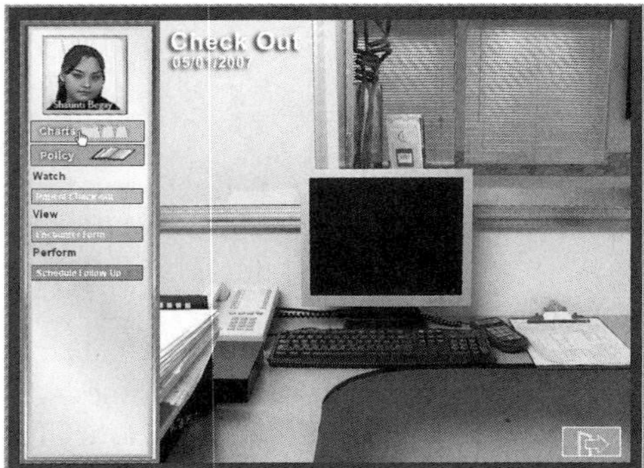

1. Click on all tabs at the top of Shaunti's chart to see what forms are included under each. Which of the tabs listed below still have no forms in them? Select all that apply.

   _____ Patient Information

   _____ Patient Medical Information

   _____ Diagnostic Tests

   _____ Hospitalization

   _____ Consultation and Referral

   _____ Workers' Comp

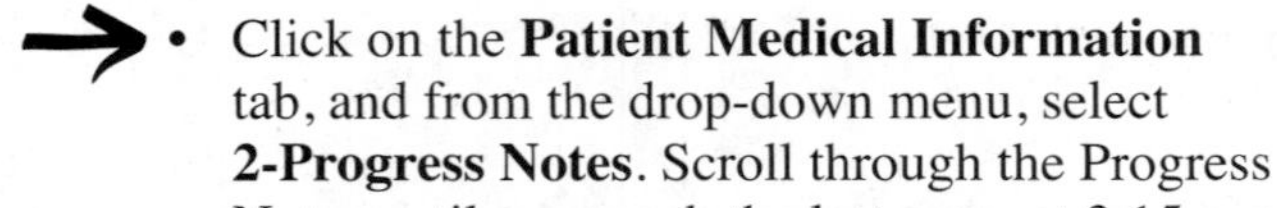

- Click on the **Patient Medical Information** tab, and from the drop-down menu, select **2-Progress Notes**. Scroll through the Progress Notes until you reach the last entry at 3:15 p.m.

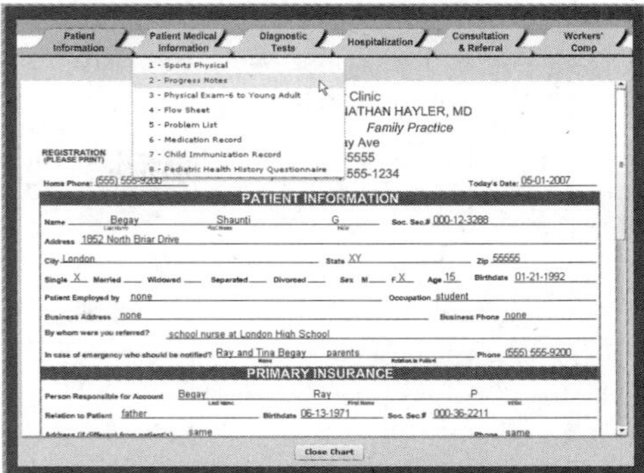

2. Indicate whether the following statement is true or false.

_____ According to the 3:15 p.m. entry in the Progress Notes, Shaunti will be scheduled to see a dermatologist who takes her insurance, Unity Health Plan.

- Click on the **Consultation & Referral** tab, and select **1-Referral Form** from the drop-down menu.
- Read through the form and note the headings of each section on the form. These sections provide all the basic information the clinic will need to arrange Shaunti's appointment, including her insurance information and the reason for the referral.

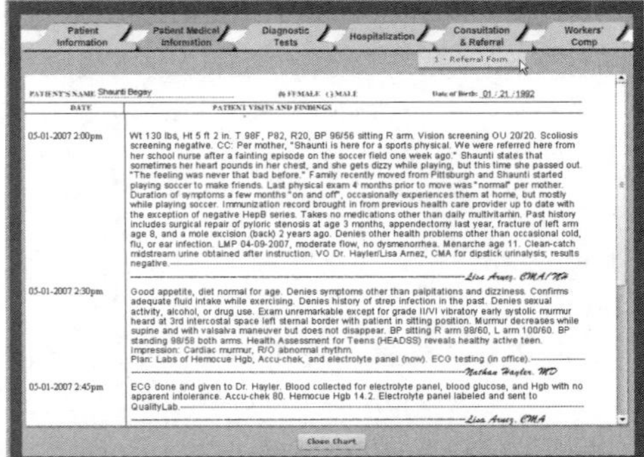

3. What condition is listed as the reason for the referral?

4. What ICD-9 diagnosis codes are listed on the referral form to indicate medical necessity of this referral to the Braeburn Cardiology Clinic?

- Click **Close Chart** at the bottom of the screen to return to the Check Out area.

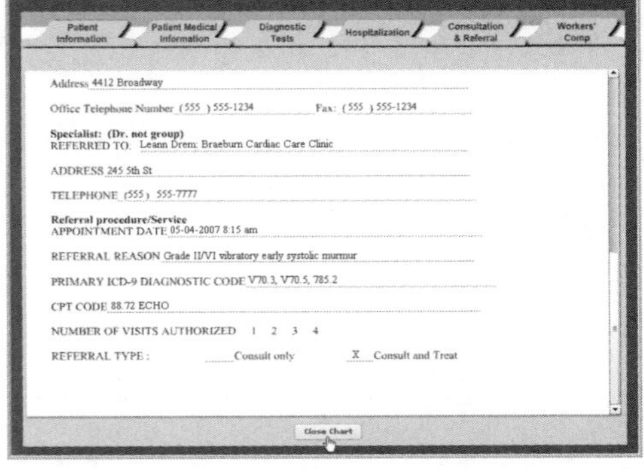

- On the room menu, click on **Patient Check-Out** under the Watch heading and watch the video of Shaunti's check-out.
- Click the **X** at the top right of the screen to close the video.

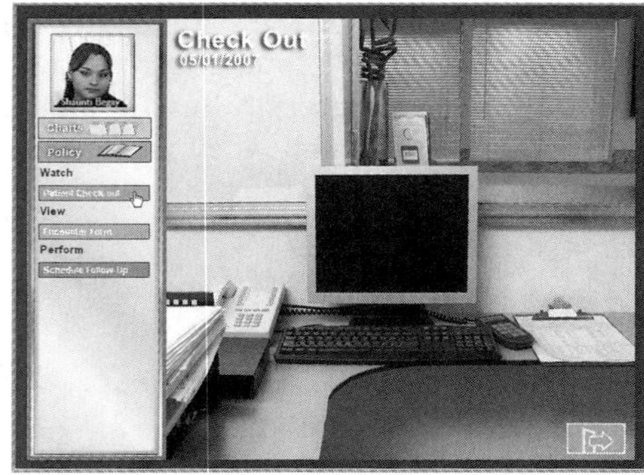

5. In this video, Mr. Begay expresses his surprise at:
   a. how much time they have had to wait for an appointment.
   b. the number of laboratory tests that the physician ordered.
   c. how quickly they are able to get an appointment with the referring provider.
   d. the amount of money due for Shaunti's examination.

6. What is offered to Mr. Begay that would provide an explanation of the charge for every services provided?

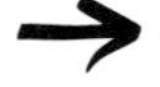

- Click on the **Encounter Form** clipboard to the right of the computer.
- Scroll through the Encounter Form and note what items were checked off for Shaunti's visit.

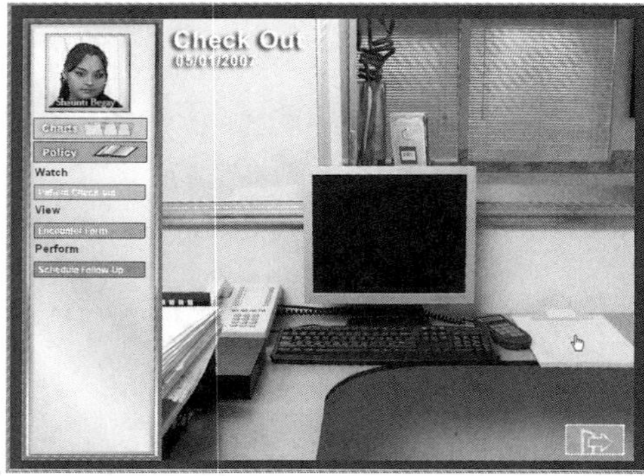

7. What are the total charges for Shaunti's visit?

8. How much did Mr. Begay pay at check-out?

9. What is the balance remaining for this visit?

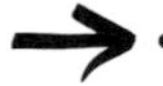

- Click **Finish** to return to the Check Out area.
- Click on the **Computer** to schedule Shaunti for her follow-up appointment.

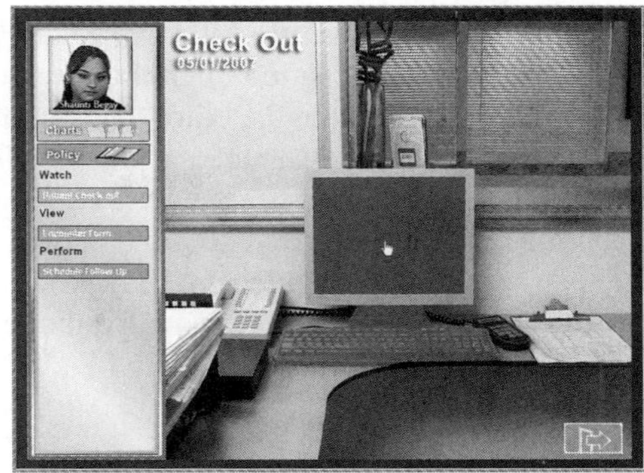

- Several steps are listed that might need to be taken to schedule a follow-up appointment for a patient. Depending on what the patient needs, you might need to select a few of these steps or you might need to select only one.
- For Shaunti, check the boxes next to **Schedule a referral to specialist**, and **Receive co-pay/ payment**. Click **Finish** to return to Check Out.

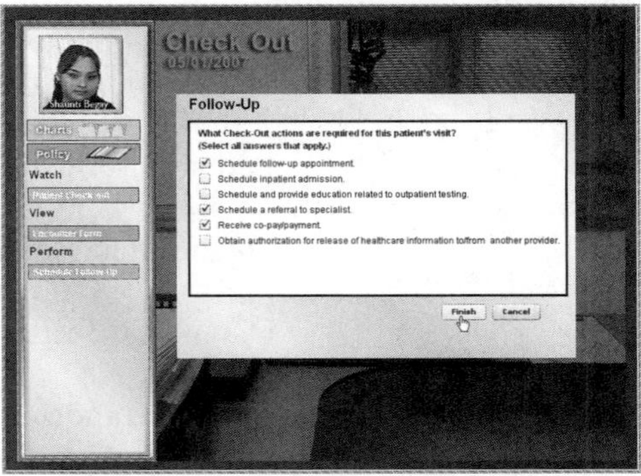

- You have completed the steps necessary for Shaunti's Check Out. Click on the exit arrow to leave the room and go to the Summary Menu.
- On the Summary Menu, click **Return to Map**. The pop-up message will inform you that all data will be lost. Click **Yes** to return to the office map and continue with Shaunti in the Billing and Coding area.

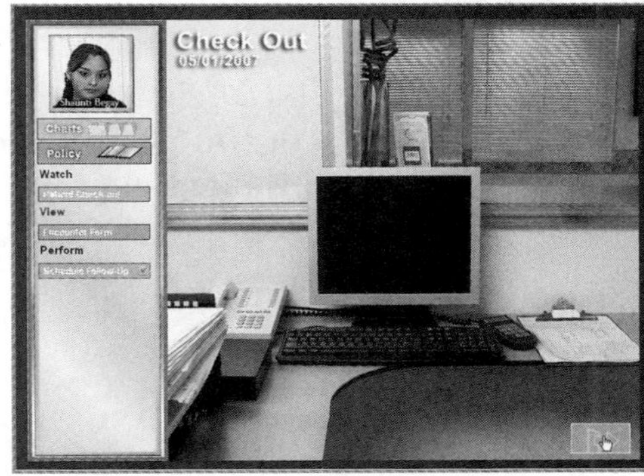

Exercise 4

Online Activity—Billing and Coding

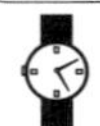

45 minutes

- Although Shaunti and her family have checked out from their appointment and have left the office, more needs to be done to process Shaunti's visit to the Mountain View Clinic.
- On the office map, click on **Billing and Coding**.

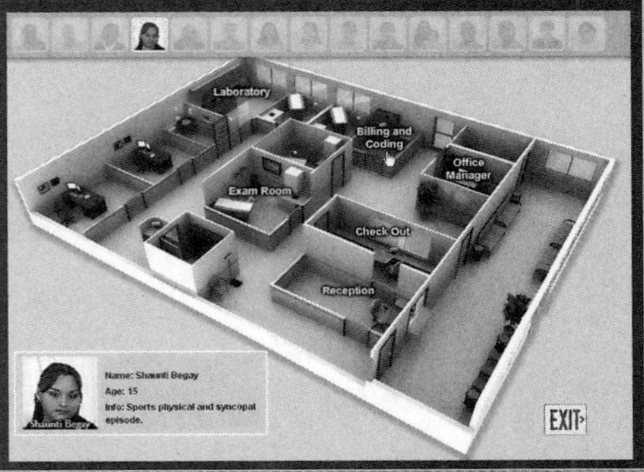

- Because we still have Shaunti selected as an active patient, her chart remains accessible in the Billing and Coding area along with the office Policy Manual. As you saw in other rooms, the chart has been updated and now contains the most current documentation. This documentation now includes not only what occurred during Shaunti's visit but also the records from her previous physician.
- Click on **Charts** to open Shaunti's medical record.

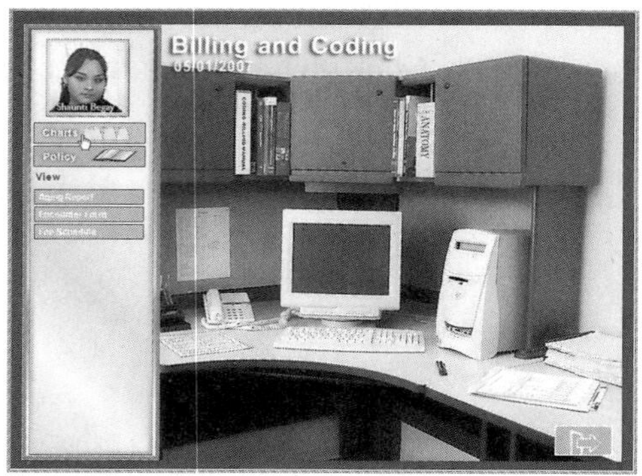

1. Click on all tabs at the top of the chart and identify which of the tabs listed below have no forms or information in them. Select all that apply.

_____ Patient Information

_____ Patient Medical Information

_____ Diagnostic Tests

_____ Hospitalization

_____ Consultation and Referral

_____ Workers' Comp

→ • Click on the **Hospitalization** tab and select **1-Operative Report**.

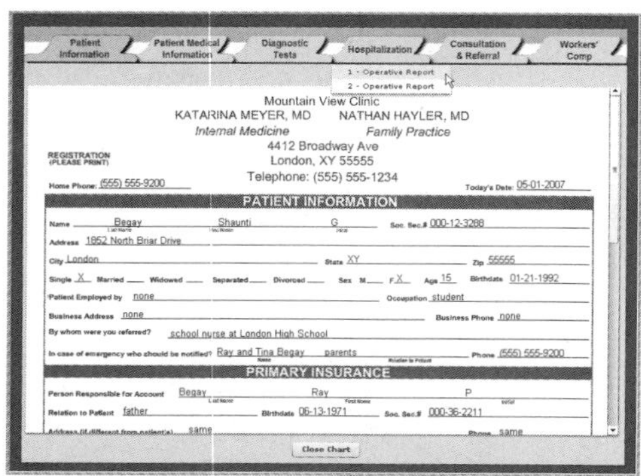

2. What is the encounter date listed on the report?

3. Read through the report. How old was Shaunti when this operation occurred?

4. What is the condition that Shaunti was being treated for?

5. What is the name of the operative procedure that was performed?

→ • Next, click on the **Consultation & Referral** tab and select **2-Office Notes** from the drop-down menu.

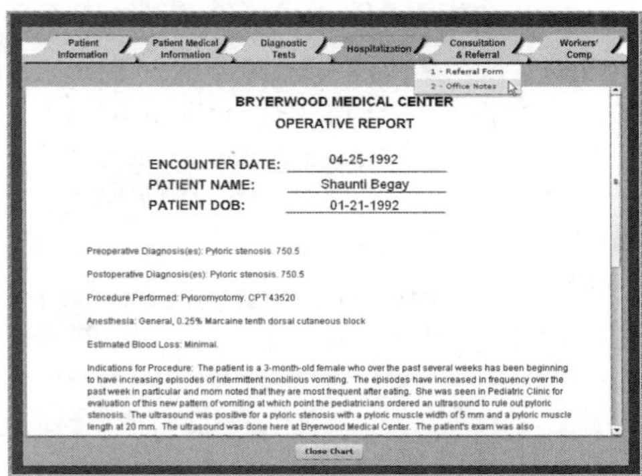

6. What is the encounter date on this report?

7. What is the name of the facility that issued this report?

8. Read through the report. How old was Shaunti at the time of this visit?

9. Why was Shaunti brought to the clinic to be seen on this date?

10. What is the name of the provider that treated Shaunti?

→ • Click on the **Patient Information** tab and select **1-Patient Information Form**.

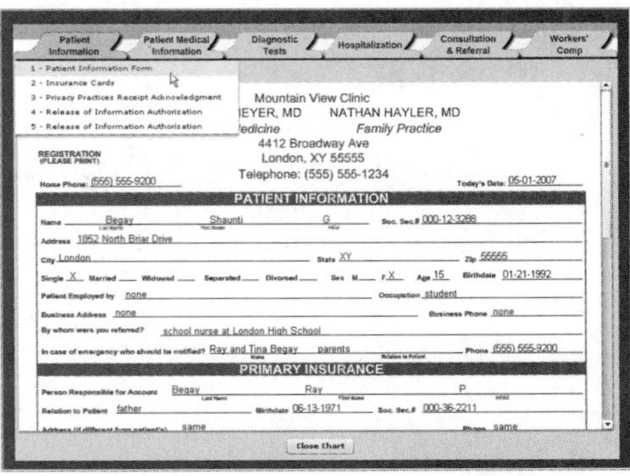

11. Medical Insurance and Billing & Coding students will be given exercises in filling out the CMS-1500 claim form. Using the information found on Shaunti's Patient Information Form, fill in the top portion of the CMS-1500 form below (blocks 2, 3, 5, 6, and 8). ***Hint:*** Blocks 2 and 5 must be entered in ALL CAPS with no punctuation.

1500

HEALTH INSURANCE CLAIM FORM

APPROVED BY NATIONAL UNIFORM CLAIM COMMITTEE 08/05

PICA | PICA | CARRIER

1. MEDICARE (Medicare #) | MEDICAID (Medicaid #) | TRICARE CHAMPUS (Sponsor's SSN) | CHAMPVA (Member ID#) | GROUP HEALTH PLAN (SSN or ID) | FECA BLK LUNG (SSN) | OTHER (ID)

1a. INSURED'S I.D. NUMBER (For Program in Item 1)

2. PATIENT'S NAME (Last Name, First Name, Middle Initial)

3. PATIENT'S BIRTH DATE MM | DD | YY SEX M F

4. INSURED'S NAME (Last Name, First Name, Middle Initial)

5. PATIENT'S ADDRESS (No., Street)

6. PATIENT RELATIONSHIP TO INSURED Self Spouse Child Other

7. INSURED'S ADDRESS (No., Street)

CITY STATE

8. PATIENT STATUS Single Married Other

CITY STATE

ZIP CODE TELEPHONE (Include Area Code) ( )

Employed Full-Time Student Part-Time Student

ZIP CODE TELEPHONE (Include Area Code) ( )

9. OTHER INSURED'S NAME (Last Name, First Name, Middle Initial)

10. IS PATIENT'S CONDITION RELATED TO:

11. INSURED'S POLICY GROUP OR FECA NUMBER

a. OTHER INSURED'S POLICY OR GROUP NUMBER

a. EMPLOYMENT? (Current or Previous) YES NO

a. INSURED'S DATE OF BIRTH MM | DD | YY SEX M F

b. OTHER INSURED'S DATE OF BIRTH MM | DD | YY SEX M F

b. AUTO ACCIDENT? PLACE (State) YES NO

b. EMPLOYER'S NAME OR SCHOOL NAME

c. EMPLOYER'S NAME OR SCHOOL NAME

c. OTHER ACCIDENT? YES NO

c. INSURANCE PLAN NAME OR PROGRAM NAME

d. INSURANCE PLAN NAME OR PROGRAM NAME

10d. RESERVED FOR LOCAL USE

d. IS THERE ANOTHER HEALTH BENEFIT PLAN? YES NO *If yes*, return to and complete item 9 a-d.

READ BACK OF FORM BEFORE COMPLETING & SIGNING THIS FORM.

12. PATIENT'S OR AUTHORIZED PERSON'S SIGNATURE I authorize the release of any medical or other information necessary to process this claim. I also request payment of government benefits either to myself or to the party who accepts assignment below.

SIGNED________ DATE________

13. INSURED'S OR AUTHORIZED PERSON'S SIGNATURE I authorize payment of medical benefits to the undersigned physician or supplier for services described below.

SIGNED________

PATIENT AND INSURED INFORMATION

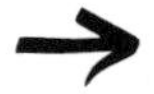

- Click **Close Chart** to return to the Billing and Coding area.
- A main source of information for Billing and Coding is the Encounter Form. Click on the **Encounter Form** file to the right of the computer to review the list of charges for Shaunti's visit.

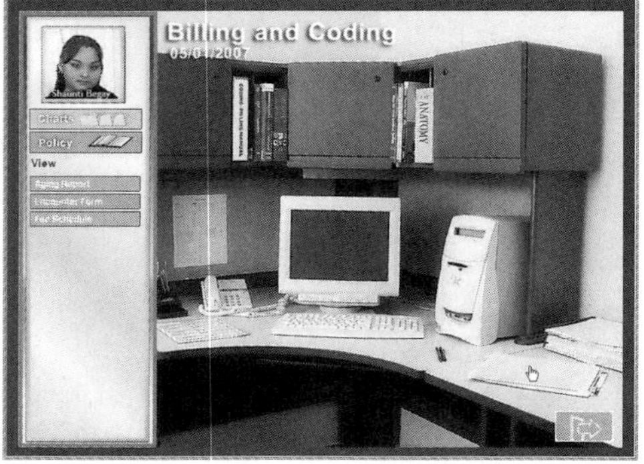

12. According to the Encounter Form, what type of insurance does Shaunti's family have?
    a. Private
    b. BCBS
    c. Medicare
    d. Medicaid
    e. HMO
    f. Tricare

13. All of the services that were provided to Shaunti are listed on the Encounter Form. List the nine services that were provided.

    (1)

    (2)

    (3)

    (4)

    (5)

    (6)

    (7)

    (8)

    (9)

- Click **Finish** to return to the Billing and Coding area.

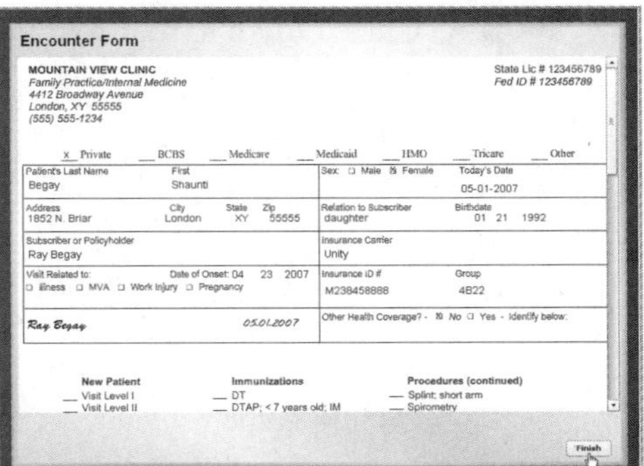

Encounter Form

MOUNTAIN VIEW CLINIC
Family Practice/Internal Medicine
4412 Broadway Avenue
London, XY 55555
(555) 555-1234

State Lic # 123456789
Fed ID # 123456789

x Private ___ BCBS ___ Medicare ___ Medicaid ___ HMO ___ Tricare ___ Other

Patient's Last Name: Begay	First: Shaunti	Sex: ☐ Male ☒ Female	Today's Date: 05-01-2007
Address: 1852 N. Briar	City: London State: XY Zip: 55555	Relation to Subscriber: daughter	Birthdate: 01 21 1992
Subscriber or Policyholder: Ray Begay		Insurance Carrier: Unity	
Visit Related to: ☐ Illness ☐ MVA ☐ Work Injury ☐ Pregnancy	Date of Onset: 04 23 2007	Insurance ID #: M238458888	Group: 4B22
Ray Begay	*05.01.2007*	Other Health Coverage? - ☒ No ☐ Yes - Identify below:	

New Patient	Immunizations	Procedures (continued)
___ Visit Level I	___ DT	___ Splint; short arm
___ Visit Level II	___ DTAP; < 7 years old; IM	___ Spirometry

Finish

- To calculate charges on the Encounter Form, you need to know what the office fee is for each service. Click on the **Fee Schedule** on the wall above the telephone to view the full list of services and charges.

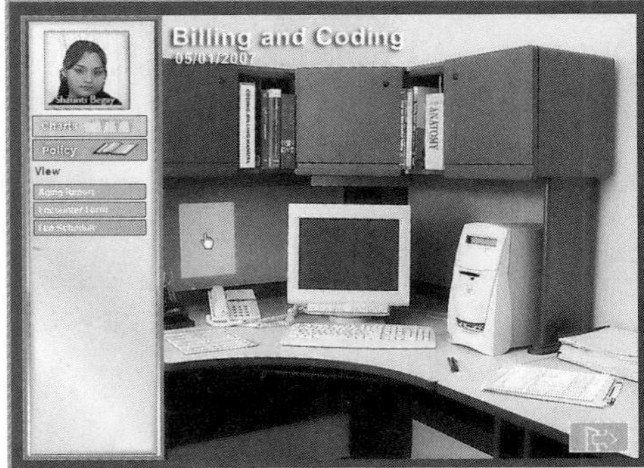

14. Determine the amount due for each of the nine services you listed in question 13 and itemize them below.

    (1)

    (2)

    (3)

    (4)

    (5)

    (6)

    (7)

    (8)

    (9)

- Click **Finish** to return to the Billing and Coding area.

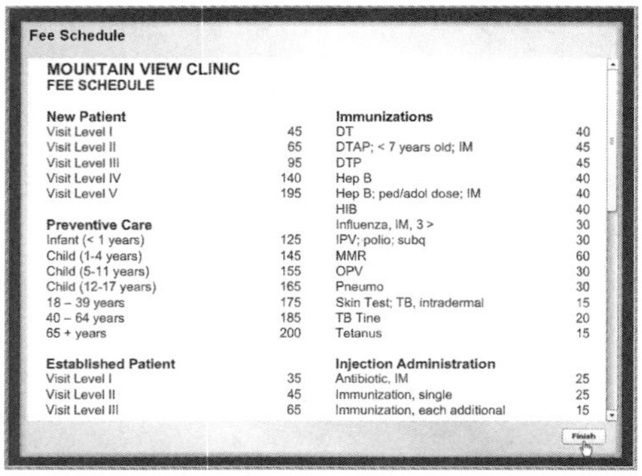

Fee Schedule

MOUNTAIN VIEW CLINIC
FEE SCHEDULE

New Patient		Immunizations	
Visit Level I	45	DT	40
Visit Level II	65	DTAP; < 7 years old; IM	45
Visit Level III	95	DTP	45
Visit Level IV	140	Hep B	40
Visit Level V	195	Hep B; ped/adol dose; IM	40
		HIB	40
Preventive Care		Influenza, IM, 3 >	30
Infant (< 1 years)	125	IPV; polio; subq	30
Child (1-4 years)	145	MMR	60
Child (5-11 years)	155	OPV	30
Child (12-17 years)	165	Pneumo	30
18 – 39 years	175	Skin Test; TB, intradermal	15
40 – 64 years	185	TB Tine	20
65 + years	200	Tetanus	15
Established Patient		**Injection Administration**	
Visit Level I	35	Antibiotic, IM	25
Visit Level II	45	Immunization, single	25
Visit Level III	65	Immunization, each additional	15

- The Aging Report is a tool used to keep track of patient accounts by recording the date and amount of the bill, as well as the date and amount of payment. The Aging Report also identifies balances that are becoming overdue, usually in increments of 30 days.
- Click on the **Aging Report** blue file to the left of the computer to view the current patient balances.

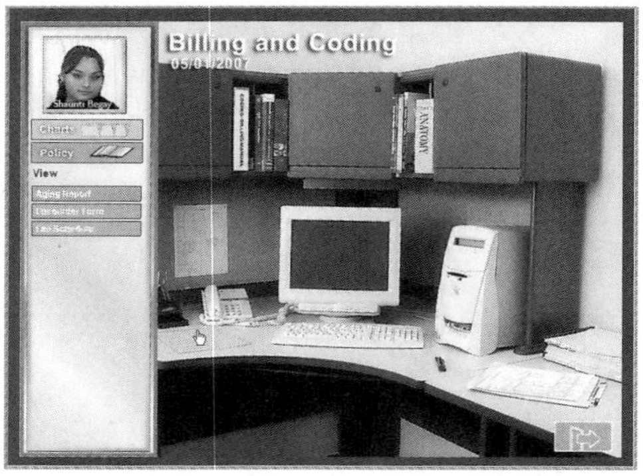

15. What are the starting and ending dates for this Aging Report?

    Starting date: Ending date:

16. The first patient on the report is Jacob Abraham. His service (99201) was billed at the rate of _______________.

17. The report indicates that Mr. Abraham made a payment of _______________ to his account.

18. The date Mr. Abraham made the cash payment was ______________.

19. What is the balance due by Mr. Abraham?

20. What is the age of the balance that Mr. Abraham owes?
    a. 31-60 days old
    b. 61-90 days old
    c. 91-120 days old
    d. Over 120 days old

→ • Scroll to the bottom of the Aging Report.

21. The total amount of the accounts receivable for both providers is ______________.

22. Of the entire accounts receivable for both providers, what percentage is over 120 days old?

→ • Click **Finish** to return to the Billing and Coding area.

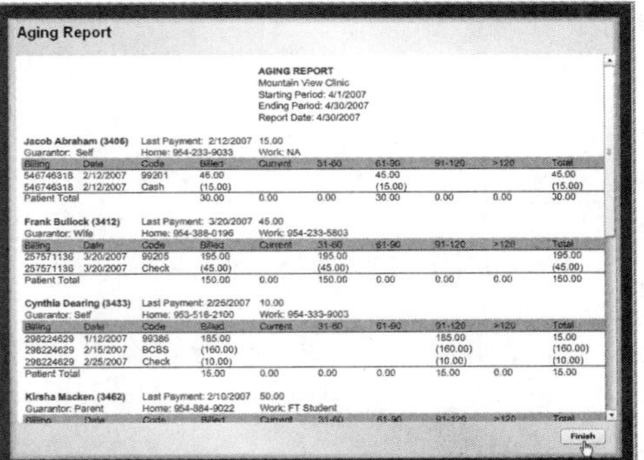

Aging Report

AGING REPORT
Mountain View Clinic
Starting Period: 4/1/2007
Ending Period: 4/30/2007
Report Date: 4/30/2007

Jacob Abraham (3406) Last Payment: 2/12/2007 15.00
Guarantor: Self Home: 954-233-9033 Work: NA

Billing	Date	Code	Billed	Current	31-60	61-90	91-120	>120	Total
546746318	2/12/2007	99201	45.00			45.00			45.00
546746318	2/12/2007	Cash	(15.00)			(15.00)			(15.00)
Patient Total			30.00	0.00	0.00	30.00	0.00	0.00	30.00

Frank Bullock (3412) Last Payment: 3/20/2007 45.00
Guarantor: Wife Home: 954-388-0196 Work: 954-233-5803

Billing	Date	Code	Billed	Current	31-60	61-90	91-120	>120	Total
257571136	3/20/2007	99205	195.00		195.00				195.00
257571136	3/20/2007	Check	(45.00)		(45.00)				(45.00)
Patient Total			150.00	0.00	150.00	0.00	0.00	0.00	150.00

Cynthia Dearing (3433) Last Payment: 2/25/2007 10.00
Guarantor: Self Home: 953-516-2100 Work: 954-333-9003

Billing	Date	Code	Billed	Current	31-60	61-90	91-120	>120	Total
298224629	1/12/2007	99386	185.00				185.00		15.00
298224629	2/15/2007	BCBS	(160.00)				(160.00)		(160.00)
298224629	2/25/2007	Check	(10.00)				(10.00)		(10.00)
Patient Total			15.00	0.00	0.00	0.00	15.00	0.00	15.00

Kirsha Macken (3462) Last Payment: 2/10/2007 50.00
Guarantor: Parent Home: 954-884-9022 Work: FT Student

Billing	Date	Code	Billed	Current	31-60	61-90	91-120	>120	Total

Finish

• You have now finished working in the Billing and Coding area. Click on the exit arrow to leave the room and go the Summary Menu.

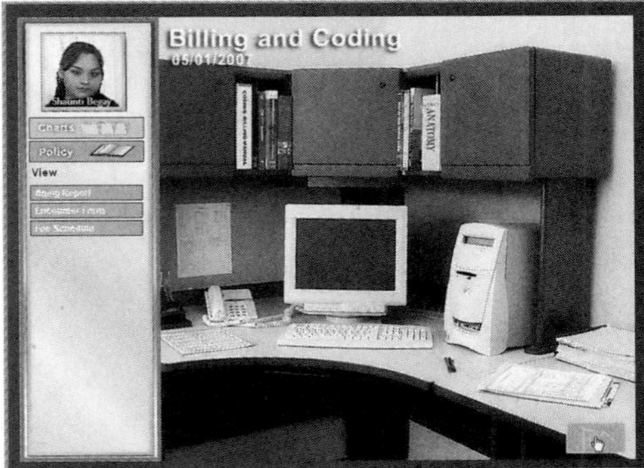

- Click **Exit the Program**. A pop-up message will inform you that all data will be lost. Click **Yes** to close the program.

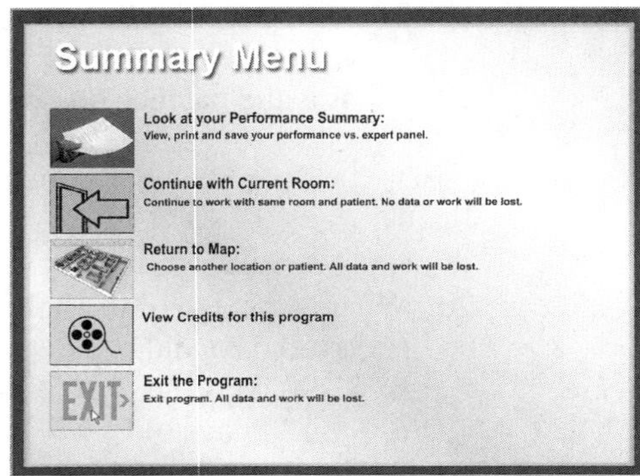

Congratulations! You have completed the *Virtual Medical Office* tours, which were designed to introduce you to the software and the various components you will be working with throughout this learning experience.

LESSON 1

Medical Law, Liability, and Ethics

Reading Assignment: Chapter 3—The Legal and Ethical Side of Medical Insurance
- Medical Law and Liability
- Insurance and Contract Law
- Medical Law and Ethics Applicable to Health Insurance
- Important Legislation Affecting Health Insurance
- Medical Ethics and Medical Etiquette

Patients: John R. Simmons, Wilson Metcalf

Learning Objectives:

- Recognize the importance of the organization's office policies as a resource in reducing potential violations in medical law, liability, or ethical issues.
- Identify the basic concepts of contract law affecting the health insurance professional.
- Understand potential liabilities and ethical issues occurring in the medical office.
- Identify breaches of medical ethics and etiquette and determine a more appropriate method of handling problematic situations.

Overview:

This lesson addresses the basic concepts of contract law, as well as important issues related to liability, medical ethics, and medical etiquette. You will access Mountain View Clinic's Policy Manual to familiarize yourself with office policies that have been established to protect the health insurance specialist from lawsuit or violations of health care laws and regulations. You will view John R. Simmons' billing records to analyze insurance information provided and identify contract laws applicable to his situation. Next, you will view Wilson Metcalf's check-in video to analyze areas in which medical ethics and etiquette have been breached. By the end of the lesson, you should be able to identify ways to protect yourself and your employer from risk.

Exercise 1

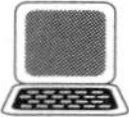

Online Activity—General Liability

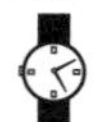

30 minutes

The primary goals of the health insurance professional are to complete and submit accurate medical insurance claims and conduct billing and collection procedures for the practice in a legal and ethical manner. Therefore the health insurance professional must be knowledgeable in the areas of medical law and liability that will affect them.

An organization's Policy Manual can serve as a foundation in protecting the health insurance professional from lawsuit or violations of health care laws and regulations. The first step that new employees should take is to thoroughly familiarize themselves with their organization's Policy Manual.

Note: Keep in mind that office policies vary from one practice to the next.

- Sign in to Mountain View Clinic and select any patient from the patient list.

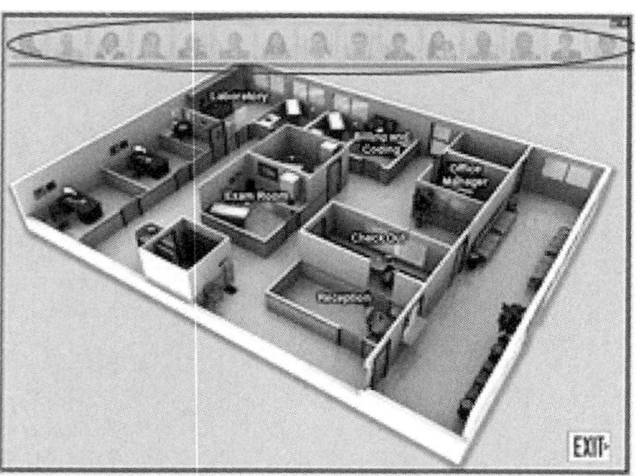

- On the office map, highlight and click on **Reception** to enter the Reception area.

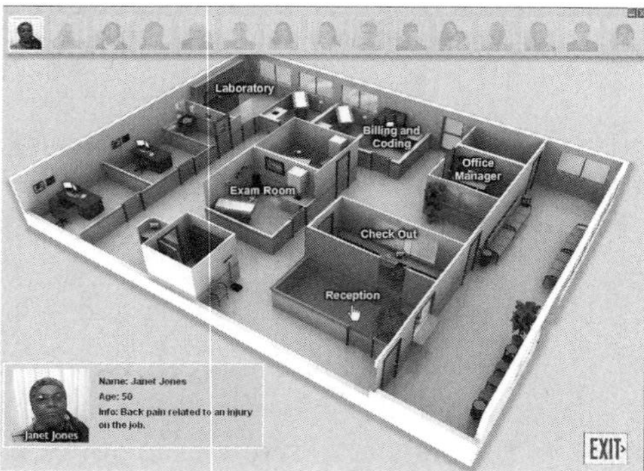

- Click on **Policy** to open the office Policy Manual.

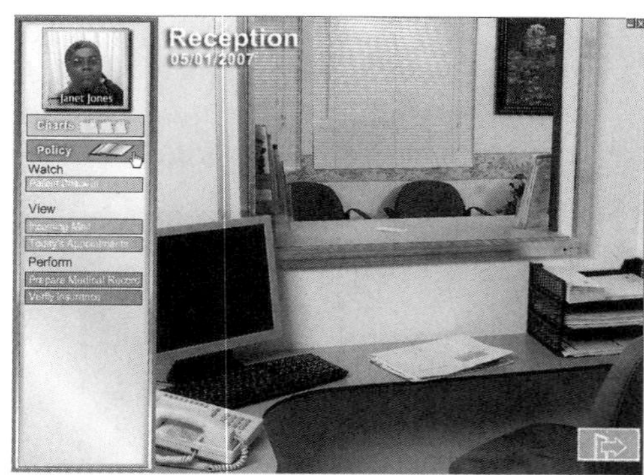

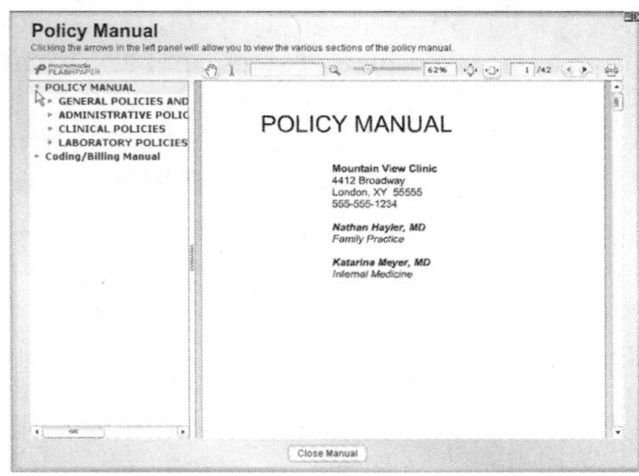

- Select the "Policy Manual" or click on the arrow to the left to open the menu of headings.
- Read through the Mountain View Clinic Policy Manual. Move through the pages by using the scroll bar on the right side of the manual or the arrow buttons at the top right side of the page. It is important to familiarize yourself with this Policy Manual because you will use this information as you complete all the exercises in the Virtual Medical Office study guide.
- Keep the Policy Manual open as you answer questions 1 through 13 below.

1. The purposes of Mountain View Clinic's Policy Manual include all of the following except:
   a. documenting standards of conduct.
   b. ensuring compliance with all health care laws and regulations.
   c. providing the health insurance professional with health care laws.
   d. identifying what behavior is expected of employees.

2. According to the job description in Mountain View Clinic's Policy Manual, what behaviors are expected health insurance professional employees?
   a. adhere to federal guidelines regarding third-party reimbursement.
   b. adhere to state guidelines regarding third-party reimbursement.
   c. adhere to third-party payer policies regarding reimbursement.
   d. adhere to federal, state, and third-party payer policies regarding third-party reimbursement.

3. According to the job description in Mountain View Clinic's Policy Manual, the health insurance professional should:
   a. report the ICD-9 and CPT codes assigned by the provider on the Encounter Form.
   b. report the ICD-9 and CPT codes assigned by the provider on the Encounter Form after verifying that they are supported in the documentation.
   c. report the ICD-9 and CPT codes that will be most likely to result in the claim being paid.
   d. report the ICD-9 and CPT codes that are most frequently used.

4. Indicate whether the following statement is true or false.

   _________ The health insurance professional at Mountain View Clinic may perform the duties of a registered or licensed practical nurse if requested to do so by the physician.

5. Assume that you are a health insurance professional working at Mountain View Clinic. A patient in the waiting room begins to show signs of a medical crisis. What should you do first?
   a. Don't get involved; it is not your responsibility since you are a health insurance professional.
   b. Request additional help by saying, "Please get the red folder!"
   c. Request additional help by saying, "Is there a doctor in the house?"
   d. Clear the waiting room.

6. Occasionally, during a phone conversation with a patient regarding a bill, the health insurance professional at Mountain View Clinic may be asked a medical question. What is the correct way to handle the patients request?
   a. Give advice based on his or her experience in the office.
   b. Give advice based on what is written in the patient's record.
   c. Instruct the patient according to the notes left by the physician.
   d. Do not give advice over the phone and take a message, or schedule an appointment for the patient.

7. You are a health insurance professional at Mountain View Clinic. A patient contacts you, identifying himself as a physician-colleague who is requesting a professional courtesy. You should:
   a. write off this patient's entire bill immediately.
   b. explain to the patient that this could be a violation of the Medicare Anti-Kickback statute and you are therefore unable to honor the request.
   c. refuse to honor the request and hang up the phone immediately.
   d. process this as an "insurance only" billing.

8. When might discounting of discounting of fees be allowed at Mountain View Clinic?
   a. Routinely, for any patient you think deserves it
   b. For all patients over age 65 and on Medicare
   c. When the physician is friends with the patient
   d. Charity or self-pay patients

9. According to Mountain View Clinic's Policy Manual, when may you, as the health insurance professional, submit a claim that is known to contain inaccurate information?
   a. When the provider tells you to submit it with inaccurate information
   b. When the charge ticket has been completed with that same inaccurate information
   c. Not until the receptionist co-signs the charge slip containing the inaccurate information
   d. Not until you have obtained guidance from the compliance leader(s) or the office administrator(s) and the resolution has been documented in writing

10. As the health insurance professional at Mountain View Clinic, if you are unsure of the rules or regulations related to any situation you are confronted with, you should:
    a. proceed with caution.
    b. stop, reconsider the situation, use your best judgment, and document it.
    c. take the advice of a co-worker with more experience.
    d. obtain guidance from the billing manager, compliance officer, or office administrator.

11. Based on your review of Mountain View Clinic's Policy Manual, do you believe the Policy Manual will assist in protecting the health insurance professional from lawsuit or violations of health care laws and regulations? Explain.

12. We are aware that physicians have a responsibility for their own actions, but what about health insurance professionals? Can the health insurance professional be a party to legal action in the event of error or omission?

13. Under the Fraud and Abuse Act, who is responsible for any allegations or violations of federal or state guidelines?

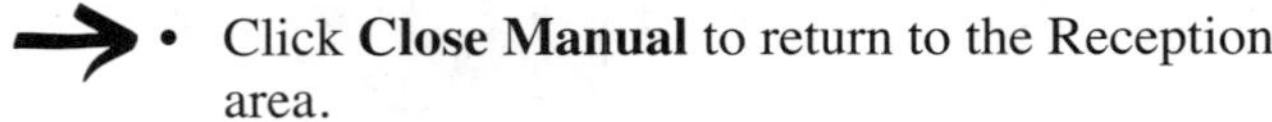

- Click **Close Manual** to return to the Reception area.

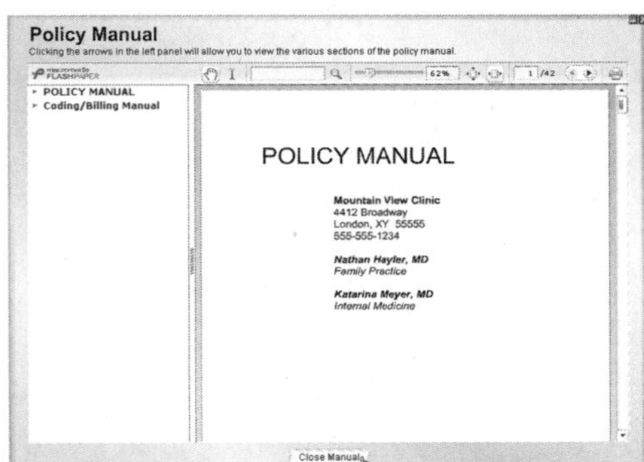

- Click the exit arrow at the lower right corner of the screen to go to the Summary Menu.

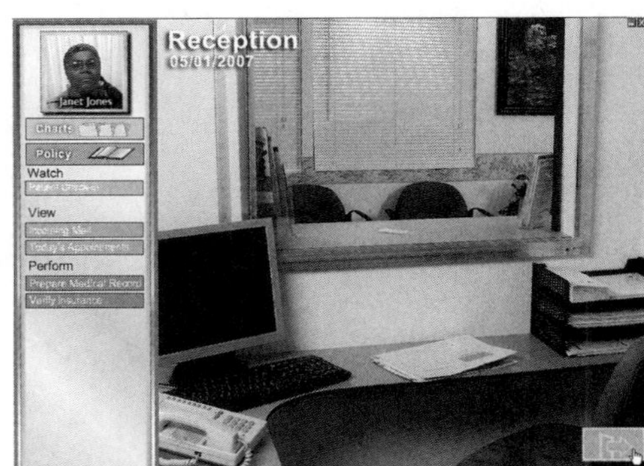

- On the Summary Menu, click **Return to Map** to continue to the next exercise.

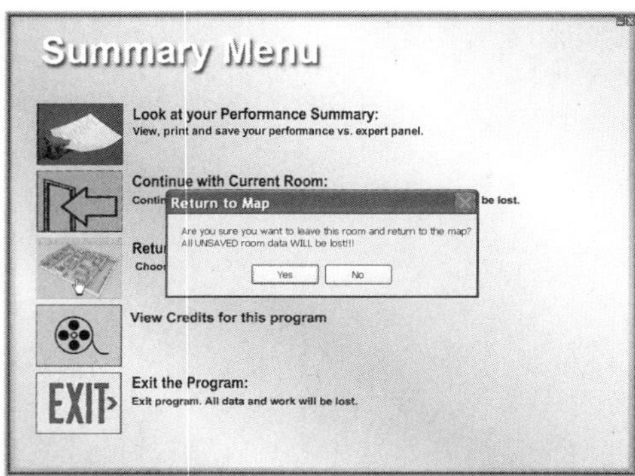

Exercise 2

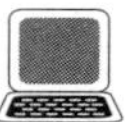

Online Activity—Understanding the Basic Concepts of Contract Law

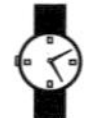

15 minutes

- Sign in to Mountain View Clinic.
- From the patient list, select **John R. Simmons**. (*Note:* If you have exited the program, sign in again to Mountain View Clinic and select John R. Simmons from the patient list.)

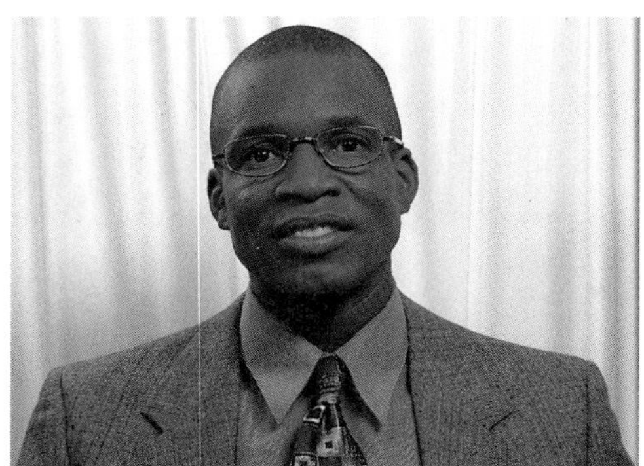

- On the office map, highlight and click on **Billing and Coding** to enter the Billing and Coding area.

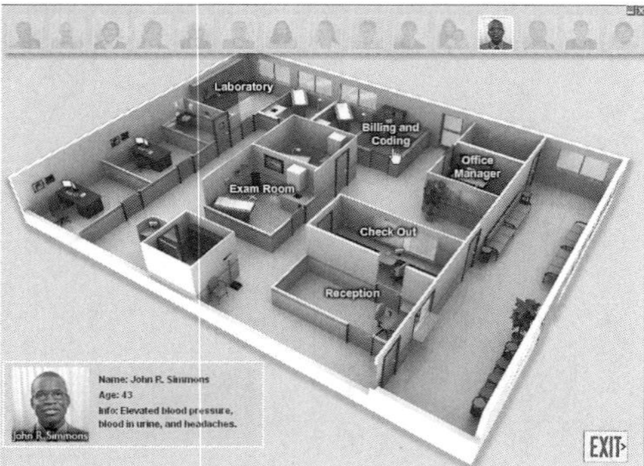

- Click on **Charts** to open Dr. Simmons' medical record.

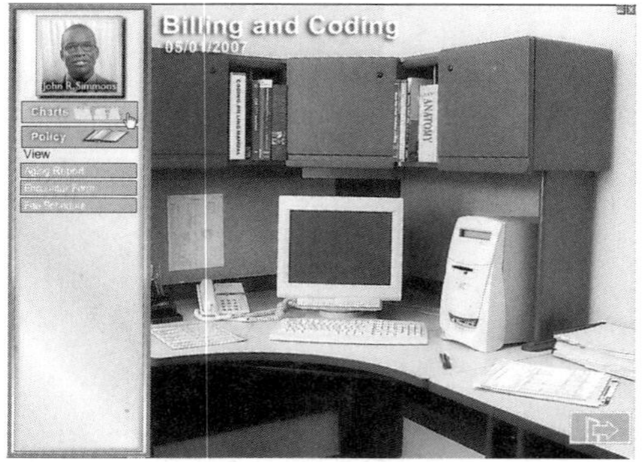

- Click on the **Patient Information** tab and select **5-Insurance Cards** from the drop-down menu.

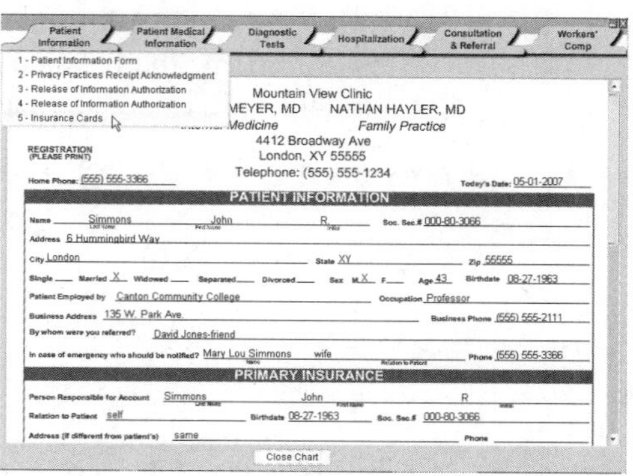

1. What type of contractual agreement exists between Dr. Simmons and his insurance carrier (Teachers' Health Group)?

2. What five elements are required to make Dr. Simmons' health insurance policy legal?

3. What type of contractual agreement exists between the health care provider and Dr. Simmons? What does that mean?

4. What is the health care provider's promise to Dr. Simmons through their contractual agreement?

5. What is Dr. Simmons' promise to the health care provider through their contact?

6. If the physician at Mountain View Clinic eventually decides to terminate his contract with Dr. Simmons, the physician must have good reason to do so and must follow specific guidelines in doing so to avoid what type of lawsuit?

7. List reasons that a physician may terminate a patient.

8. In the contractual agreement between Dr. Simmons and Mountain View Clinic, Dr. Simmons (the patient) is referred to as the first party and Mountain View Clinic is referred to as the second party. Who is the third party?

→ • Select **Close Chart** to return to the Billing and Coding area.

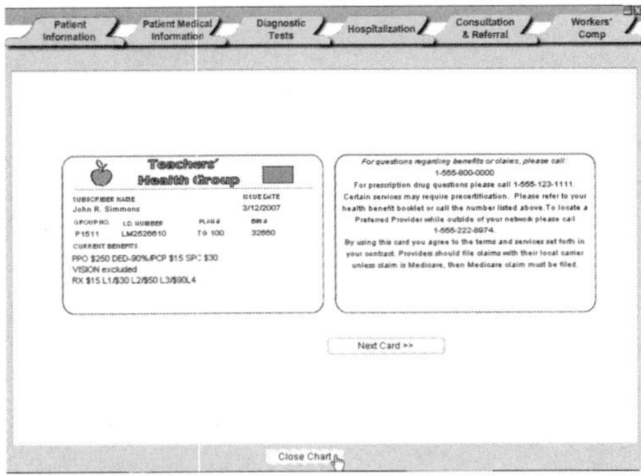

- Click the exit arrow at the lower right corner of the screen to go to the Summary Menu.
- On the Summary Menu, click **Return to Map** to continue to the next exercise.

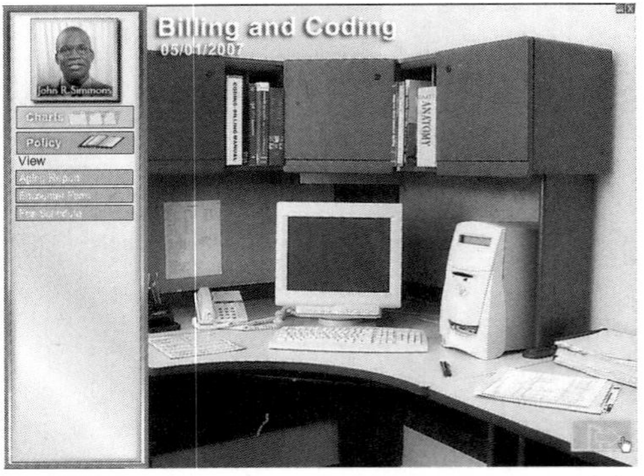

Exercise 3

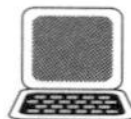

Online Activity—Identifying Potential Liability, Ethical Issues, and Possible Solutions

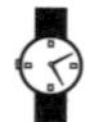

15 minutes

The health insurance professional will have both direct and indirect contact with patients, physicians, clinical staff members, business staff members, and insurance carriers. No matter what position an employee holds or how much education he or she has had, direct and indirect patient contact involves ethical and legal responsibility. The health insurance professional is expected to follow the codes of conduct in health care referred to as medical ethics and medical etiquette.

- Sign in to Mountain View Clinic.
- From the patient list, select **Wilson Metcalf**. (*Note:* If you have exited the program, sign in again to Mountain View Clinic and select Wilson Metcalf from the patient list.)

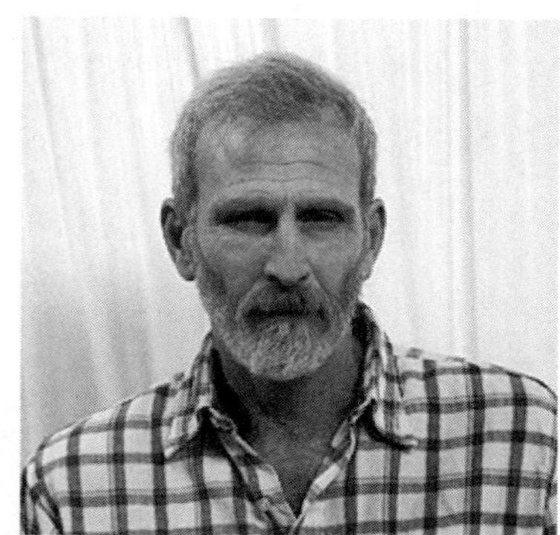

- On the office map, highlight and click on **Reception** to enter the Reception area.

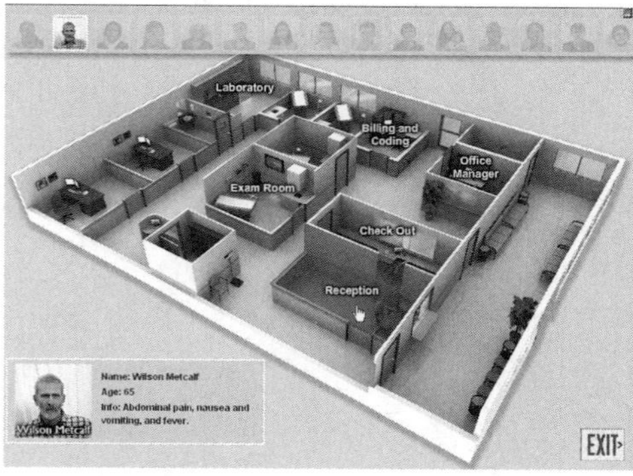

- Click on **Policy** to open the office Policy Manual.

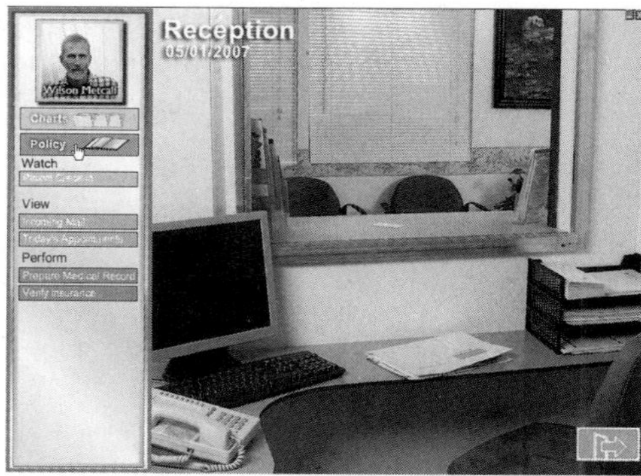

- From the menu on the left side of the screen, click on the arrow next to Policy Manual to expand the menu.

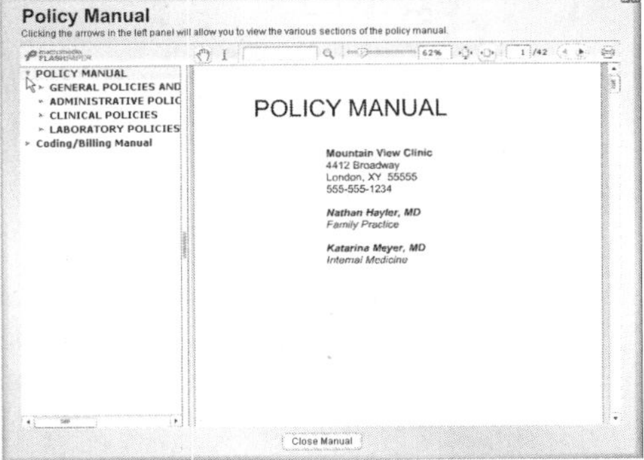

- Click on **Administrative Policies** and then on **Emergency Office Guidelines**. Read from pages 17 through 19 of the Policy Manual.

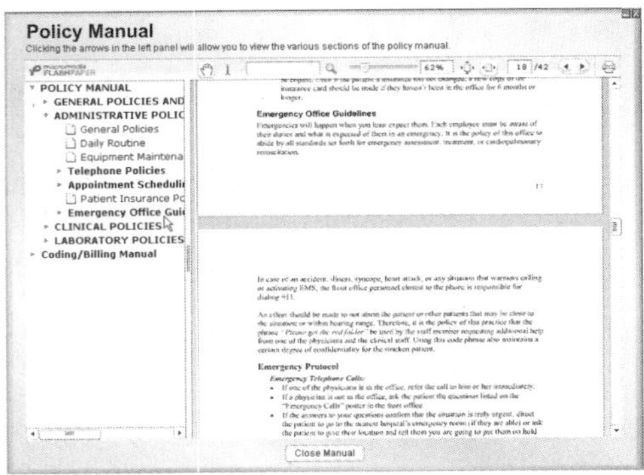

- Click on **Close Manual** to return to the Reception area.
- Under the Watch heading, click on **Patient Check-In** and view the video.

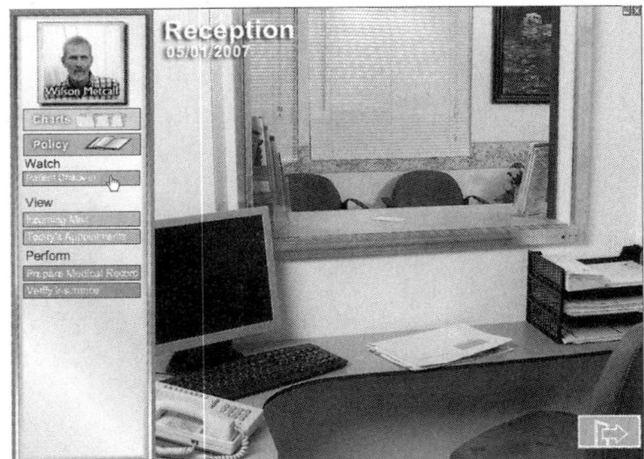

1. Regardless of the health insurance professional's job description or what area of the clinic he or she works from, the health insurance professional must be aware of how to respond to all types of ethical situations that may occur at any location in the office. As you watched the video, what did you observe about Mr. Metcalf's condition?

2. Based on your observations, if you had been assisting Mr. Metcalf, would you have kept him at the counter as Kristin did while she completed the check-in process? Explain your answer.

3. Did Kristin leave herself and the practice open to any potential liability issue(s) in this scene? If so, describe the issue(s) you identified.

4. If Mr. Metcalf had been injured as a result of his fall and the subsequent treatment by the office staff and he chose to pursue legal action against the practice, who would be at risk for liability?
   a. The physicians, the practice, and all three medical assistants
   b. The practice, Charlie, and Kristin
   c. Only Charlie and Kristin
   d. Only Kristin

5. Under the "Work Ethics" heading in Mountain View Clinic's Policy Manual, it states that each employee will act as a "team player" in all areas of the office practice. Imagine that you, as a health insurance professional, were working at Mountain View Clinic and present during the events that occurred in Mr. Metcalf's check-in video. As a team player, what actions could you have taken that may have helped to avoid the liability issues that occurred in this case?

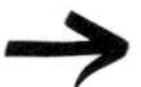

- At the end of the video, click **Close** to return to the Reception area.
- Remain in the Reception area and continue to the next exercise.

Exercise 4

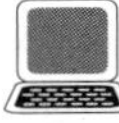

Online Activity—Breaches of Medical Ethics and Medical Etiquette

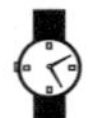

15 minutes

- Click on **Policy** to open the office Policy Manual. (*Note:* If you have exited the program, sign in again to Mountain View Clinic, select Wilson Metcalf from the patient list, and enter the Reception area.)

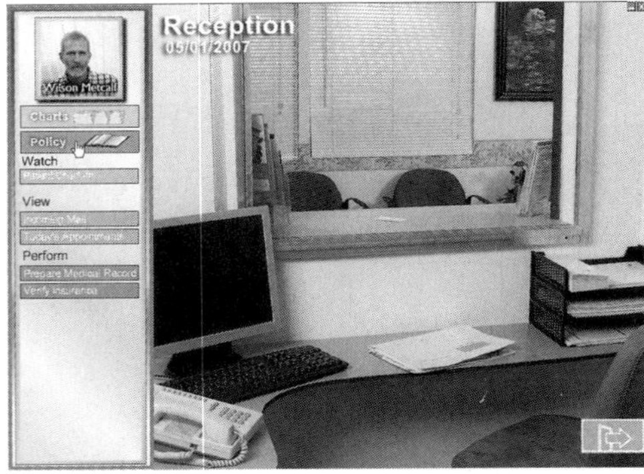

- Type "ethics" in the search bar and click on the magnifying glass.
- Read the section in the Policy Manual concerning "Work Ethics and Professional Behavior."
- Keep the Policy Manual open to answer the following questions.

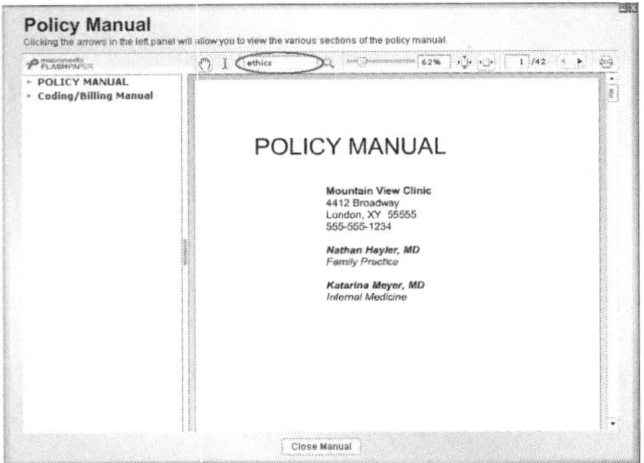

1. The "Work Ethics and Professional Behavior" section in the Policy Manual notes that employees are to show compassion and care toward patients. Based on these guidelines, describe how Kristin's interaction with Mr. Metcalf fell short of those guidelines. (*Note:* If necessary, click **Close Manual** to return to Reception and review the Patient Check-In video again.)

Questions 2 through 7 list some of the medical ethics and etiquette problems that were identified in Wilson Metcalf's Patient Check-In video. In the blank preceding each statement, identify the problem as an issue of medical ethics or medical etiquette (write "Ethics" or "Etiquette" in the blank). In the space below each statement, describe a more appropriate manner to handle the situation.

2. _________ Kristin does not acknowledge Mr. Metcalf's obvious distress.

3. _________ Kristin has Mr. Metcalf stand longer than necessary.

4. _________ Kristin asks for insurance information before establishing the true nature of Mr. Metcalf's medical condition.

5. _________ Kristin asks Mr. Metcalf to update his insurance information instead of first addressing his discomfort.

6. _________ In front of Mr. Metcalf and other patients, Kristin suggests to Charlie that Mr. Metcalf needs soap.

7. _________ Kristin shouts loudly to the other assistants for help and to bring the red folder rather than using the intercom or asking someone personally to get the folder.

8. In addition to Kristin's comments about Mr. Metcalf needing soap, what did you notice about her nonverbal communications throughout the video?

9. Explain why it is important for the health insurance professional, as a team player, to be aware of all situations occurring in the office and to be prepared to address them, regardless of his or her job description.

→ • Click the exit arrow at the lower right corner of the screen to go to the Summary Menu.
• On the Summary Menu, click **Return to Map** to continue to the next lesson or click **Exit the Program**.

LESSON 2

The Medical Record

Reading Assignment: Chapter 3—The Legal and Ethical Side of Medical Insurance
- The Medical Record
- Documentation of Patient Medical Record

Patient: Wilson Metcalf

Learning Objectives:

- Recognize the importance of the organization's medical record policies as a resource in meeting federal, state, local, and practice guidelines related to the medical record.
- Identify the elements of a medical record and locate them in the chart.
- Correctly update patient information in the medical record.
- Identify specific details of documentation within the medical record to support services billed.
- Identify the physician's diagnosis(es) in the medical record.

Overview:

This lesson addresses the essential components and general guidelines associated with medical records. You will view Mountain View Clinic's Policy Manual to familiarize yourself with office policies that serve as a foundation in adherence with federal, state, local, and practice guidelines related to the medical record. You will also view Wilson Metcalf's medical record to recognize and identify various components of the medical record. Next, you will view Mr. Metcalf's check-in video and practice updating insurance information in the medical record. By the end of the lesson, you should be able to locate basic patient medical information and the physician's diagnoses.

Exercise 1

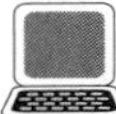

Online Activity—General Medical Record Guidelines

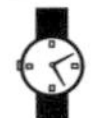

15 minutes

The medical record serves many purposes in the medical practice. It is the source of information used for the health insurance professional to submit accurate insurance claims. Therefore the health insurance professional must be knowledgeable of all federal, state, and local regulations related to medical records. Keep in mind that policies will vary from practice to practice and state to state. A critical step in the proper handling of medical records begins with the health insurance professional becoming familiar with the medical facility's medical record policies.

- Sign in to Mountain View Clinic.
- Select **Wilson Metcalf** from the patient list.

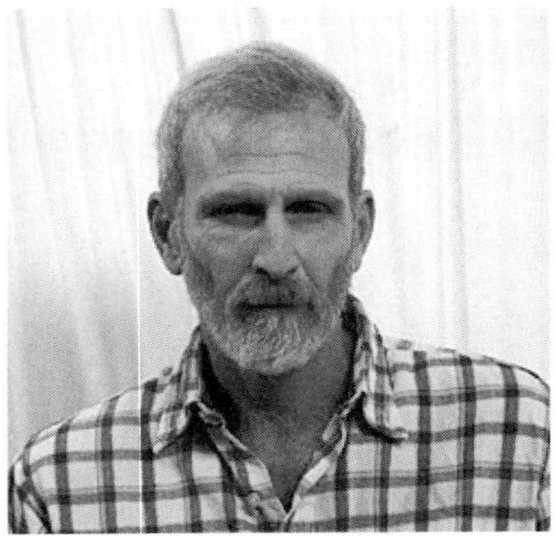

- On the office map, highlight and click on **Billing and Coding** to enter the Billing and Coding area.

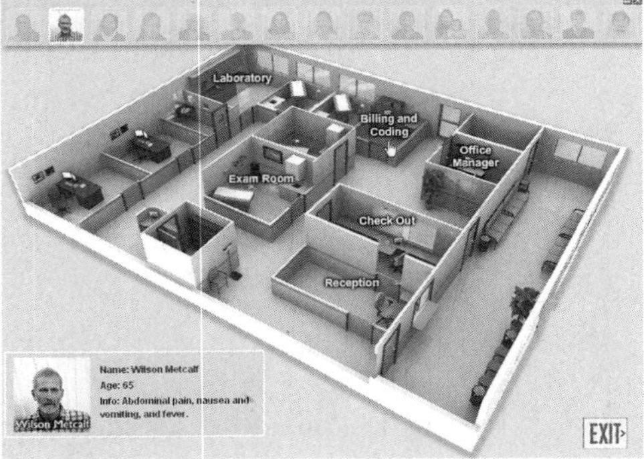

- Click on **Policy Manual** to open the office Policy Manual.

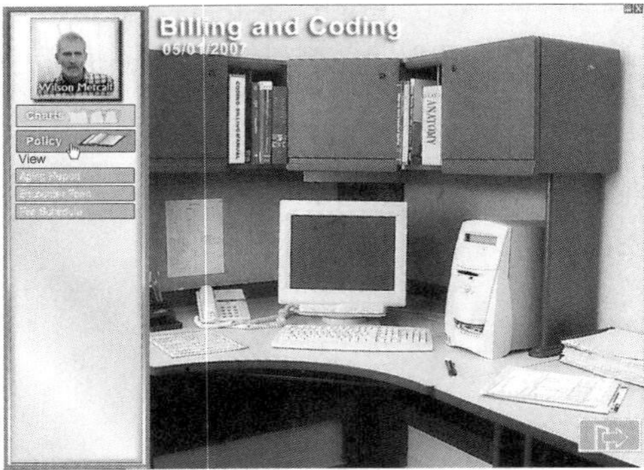

- Review all of Mountain View Clinic's policies regarding medical records
- Use the information provided in Mountain View Clinic's Policy Manual to answer the following questions.
- *Note:* Use the search bar in the Policy Manual to search for key terms in the questions to help find the appropriate information.

1. According to Mountain View Clinic's Policy Manual, what step should you, as the health insurance professional, take to ensure continuity of patient care when medical records are used? (*Hint:* Search in the Administrative Policies section under General Policies for this answer.)
   a. Tell the receptionist that you have taken the patient's record.
   b. Sign out any patient record you have taken.
   c. Return the chart within 24 hours.
   d. Just use common sense.

2. At Mountain View Clinic, a medical record progress note must be completed by the physician and placed in the chart:
   a. as soon as the patient leaves the office.
   b. as soon as the dictation has been transcribed.
   c. within 24 hours from the date of service.
   d. within 14 days from the date of service.

3. According to Mountain View Clinic's Policy Manual, the health insurance professional should ask for clarification regarding charges and associated documentation submitted by a physician:
   a. within 14 days from the date of service.
   b. after the claim has been billed.
   c. upon the request for clarification from the insurance carrier.
   d. never; there is no need for clarification because reporting of charges and associated documentation is the physician's responsibility.

4. What is the length of time for maintaining an adult patients medical record at Mountain View Clinic?
   a. For as long as the adult is a patient at the clinic
   b. For a period of 3 years from the last date of service
   c. For a period of 15 years from the last date of service
   d. For a period of 15 years from the time the adult leaves the practice

5. After the minimum retention time has been met, outside vendors to Mountain View Clinic should dispose of records by:
   a. returning them to the clinic.
   b. dropping them off at the local recycling center.
   c. putting them in a garbage pickup area.
   d. shredding or burning them.

→ • Click **Close Manual** to return to the Billing and Coding area.

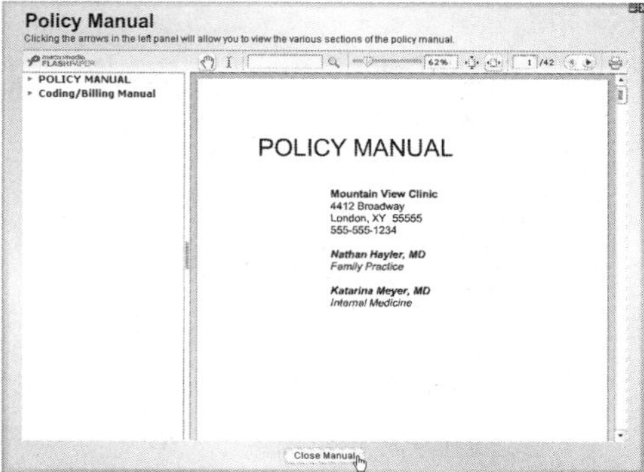

- Click the exit arrow at the lower right corner of the screen to go to the Summary Menu.
- On the Summary Menu, click **Return to Map** to continue to the next exercise.

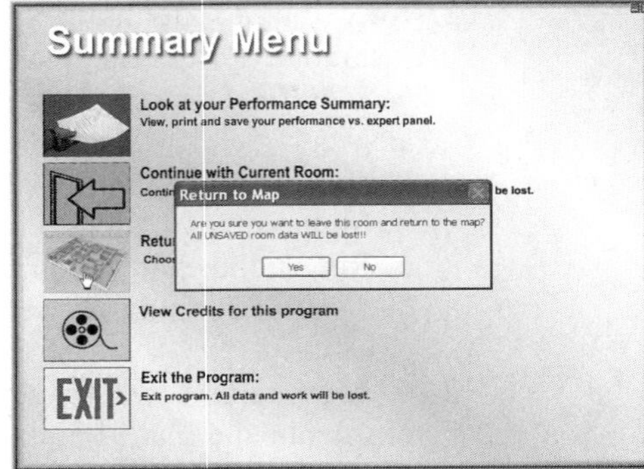

Exercise 2

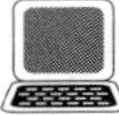

Online Activity—Components of the Medical Record: Patient Information

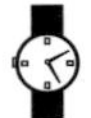

15 minutes

It is essential for the health insurance professional to be familiar with all components of the medical record and where they are placed.

- From the patient list, select **Wilson Metcalf**. (*Note:* If you have exited the program, sign in again to Mountain View Clinic, select Wilson Metcalf from the patient list, and enter the Reception area.)

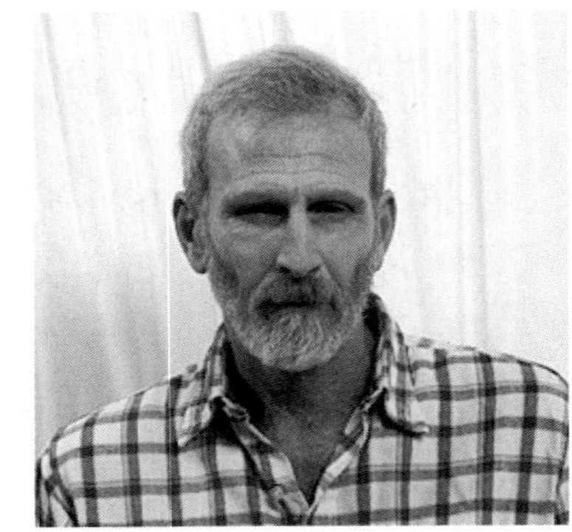

- On the office map, highlight and click on **Check Out** to enter the Check Out area.

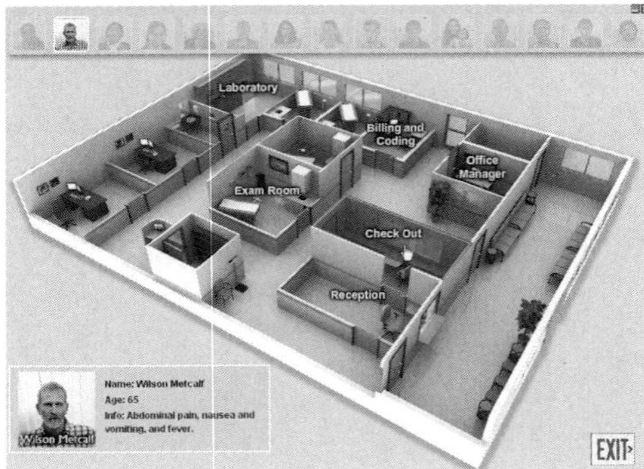

- Click on **Charts** to open Mr. Metcalf's medical record.

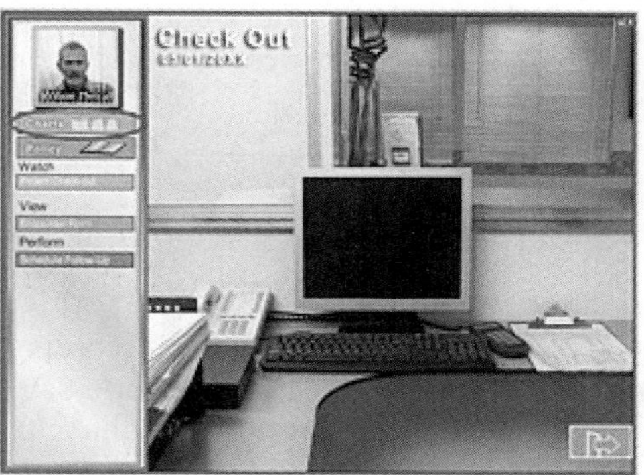

- At the top of the chart, there are a series of tabs separating the different sections of the medical record. Click on the various tabs to explore what parts of the medical record are included under each tab.

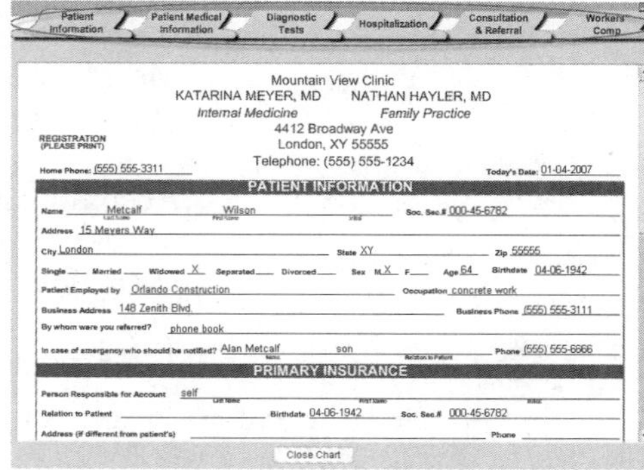

Maneuver within Mr. Metcalf's chart to answer the following questions. (*Hint:* Look closely at the drop-down list from the tabs while answering the questions.)

1. Copies of the patient's insurance card(s) are included under which tab?
   a. Patient Information
   b. Patient Medical Information
   c. Hospitalization
   d. Workers' Comp

2. The patient's medication record is included under which tab?
   a. Patient Information
   b. Patient Medical Information
   c. Diagnostic Tests
   d. Hospitalization

3. Which tab or section does not contain forms at the present time?
   a. Patient Medical Information
   b. Diagnostic Tests
   c. Hospitalization
   d. Workers' Comp

4. Inpatient Progress Notes are listed twice under the Hospitalization tab because:
   a. the record has been duplicated in error.
   b. another patient's record has been filed in Mr. Metcalf's chart in error.
   c. there are two different dates of service.
   d. there are two different records from two different physicians.

5. Using all information and forms found under the Patient Information tab of Mr. Metcalf's chart, identify whether each of the following statements is true or false.

   a. _________ There are two Patient Information Forms in Wilson Metcalf's chart.

   b. _________ Based on patient registration information available on 1/4/2007, the patient's mailing address is 148 Zenith Blvd., London, XY 55555.

   c. _________ According to the Primary Insurance section of the Patient Information Form dated 1/4/2007, Mr. Metcalf's primary insurance is Independent Contractor's Group.

   d. _________ Mr. Metcalf has one insurance card on file at Mountain View Clinic.

   e. _________ Mr. Metcalf's Medicare insurance card states that his coverage became effective on 4/6/2007.

   f. _________ According to Mr. Metcalf's updated Patient Information Form dated 5/1/2007, his primary insurance is Independent Contractor's Group insurance.

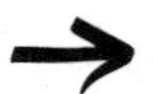

- When you are finished, click **Close Chart** to return to the Check Out area.
- Click the exit arrow and select **Return to Map** from the Summary Menu.

Exercise 3

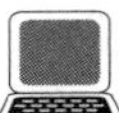

Online Activity—Updating Patient Information in the Medical Record

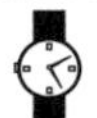

15 minutes

- Keep Wilson Metcalf as your patient and click on **Reception**. (*Note:* If you have exited the program, sign in again to Mountain View Clinic, select Wilson Metcalf from the patient list, and enter the Reception area.)
- Under the Watch heading, click on **Patient Check-In** to view the video.

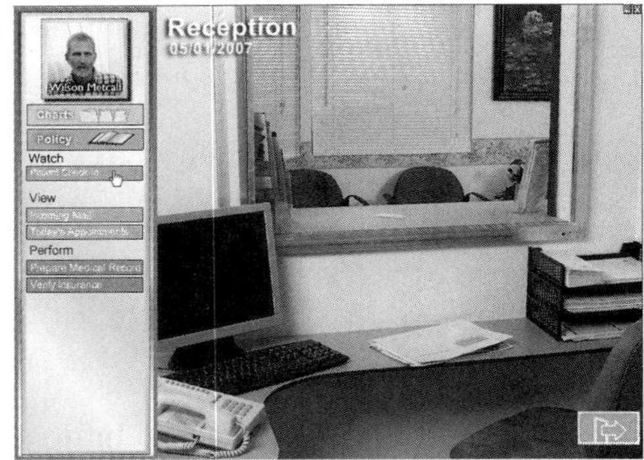

- When Mr. Metcalf begins to look for his insurance card, click on the pause or stop button at the lower left hand corner of the video screen.
- Click **Close** to return to the Reception area.
- Click on **Charts** to open Mr. Metcalf's medical record.

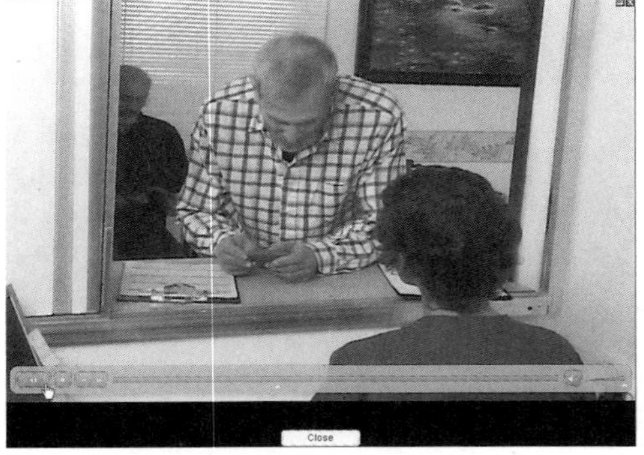

1. Using the new insurance card in Mr. Metcalf's chart, update the Primary Insurance section of his Patient Information Form below.

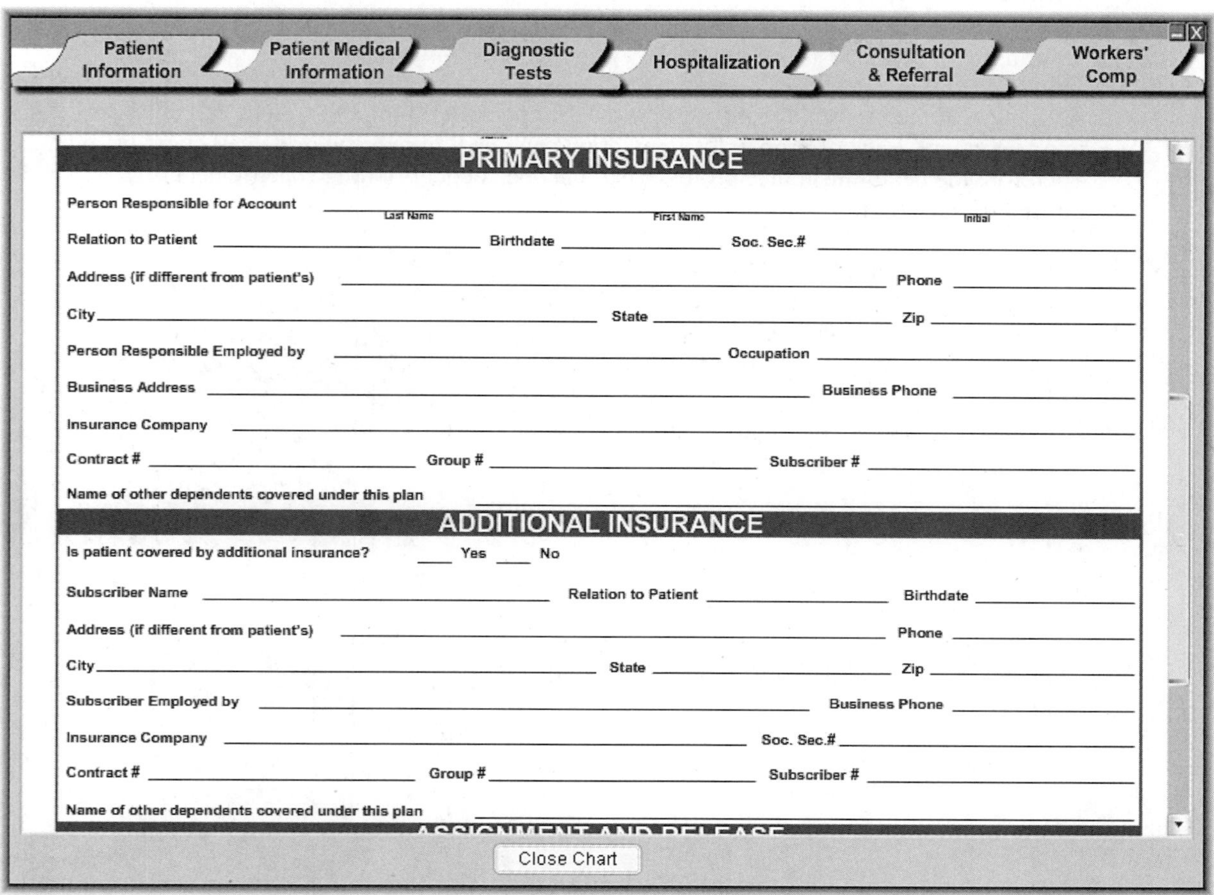
Patient Information | Patient Medical Information | Diagnostic Tests | Hospitalization | Consultation & Referral | Workers' Comp

PRIMARY INSURANCE

Person Responsible for Account ____ Last Name ____ First Name ____ Initial

Relation to Patient ____ Birthdate ____ Soc. Sec.# ____

Address (if different from patient's) ____ Phone ____

City ____ State ____ Zip ____

Person Responsible Employed by ____ Occupation ____

Business Address ____ Business Phone ____

Insurance Company ____

Contract # ____ Group # ____ Subscriber # ____

Name of other dependents covered under this plan ____

ADDITIONAL INSURANCE

Is patient covered by additional insurance? ___ Yes ___ No

Subscriber Name ____ Relation to Patient ____ Birthdate ____

Address (if different from patient's) ____ Phone ____

City ____ State ____ Zip ____

Subscriber Employed by ____ Business Phone ____

Insurance Company ____ Soc. Sec.# ____

Contract # ____ Group # ____ Subscriber # ____

Name of other dependents covered under this plan ____

Close Chart

2. Kristin, the receptionist, asks Mr. Metcalf whether there has been a change in his insurance. What is his response?

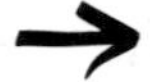

- Click **Close Chart** to return to the Reception area.
- Click the exit arrow to go to the Summary Menu.
- On the Summary Menu, click **Return to Map** and continue to the next exercise.

Exercise 4

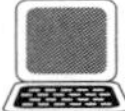

Online Activity—Other Components of the Medical Record

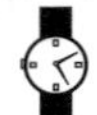

15 minutes

A function of the medical record is to provide support for billing of services and third-party reimbursement. Lack of proper documentation can result in reduced or denied claim payment. Therefore the health insurance professional must be adept at finding specific details of information within the medical record.

- From the patient list, select **Wilson Metcalf**. (*Note:* If you have exited the program, sign in again to Mountain View Clinic, select Wilson Metcalf from the patient list, and enter the Exam Room.)
- On the office map, highlight and click on **Exam Room** to enter the Exam Room.

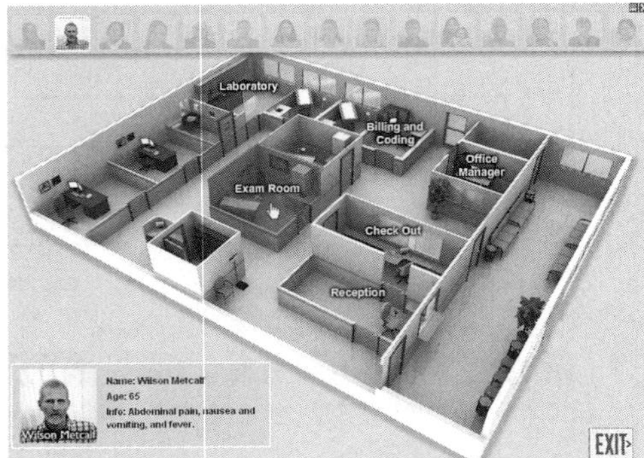

- Click on **Charts** to open Mr. Metcalf's medical record and review all components of the medical record.

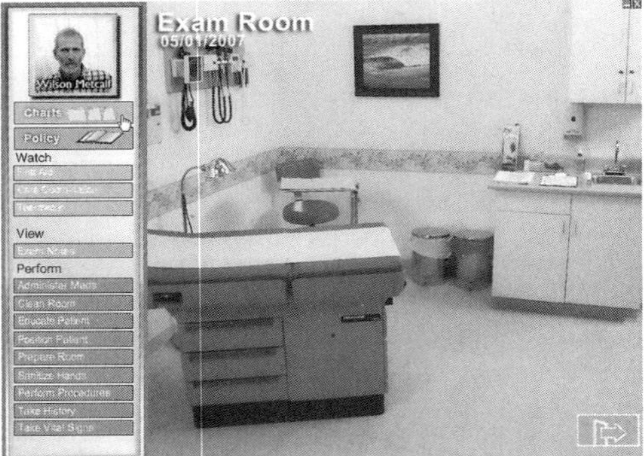

- When you have finished reviewing, click on **Close Chart** to return to the Exam Room.
- Under the View heading, click on **Exam Notes** and read the documentation regarding Mr. Metcalf's visit.

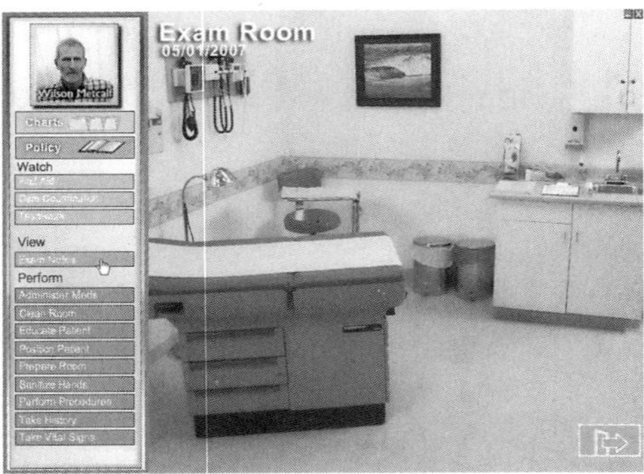

1. On what date was Mr. Metcalf's General Health History taken?

2. According to Mr. Metcalf's General Health History, what was his mother's cause of death? (*Hint:* Use the arrow buttons to scroll back and forth in the record as needed.)

3. What three medications was Mr. Metcalf taking when he came to the practice on 1/4/2007?

4. Did Mr. Metcalf have any previous diagnostic tests performed? If so, what test(s) and when?

5. According to Mr. Metcalf's records, how many previous visits to the hospital has he had?

6. Why was Mr. Metcalf admitted to the hospital on 4/9/1994?

7. Whose signature appears at the end of the Progress Note dated 5/1/2007?

8. What was the chief complaint documented in Dr. Meyer's Exam Note of 5/1/2007?

9. What is the final diagnosis documented in Dr. Meyer's Exam Note of 5/1/2007?

10. Where would an itemization of the services billed on 5/1/2007 be located in the medical record?

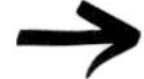

- Click **Finish** to return to the Exam Room.
- Click the exit arrow at the lower right corner of the screen to go to the Summary Menu.
- On the Summary Menu, click **Return to Map** to continue to the next lesson or click **Exit the Program**.

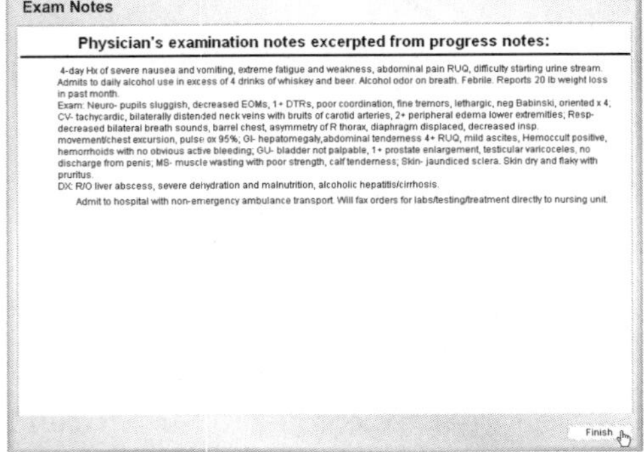

LESSON 3

Confidentiality and Privacy

Reading Assignment: Chapter 3—The Legal and Ethical Side of Medical Insurance
- Health Insurance Portability and Accountability Act
- Compliance, Confidentiality, and Privacy

Patients: Wilson Metcalf, Teresa Hernandez

Learning Objectives:

- Recognize the importance of the organization's policies as a resource in meeting confidentiality and privacy guidelines.
- Identify the forms used to protect patient privacy.
- Identify medical practice confidentiality and privacy issues.

Overview:

This lesson addresses the issues of privacy and confidentiality as they relate to the patient's authorization to release private health information. You will view Mountain View Clinic's Policy Manual to familiarize yourself with office policies that serve as a foundation in adherence to confidentiality and privacy guidelines. You will review Wilson Metcalf's chart and identify forms required under HIPAA to ensure compliance with the Privacy Rule. Then you will review Teresa Hernandez's check-in and check-out video to identify any potential confidentiality issues. By the end of the lesson, you should understand the importance of patient confidentiality and the steps that must be taken to protect a patient's privacy.

Exercise 1

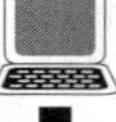

Online Activity—General Confidentiality and Privacy Guidelines

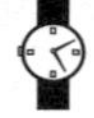

15 minutes

The health insurance professional has a responsibility to treat all patient information with the highest degree of confidentiality and in accordance with state and federal privacy laws. To ensure compliance with privacy laws, the health insurance professional should be knowledgeable of all federal and state privacy laws. Health insurance professionals should also familiarize themselves with the medical facility's privacy policies.

Note: Keep in mind that privacy policies will vary from practice to practice.

- Sign in to Mountain View Clinic.
- From the patient list, select **Wilson Metcalf**.

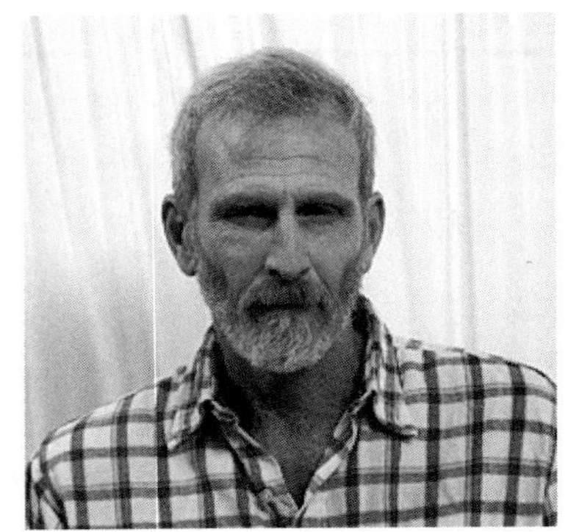

- On the office map, highlight and click on **Exam Room** to enter the Exam Room.

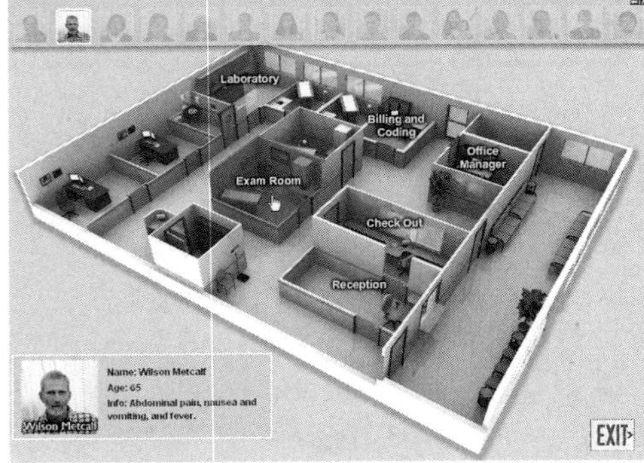

- Click on **Policy** to open the office Policy Manual.
- Type "HIPAA" in the search bar and click on the magnifying glass.
- Read the information in the Policy Manual related to HIPAA.
- Click **Close Manual** to return to the Exam Room area.

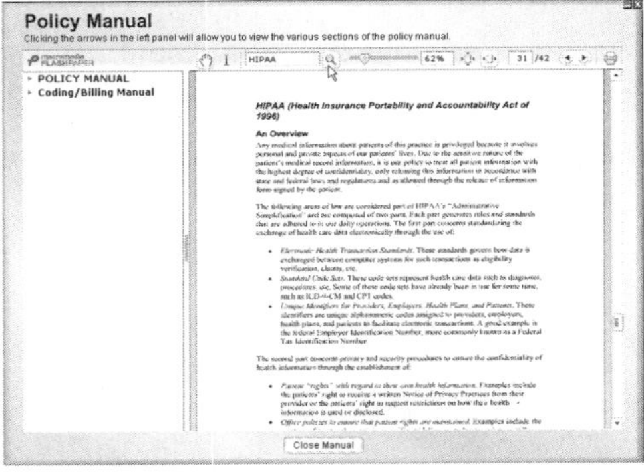

- Under the Watch heading, click on **Care Coordination** and view the video.

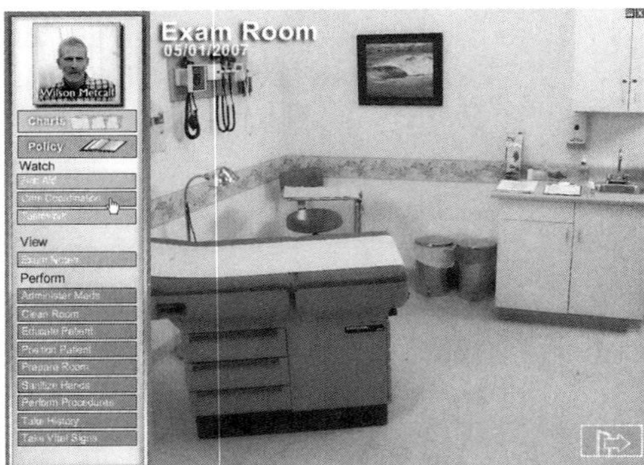

- At the end of the video, click **Close** to return to the Exam Room.
- Click on **Charts** to open Mr. Metcalf's medical record.

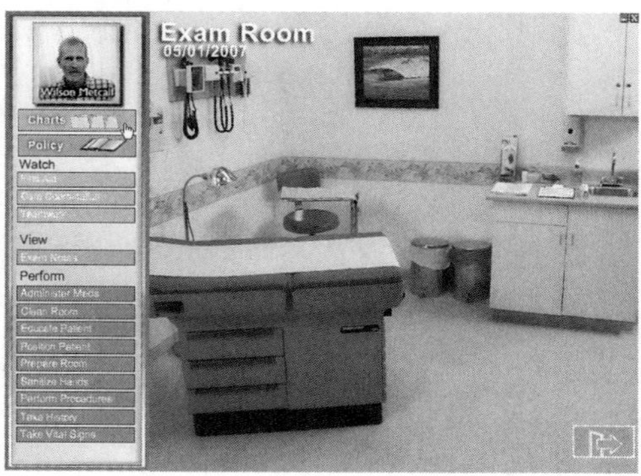

- Use the chart and what you observed in the video to answer the following questions.

1. According to Mountain View Clinic's Policy Manual, there are six forms that are used with patients in order to implement the HIPAA Privacy Rule. List these six forms.

2. Under what tab in Mr. Metcalf's chart would HIPAA forms allowing release of information for referral purposes be filed?
   a. Patient Information
   b. Patient Medical Information
   c. Hospitalizations
   d. Consultations and Referrals

3. What form was provided to Mr. Metcalf that informed him of his right to privacy under HIPAA and outlined the complete description of how his health information would be used and/or disclosed?
   a. Notice of Privacy Practices
   b. Acknowledgement of Receipt of Notice of Privacy Practices
   c. Protected Health Information Disclosure Record
   d. Right to Request Confidential Communication Notice

4. What form in Mr. Metcalf's chart was signed by him, ensuring that he has been advised of the office's privacy policies and how his health information will be handled?
   a. Notice of Privacy Practices
   b. Acknowledgement of Receipt of Notice of Privacy Practices
   c. Authorization for Release of Information
   d. Right to Request Confidential Communication Notice

5. What form in Mr. Metcalf's chart was signed and allows the practice to release his information to the hospital?
   a. Acknowledgement of Receipt of Notice of Privacy Practices
   b. Authorization for Release of Information
   c. Protected Health Information Disclosure Record
   d. Request for Correction/Amendment of Protected Health Information

6. On 1/4/2007, Mr. Metcalf agreed to have the practice provide his son Alan with information from the medical record. What information was included in this authorization for release?
   a. His entire medical record
   b. All Progress Notes
   c. Mental health/alcohol and drug abuse treatment
   d. Statement of charges/payments

7. To what other records does Mr. Metcalf's son Alan have access?

8. On 1/4/2007, Mr. Metcalf agreed to allow Bristol Medical Center to release information to Dr. Meyer for the purpose of:
   a. continued patient care.
   b. disability determination.
   c. legal purposes.
   d. submission of insurance claims.

9. To what records does Dr. Meyer have access, according to the same release?

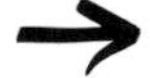

- Click **Close Chart** to return to the Exam Room.
- Click the exit arrow at the lower right corner of the screen to go to the Summary Menu.
- On the Summary Menu, click **Return to Map** and continue to the next exercise.

Exercise 2

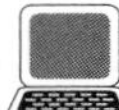

Online Activity—Keeping Compliant

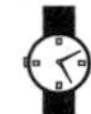

15 minutes

- From the patient list, select **Teresa Hernandez**. (*Note:* If you have exited the program, sign in again to Mountain View Clinic, and select Teresa Hernandez from the patient list.)

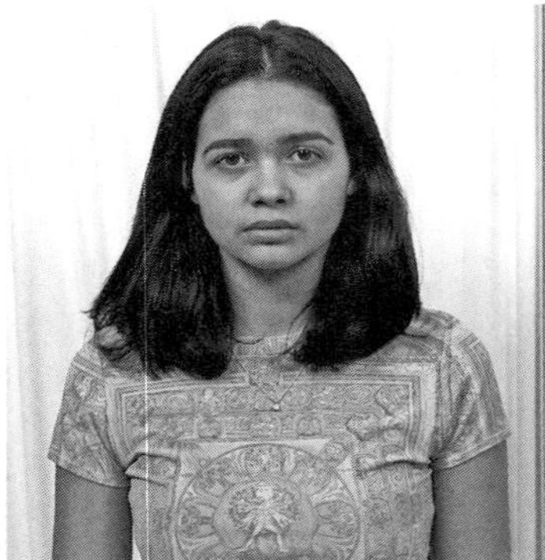

- On the office map, highlight and click on **Reception** to enter the Reception area.

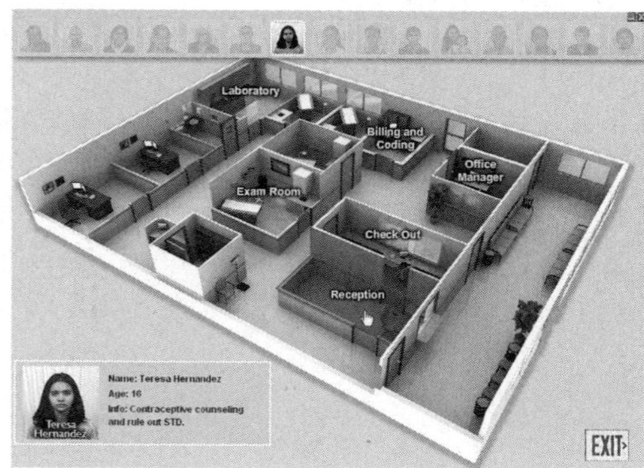

- Under the Watch heading, click on **Patient Check-In** to view the video.
- At the end of the video, click **Close** to return to the Reception area.
- Click the exit arrow at the lower right corner of the screen to go to the Summary Menu.
- On the Summary Menu, click **Return to Map**.

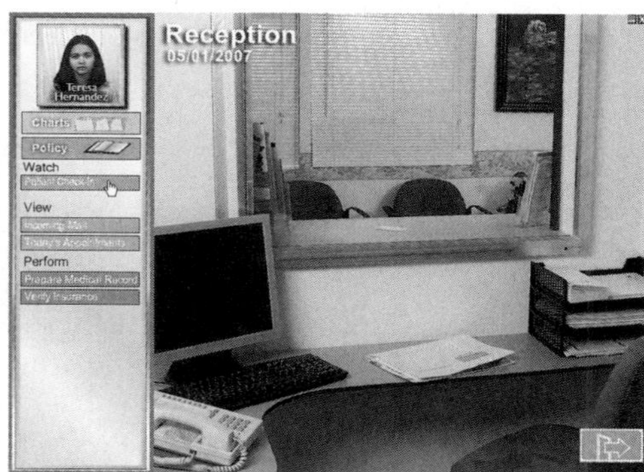

- On the office map, highlight and click on **Check Out** to enter the Check Out area.

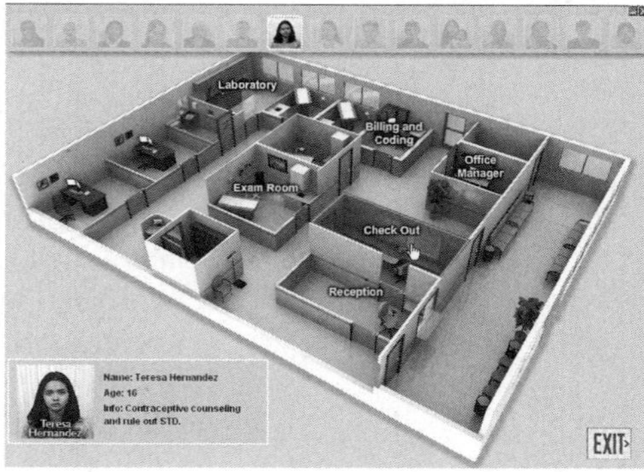

- Under the Watch heading, click on **Patient Check-Out** to view the video.
- At the end of the video, click **Close** to return to the Check Out area.
- Click on **Encounter Form** to view the Encounter Form.
- Select **Finish**.

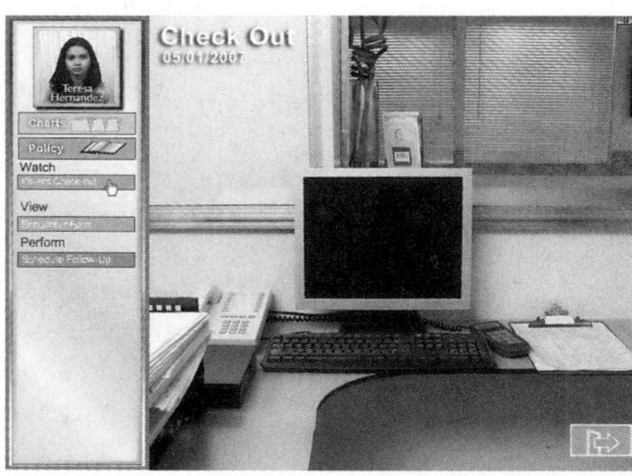

- Now click on **Charts** to open Teresa's medical record.
- Select **Progress Notes** from the **Patient Medical Information** tab.

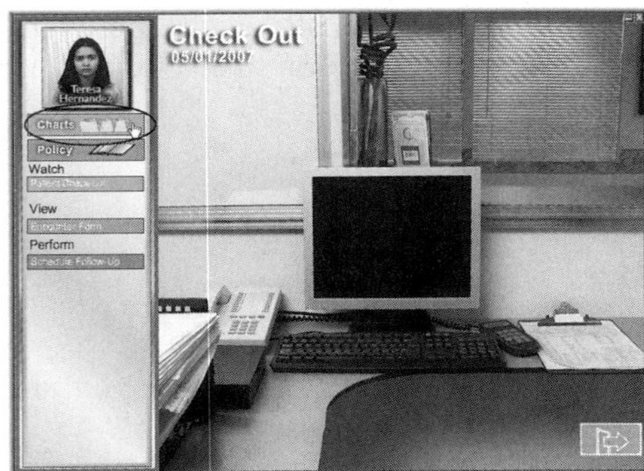

1. What is the purpose of Teresa's visit to the clinic on 5/1/2007?

2. Confirm the effectiveness of the actions taken by the staff in protecting the privacy of the Teresa's visit by indicating whether each of the following statements is true or false.

   a. _________ The receptionist at Mountain View Clinic provided the patient with an explanation of her privacy rights, and the patient was confident that her health information would be protected as she requested.

   b. _________ The patient was given a Notice of Privacy Practices stating how her health information would be used.

   c. _________ Upon notification by the patient that she did not want her father to receive any information regarding this visit, the receptionist provided the patient with an opportunity to state her request in writing and it was filed in the patient's chart.

   d. _________ Because of the confidential nature of the patient's conversation with the receptionist, care was taken to ensure that other patients in the waiting room were not within hearing range of the conversation.

   e. _________ The physician made a notation on the patient's Encounter Form to remind the health insurance specialist that special privacy precautions should be taken in submitting the claim to the insurance carrier to prevent the patient's parents from receiving information.

   f. _________ Upon check-out, the patient was advised that although the practice would not release any confidential information to the parents, the insurance carrier would send the parents an explanation of benefits; thus it was suggested that the patient provide an alternative address where the EOB could be sent.

   g. _________ The alternative address that the patient requested be used to protect her privacy was documented in the chart.

3. Based on this exercise, are you confident that Teresa Hernandez's father will not receive any information regarding her visit to Mountain View Clinic and that the staff has taken all necessary precautions to protect her health information?

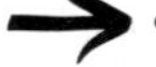

- Click **Close Chart** to return to the Exam Room.
- Click the exit arrow at the lower right corner of the screen to go to the Summary Menu.
- On the Summary Menu, click **Return to Map** to continue to the next lesson or click **Exit the Program**.

LESSON 4

Types of Health Insurance

Reading Assignment: Chapter 4—Types and Sources of Health Insurance
- Types of Health Insurance
- Sources of Health Insurance
- Other Terms Common to Third-Party Carriers

Patients: All

Learning Objectives:

- Identify Mountain View Clinic's billing and collection policies related to participating and nonparticipating insurance carriers.
- Identify the sources of health insurance used by Mountain View Clinic patients.
- Determine which, if any, Mountain View Clinic patients are affected by coordination of benefits, or the "birthday rule."
- Determine appropriate actions the health insurance professional can take to help patients avoid costly outcomes as they deal with new insurance policies.

Overview:

This lesson addresses the basic types of health insurance plans—indemnity (fee-for-service) and managed care—as well as the various sources from which patients can acquire health insurance coverage (Medicare, Blue Cross/Blue Shield, etc.). You will view Mountain View Clinic's Policy Manual to identify the various types of health insurance, and learn how to identify the patient's primary insurance source, as well as how to determine whether the patient has secondary coverage. You will learn to apply coordination of benefit rules and the birthday rule. You will also review Shaunti Begay's check-in and check-out video to determine the appropriate steps that should be taken to assist patients who have insurance coverage through a nonparticipating insurance.

Exercise 1

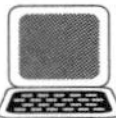

Online Activity—Types of Health Insurance

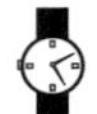

15 minutes

- Sign in to Mountain View Clinic and select any patient from the patient list.

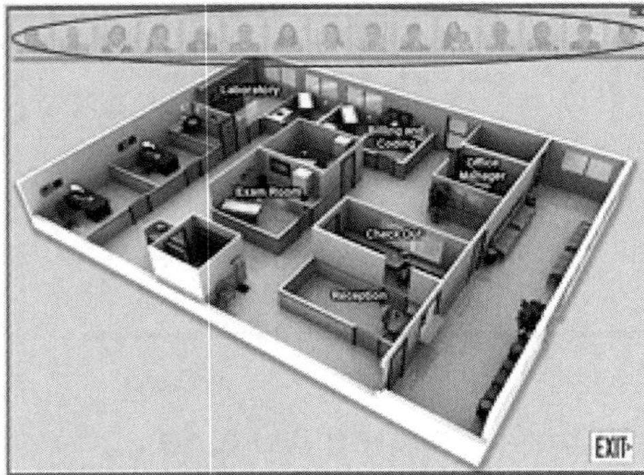

- On the office map, highlight and click on **Reception** to enter the Reception area.
- Click on **Policy** to open the office Policy Manual.
- Search for and read the sections on Financial Policy, Accepted Insurance Carriers, and Managed Care Plans (beginning on page 32). Also search Patient insurance Policies and read the information under that heading.

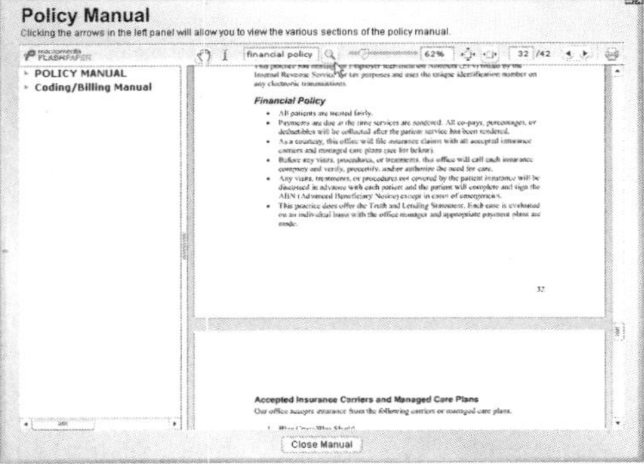

1. According to Mountain View Clinic's Policy Manual, when should the patient be told whether the provider participates with the patient's insurance carrier?
   a. Before the patient schedules the appointment
   b. When the patient checks in for his or her appointment
   c. When the patient checks out from his or her appointment
   d. When a statement is sent to the patient for payment of the services provided

2. If the physician at Mountain View Clinic does not participate with the patient's insurance plan, the patient should be informed that the office does not accept the insurance and:
   a. the patient should leave and find services elsewhere.
   b. the patient may schedule an appointment, but payment is expected at the time of service.
   c. the patient may schedule an appointment and the patient will be billed within 30 days from the date of service.
   d. the patient should be advised to drop the current insurance and find a carrier that the provider participates with.

3. Which health insurance plans does Mountain View Clinic participate with? Select all that apply.

   _____ Blue Cross/Blue Shield

   _____ Medicare

   _____ Liberty Bell Mutual

   _____ Teachers' Health Group

   _____ Acme Auto

   _____ Workers' Compensation

   _____ Small Business Owners' Health

   _____ Metropolitan Assurance

   _____ Unity Health Care

4. You have just been hired as a health insurance professional at Mountain View Clinic. A staff member at the clinic tells you that insurance cards should be photocopied if the patient's insurance has changed or if the patient has not been in the office for 6 months or longer. You know that this is:
   a. correct only if the office accepts the insurance.
   b. correct even if the office does not accept the insurance.
   c. never correct; it is unnecessary as long as you have updated the information on the Patient Information Form.

5. Does Mountain View Clinic offer Truth in Lending Statements for patients who cannot pay at the time of service? What is the policy for patients who have an emergency situation and need to be seen, but cannot pay?

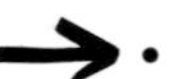

- Click **Close Manual** to return to the Reception area.
- Click the exit arrow at the lower right corner of the screen to go to the Summary Menu.
- On the Summary Menu, click **Return to Map** to continue to the next exercise.

Exercise 2

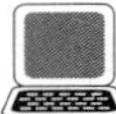

Online Activity—Identifying Sources of Patient Insurance Coverage

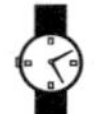

30 minutes

- From the patient list, select Janet Jones. In this exercise, you'll review the insurance coverage for *each patient*.
- On the office map, highlight and click on **Check Out** to enter the Check Out area.

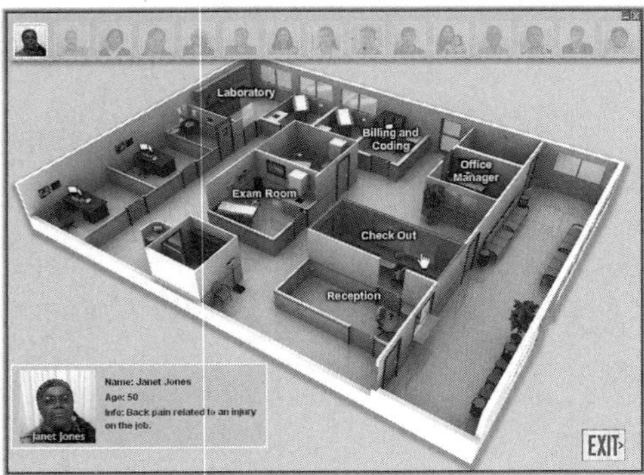

- Click on **Charts** to open the patient's medical record.
- Review the insurance section of the *most recent* Patient Information Form.
- You can also select **Insurance Cards** from under the **Patient Information** tab to verify the patient's primary and secondary coverage.

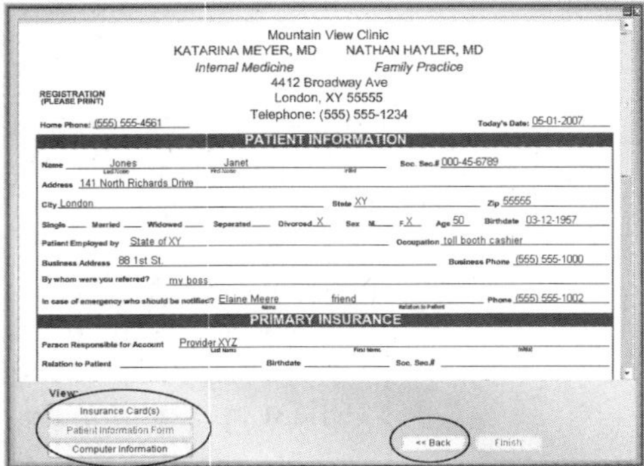

- To complete the following table, you will need to close the patient's chart, click the exit arrow, and return to the map to select the next patient.

1. For each patient listed in the left column below, enter the name of the patient's primary insurer and secondary insurer, if any (in the second and third columns). In the last column, write "Yes" or "No" to indicate whether or not the clinic will file the patient's insurance claim(s).

Patient Name	Primary Insurance	Secondary Insurance	Will Clinic File Claim?
Janet Jones			
Wilson Metcalf			
Rhea Davison			
Shaunti Begay			
Jean Deere			
Renee Anderson			
Teresa Hernandez			
Louise Parlet			
Tristan Tsosie			
Jose Imero			
Jade Wong			
John R. Simmons			
Hu Huang			
Kevin McKinzie			
Jesus Santo			

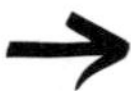

- After completing the table for all the patients, click **Close Chart** to return to the Check Out area.
- Click the exit arrow at the lower right corner of the screen to go to the Summary Menu.
- On the Summary Menu, click **Return to Map** and continue to the next exercise.

Exercise 3

Writing Activity—Coordination of Benefits/Birthday Rule

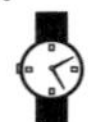

5 minutes

In the event that a patient is covered by two insurance policies, the health insurance professional must rely on the patient to state which policy is primary. This is known as coordination of benefits.

1. Listed in the left below are the five patients from the previous exercise who have two insurance carriers. Based on your knowledge of coordination of benefits, the definition of supplemental insurance, and the meaning of the birthday rule, provide an explanation for the sequencing of primary and secondary insurance coverage.

Patient	Primary	Secondary	Explanation for Coordination of Benefits
Jean Deere	Medicare A, B	Oasis Health Supplement	
Louise Parlet	Teachers' Health Group	Blue Cross/ Blue Shield	
Tristan Tsosie	Blue Cross	Mutual Health	
John Simmons	Teachers' Health Group	Small Business Owner's Group	
Hu Huang	Medicare A, B	Oasis Health Supplement	

Exercise 4

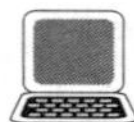

Online Activity—Participating Versus Nonparticipating Provider

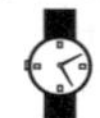

5 minutes

- From the patient list, select **Shaunti Begay**.

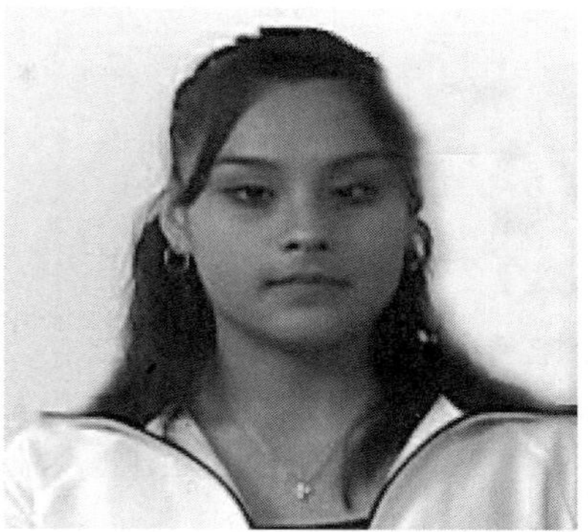

- On the office map, highlight and click on **Reception** to enter the Reception area.

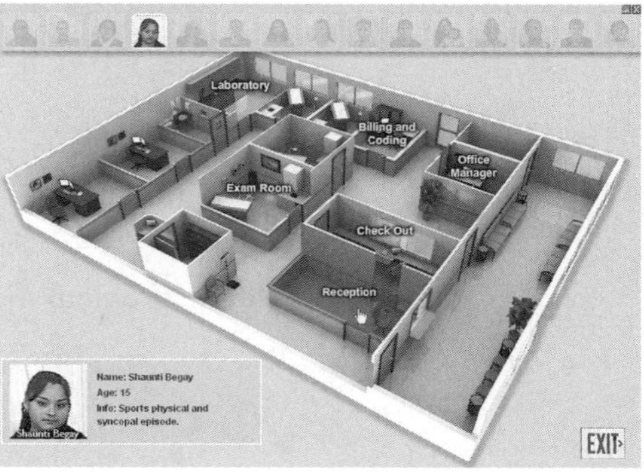

- Under the Watch heading, click on **Patient Check-In** to view the video.

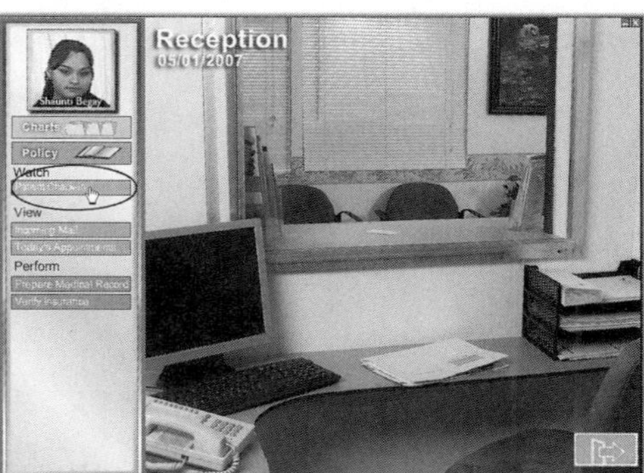

- At the end of the video, click **Close** to return to the Reception area.
- Click the exit arrow at the lower right corner of the screen to go to the Summary Menu.
- On the Summary Menu, click **Return to Map**.
- On the office map, highlight and click on **Check Out** to enter the Check Out area.

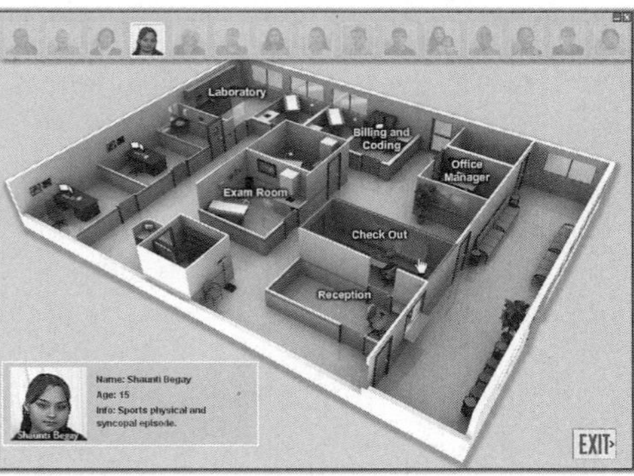

- Under the Watch heading, click on **Patient Check-Out** to view the video.

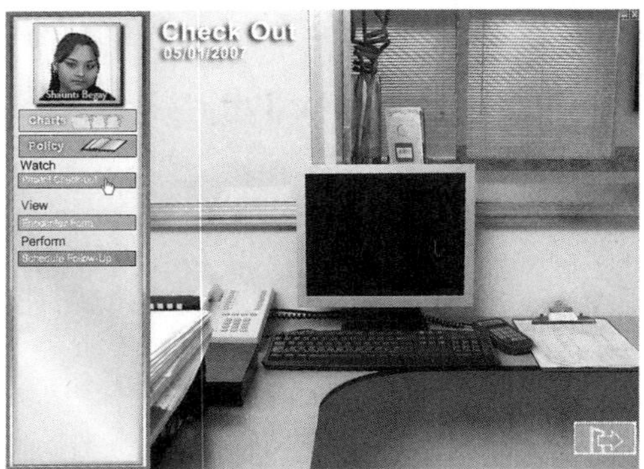

- At the end of the video, click **Close** to return to the Check Out area.
- Click on the **clipboard** to view the Encounter Form completed for Shaunti's visit.

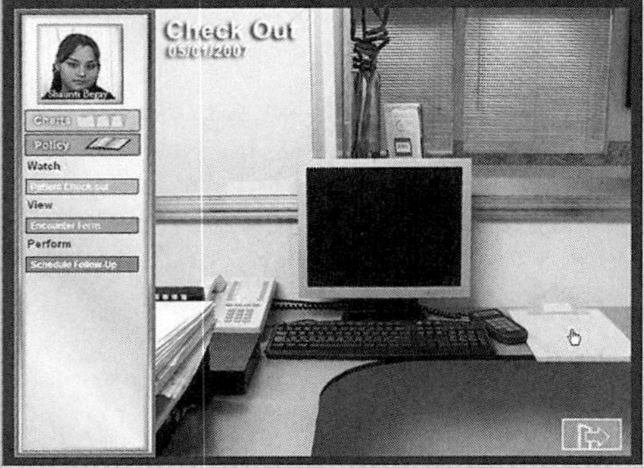

1. How could the problem in the video regarding the patient's insurance plan have been avoided?

2. What information does Kristin give to Shaunti's parents regarding their insurance carrier?

3. What does Kristin offer to do to assist Shaunti's parents with this unfortunate situation?

4. Where would Kristin find the phone number to contact the insurance plan?

5. In the Check-Out video, the Mountain View Clinic staff member had to determine the total fees for the services provided to Shaunti. Where would she locate this information? How much was she required to ask Mr. Begay to pay?

- Click **Finish** to close the Encounter Form and return to the Check Out area.
- Click the exit arrow at the lower right corner of the screen to go to the Summary Menu.
- On the Summary Menu, click **Return to Map** to continue to the next exercise or click **Exit the Program**.

LESSON 5

Introduction to the Universal Claim Form

Reading Assignment: Chapter 5—Claim Submission Methods
- The Universal Insurance Claim Form
- Essential Information for Claims Processing

Patient: Renee Anderson

Learning Objectives:

- Identify Mountain View Clinic's policies for verifying a patient's insurance coverage.
- Verify a patient's insurance coverage.
- Prepare documents needed to complete a CMS-1500 claim form.
- Complete the patient ledger card.

Overview:

In this lesson you will be introduced to the CMS-1500 claim form, along with the information and the source documents required to complete the claim form. You will view Mountain View Clinic's Policy Manual to identify all policies that will serve as a resource in following appropriate steps for verification of patient's insurance coverage. After watching Renee Anderson's check-in video, you will identify the appropriate actions to perform when verifying the patient's insurance coverage. You will also identify insurance information required to complete a CMS-1500 claim form. Next, you will view Renee Anderson's encounter form and Mountain View Clinic's Fee Schedule to identify the services provided and the process for assigning fees to those services. From the Encounter Form, a ledger card will be generated, correlating appropriate clinic fees with the procedures/services rendered. By the end of the lesson, you will be familiar with the CMS-1500 claim form and understand the process for collecting information and preparing documents needed to complete the claim.

Exercise 1

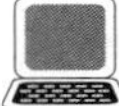

Online Activity—Verify Patient's Insurance Coverage

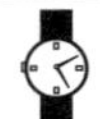

10 minutes

- Sign in to Mountain View Clinic.
- From the patient list, select **Renee Anderson**.

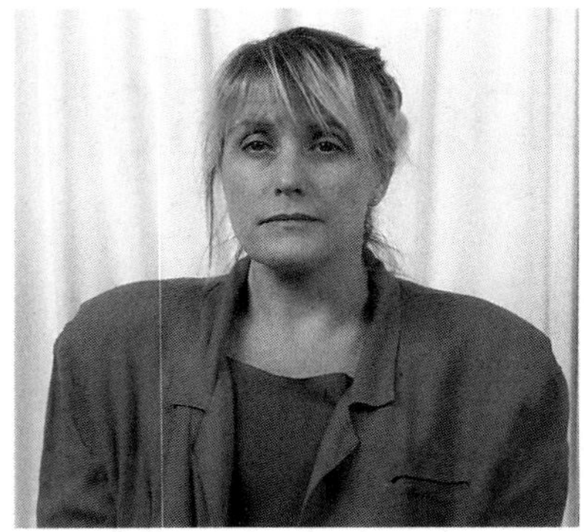

- On the office map, highlight and click on **Reception** to enter the Reception area.

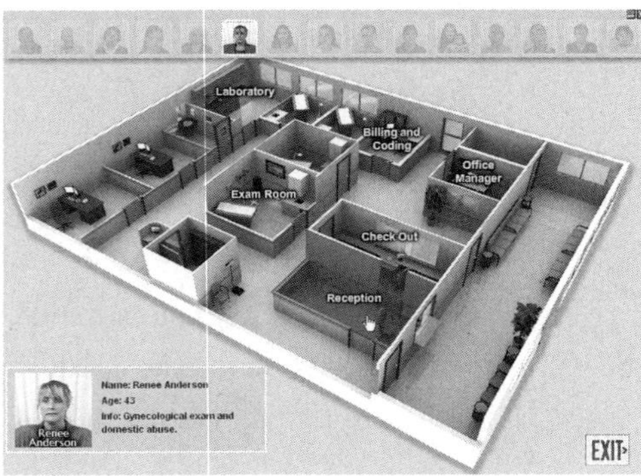

- Click on **Policy** to open the office Policy Manual.

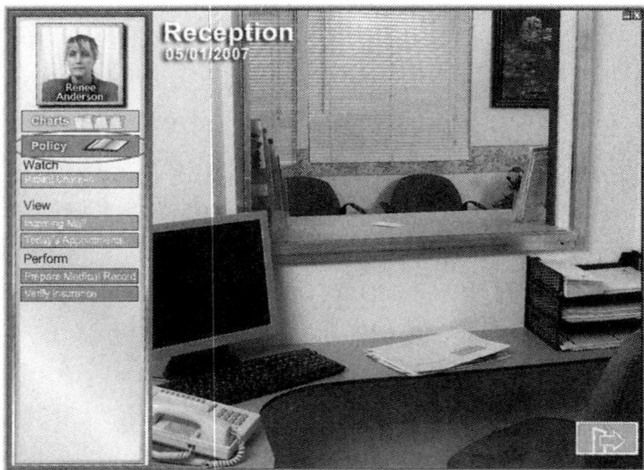

- Using the arrows at the top right of the page, navigate to page 17 and read the section titled "Patient Insurance Policies."

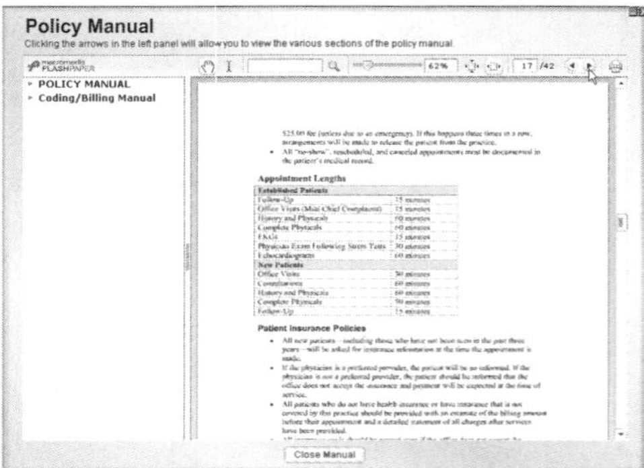

- Click **Close Manual** to return to the Reception area.
- Under the Watch heading, click on **Patient Check-In** to view the video.
- At the end of the video, click **Close** to return to the Reception area.

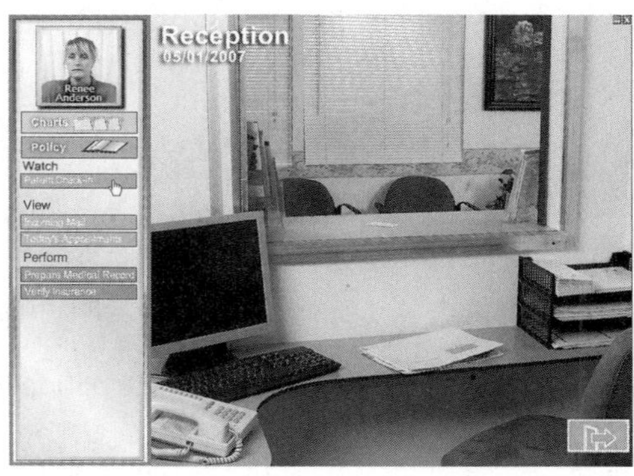

1. According to the Mountain View Clinic Policy Manual, when should the administrative employee inquire about the status of insurance benefits?
   a. When the appointment is scheduled
   b. At the time the patient is checked in
   c. During patient examination
   d. During patient check-out

2. In addition to asking the patients to verify their insurance coverage at the time of check-in, Mountain View Clinic staff members are expected to verify insurance coverage by:
   a. asking anyone accompanying the patient to verify insurance coverage.
   b. asking the patient to complete the Patient Information Form.
   c. asking the patient to recite his or her insurance identification number.
   d. asking to see the patient's insurance card and copying both sides of it.

3. The Mountain View Clinic Policy Manual expects staff members to obtain correct insurance information upon registration. This will enable the health insurance professional to submit:
   a. a clean claim.
   b. a neat claim.
   c. more claims per hour.
   d. more accurately coded claims.

4. Which actions should be performed during Renee Anderson's insurance verification process? Select all that apply.

   _____ Ask the patient to complete a registration form.

   _____ Ask the patient for her insurance identification card.

   _____ Make a copy of the ID card for the patient record.

   _____ Inform the patient that the entire fee will be due and payable at check-out.

   _____ Inform the patient that the copay will be payable at check-out.

   _____ Inform the patient that she must complete the insurance claim form herself.

5. Which of the following actions did Kristin perform during the registration process for Ms. Anderson to verify her insurance coverage?

_____ Ask the patient to complete a registration form.

_____ Ask the patient for her insurance identification card.

_____ Make a copy of the ID card for the patient record.

_____ Inform the patient that the entire fee will be due and payable at check-out.

_____ Inform the patient that the copay will be payable at check-out.

_____ Inform the patient that she must complete the insurance claim form herself.

→ • Click on the **Insurance Card** to open the Verify Insurance window.

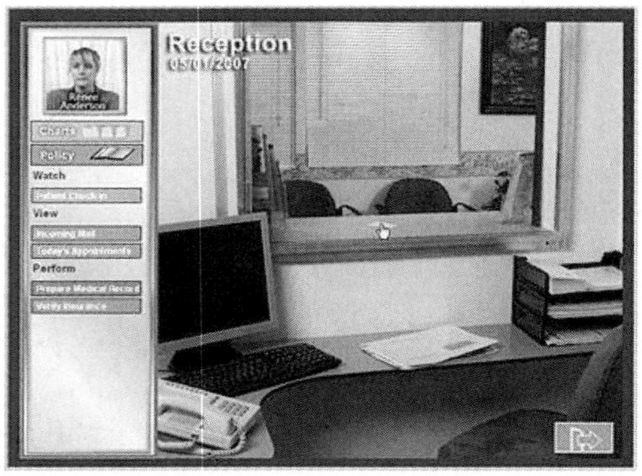

• Click on **Ask** next to the question "Do you have insurance?"
• Under View, click on **Insurance Card(s)**.

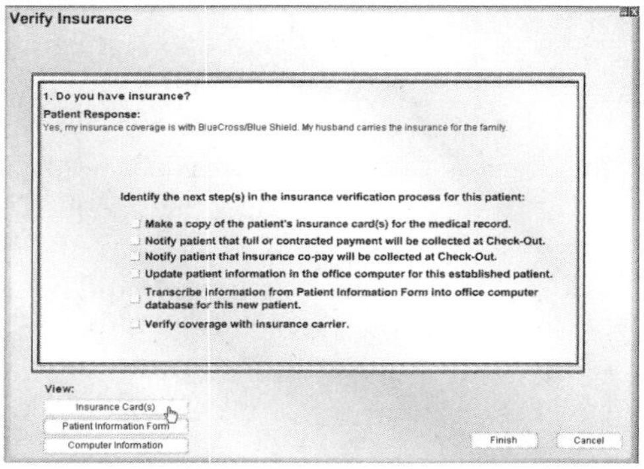

6. Below, provide the requested information from Ms. Anderson's insurance card.

Insurance Carrier:

Subscriber:

Plan #:

Group #:

ID #:

Issue Date:

Copay for PCP:

Copay for Specialist:

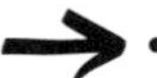

- Click the **Back** button.
- Click **Finish** to return to the Reception area.
- Click the exit arrow at the lower right corner of the screen to go to the Summary Menu.
- On the Summary Menu, click **Return to Map** and continue to the next exercise.

Exercise 2

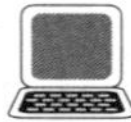

Online Activity—Essential Information for Claims Processing

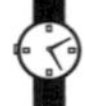

10 minutes

- Keep Renee Anderson as your patient. (*Note:* If you have exited the program, sign in again to Mountain View Clinic and select Renee Anderson from the patient list.)
- On the office map, highlight and click on **Check Out** to enter the Check Out area.

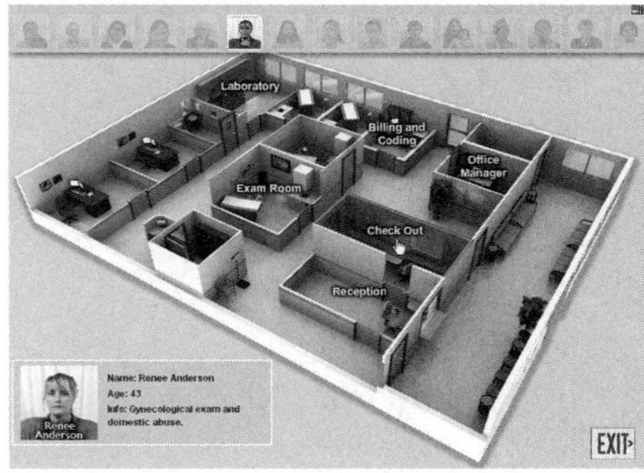

- Under the Watch heading, click on **Patient Check-Out** to view the video.

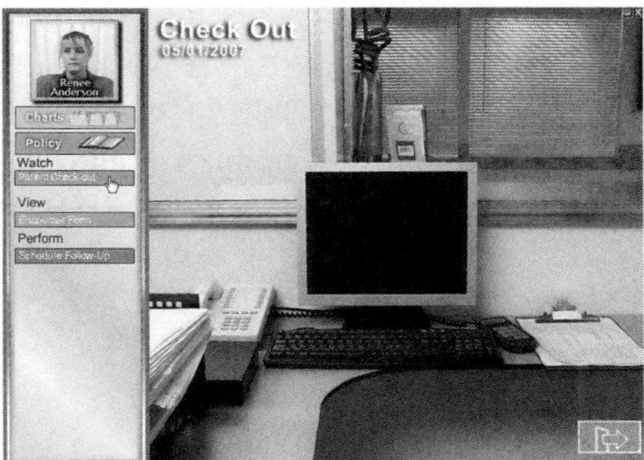

- At the end of the video, click **Close** to return to the Check Out area.
- Under the View heading, click on **Encounter Form** and review the charges for Ms. Anderson's visit.

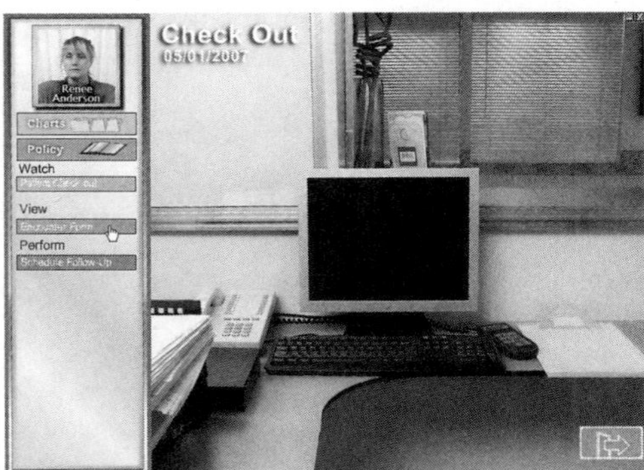

1. Below, provide the information that will be obtained from Ms. Anderson's Encounter Form to complete the CMS-1500 form.

Date of Service:

Date of Birth:

Procedures Performed:

Diagnosis:

Diagnosis:

Diagnosis:

Performing Physician:

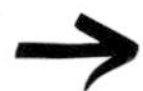

- Click **Finish** to close the Encounter Form and return to the Check Out area.
- Click the exit arrow at the lower right corner of the screen to go to the Summary Menu.
- On the Summary Menu, click **Return to Map**.
- On the office map, highlight and click on **Billing and Coding** to enter the Billing and Coding area.

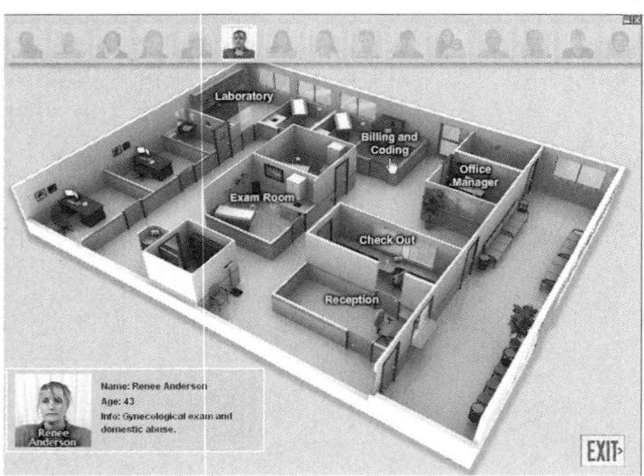

- Click on **Fee Schedule** to review Mountain View Clinic's list of charges for services.

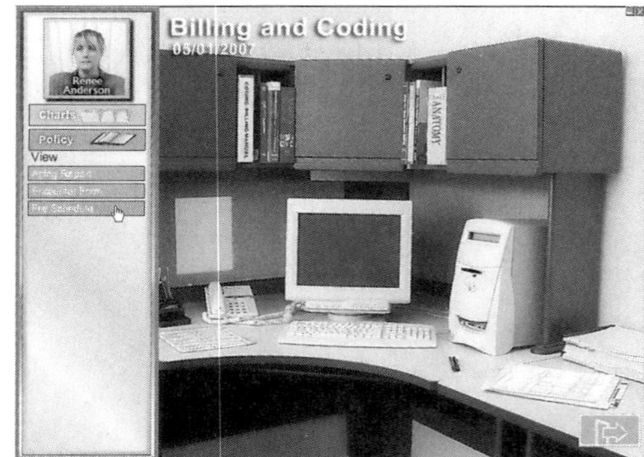

2. Using Mountain View Clinic's Fee Schedule, itemize the fee for each service performed and verify that the amount indicated as the total amount charged on the Encounter Form is correct.

3. What is the amount received from Ms. Anderson, and why did she pay this amount?

4. How much will Mountain View Clinic bill Ms. Anderson by sending her a monthly statement?
   a. $0
   b. $15
   c. $260
   d. $275

→ • Keep the Fee Schedule open and continue to the next exercise.

Exercise 3

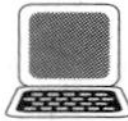

Online Activity—Completing a Patient Ledger Card

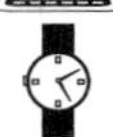

15 minutes

- The following questions refer to Renee Anderson's Fee Schedule. (*Note:* If you have exited the program, sign in again to Mountain View Clinic, select Renee Anderson from the patient list, enter the Billing and Coding area, and open the Fee Schedule.)

1. Using the information you obtained and recorded in Exercise 2, complete the following ledger card for Ms. Anderson. Include the copayment she made at check-out.

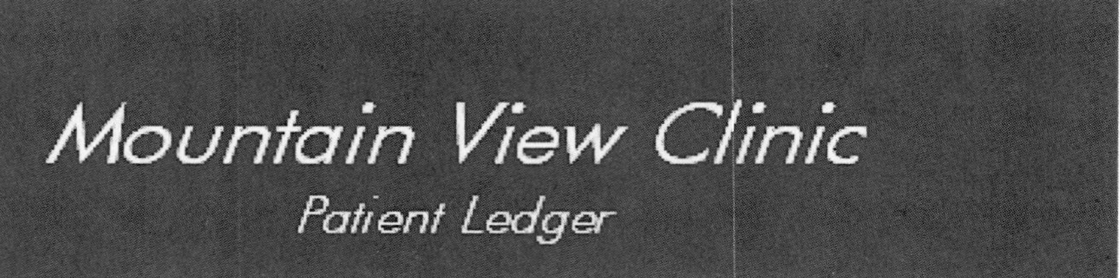

Patient Name:
Insurance Type:

Date	Professional Service	Fee ($)	Payment ($)	Adj. ($)	Prev. Bal. ($)	New Balance ($)
	Totals:					

2. Which documents generated during Ms. Anderson's visit will you need for completing the CMS-1500 claim form? Select all that apply.

_____ Patient Information Form

_____ Insurance ID Card

_____ General Health History Questionnaire

_____ Medication Record

_____ Encounter Form

_____ Ledger Card

_____ Fee Schedule

- Click **Finish** to close the Fee Schedule and return to the Billing and Coding area.
- Click the exit arrow at the lower right corner of the screen to go to the Summary Menu.
- On the Summary Menu, click **Return to Map** to continue to the next lesson or click **Exit the Program**.

LESSON 6

Completing the CMS-1500 Paper Form

Reading Assignment: Chapter 5—Claim Submission Methods
- Claim Form Completion Instructions
- Optical Character Recognition

Patient: Renee Anderson

Resources Needed: Optical Character Recognition (OCR) Formatting Rules

Learning Objectives:

- Identify Mountain View Clinic's policies related to completion of CMS-1500 claim forms.
- Complete the patient/insured (top) section of the CMS-1500 claim form.
- Use appropriate optical character recognition (OCR) formatting to complete the form.
- Complete the physician/supplier section of the CMS-1500 claim form.

Overview:

This lesson focuses on completing the universal claim form—the CMS-1500—using appropriate OCR formatting rules. You will view Mountain View Clinic's Policy Manual to identify all policies that will serve as a resource in completing a CMS-1500 claim form. Next, you will review the medical chart and any other relevant documents to gather the information necessary to complete the CMS-1500 claim form for Renee Anderson. After you complete this lesson, you will understand the importance of a "clean" claim.

Exercise 1

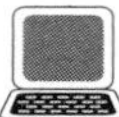

Online Activity—General Guidelines for Completing CMS-1500 Form

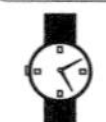

15 minutes

- Sign in to Mountain View Clinic.
- From the patient list, select **Renee Anderson**.

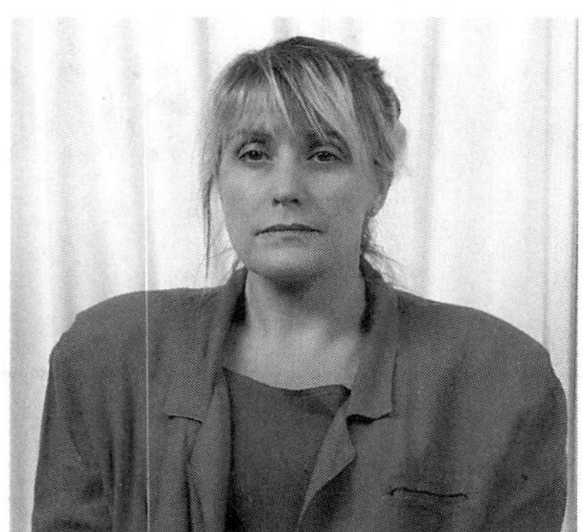

- On the office map, highlight and click on **Billing and Coding** to enter the Billing and Coding area.

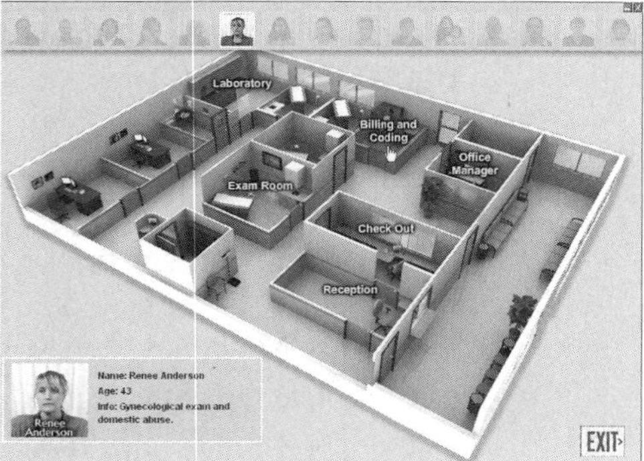

- Click on **Policy** to open the office Policy Manual.
- Review all of Mountain View Clinic's policies regarding completion of the CMS-1500 claim form.
- Answer the following questions, using the information provided in Mountain View Clinic's Policy Manual.

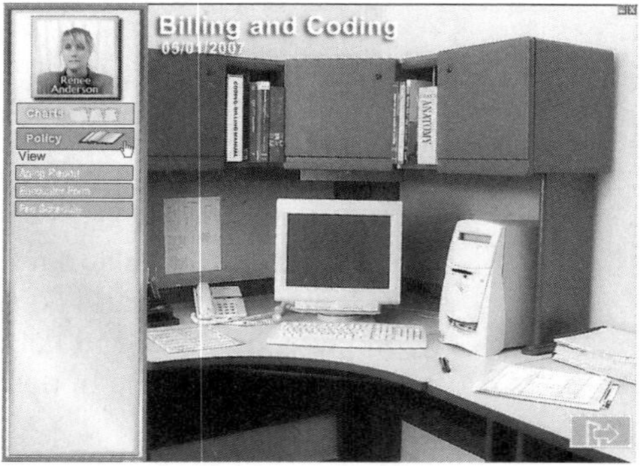

1. According to Mountain View Clinic's Policy Manual, the health insurance professional should file all CMS-1500 claim forms:
   a. according to Mountain View Clinic's guidelines.
   b. according to appropriate third-party guidelines.
   c. according to the guidelines of the state in which the practice is located.
   d. according to federal guidelines.

2. The health insurance professional is responsible for ensuring that the information reported on the CMS-1500 claim form is accurate. According to Mountain View Clinic's Policy Manual, "submission of a claim for services that were not actually provided" would be considered:
   a. a simple mistake.
   b. a false claim.
   c. a claim with an error.
   d. an incidental error.

3. The Mountain View Clinic Policy Manual states that "submission of a claim for services that are not adequately documented in the medical record" could be perceived as:
   a. an oversight.
   b. abusive billing activity.
   c. fraudulent billing activity.
   d. the physician's responsibility.

4. When reporting ICD-9 and CPT code information on the CMS-1500 to a health care benefit program, health insurance professionals should be aware that criminal convictions for any health care fraud:
   a. cannot be brought against them because they are just reporting the information provided to them by the physician.
   b. can be brought against them if they knowingly and willfully report information that is incorrect.
   c. can be brought against them if they mistakenly submit incorrect information.
   d. cannot be brought against them if they do not sign the claim form.

5. According to the Mountain View Clinic Policy Manual, if health insurance professionals are in doubt as to how to report information provided for a particular service on the CMS-1500 claim form, they should:
   a. not submit the claim until they have been told what to do by the physician.
   b. not submit the claim until they have received the appropriate guidance in writing.
   c. submit the claim with the information provided and see whether the claim is denied.
   d. submit the claim with the information provided and refund the money later if necessary.

- Click **Close Manual** to return to the Billing and Coding area.
- Remain in the Billing and Coding area with Renee Anderson as your patient and continue to the next exercise.

Exercise 2

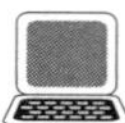

Online Activity—Completing the Patient/Insured Section of the CMS-1500 Form

15 minutes

- Click on **Charts** to open Renee Anderson's medical record. (*Note:* If you have exited the program, sign in again to Mountain View Clinic, select Renee Anderson from the patient list, enter the Billing and Coding area, and open the patient's chart.)

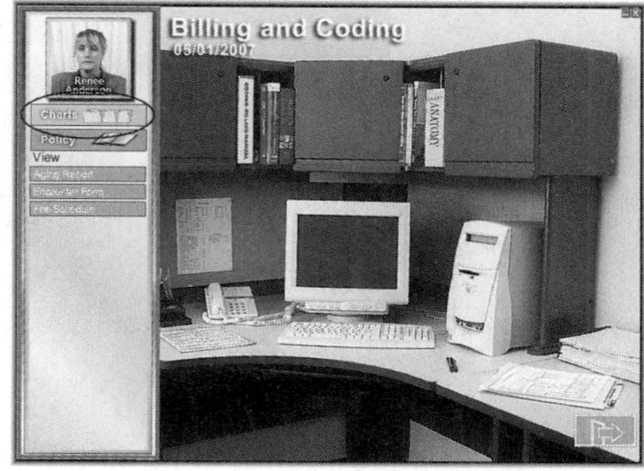

1. Using the correct OCR formatting rules, complete blocks 1 through 13 of the claim form below. Refer to Ms. Anderson's Patient Information Form and the copy of her insurance card(s). The registration form includes the number 1851 as the contract number. This should be placed in block 11 for policy group or FECA.

1. MEDICARE (Medicare#) ☐ MEDICAID (Medicaid#) ☐ TRICARE (ID#DoD#) ☐ CHAMPVA (Member ID#) ☐ GROUP HEALTH PLAN (ID#) ☐ FECA BLK LUNG (ID#) ☐ OTHER (ID#) ☐		1a. INSURED'S I.D. NUMBER (For Program in Item 1)
2. PATIENT'S NAME (Last Name, First Name, Middle Initial)	3. PATIENT'S BIRTH DATE MM DD YY SEX M ☐ F ☐	4. INSURED'S NAME (Last Name, First Name, Middle Initial)
5. PATIENT'S ADDRESS (No., Street)	6. PATIENT RELATIONSHIP TO INSURED Self ☐ Spouse ☐ Child ☐ Other ☐	7. INSURED'S ADDRESS (No., Street)
CITY / STATE	8. RESERVED FOR NUCC USE	CITY / STATE
ZIP CODE / TELEPHONE (Include Area Code) ( )		ZIP CODE / TELEPHONE (Include Area Code) ( )
9. OTHER INSURED'S NAME (Last Name, First Name, Middle Initial)	10. IS PATIENT'S CONDITION RELATED TO:	11. INSURED'S POLICY GROUP OR FECA NUMBER
a. OTHER INSURED'S POLICY OR GROUP NUMBER	a. EMPLOYMENT? (Current or Previous) ☐ YES ☐ NO	a. INSURED'S DATE OF BIRTH MM DD YY SEX M ☐ F ☐
b. RESERVED FOR NUCC USE	b. AUTO ACCIDENT? ☐ YES ☐ NO PLACE (State)	b. OTHER CLAIM ID (Designated by NUCC)
c. RESERVED FOR NUCC USE	c. OTHER ACCIDENT? ☐ YES ☐ NO	c. INSURANCE PLAN NAME OR PROGRAM NAME
d. INSURANCE PLAN NAME OR PROGRAM NAME	10d. CLAIM CODES (Designated by NUCC)	d. IS THERE ANOTHER HEALTH BENEFIT PLAN? ☐ YES ☐ NO *If yes,* complete items 9, 9a, and 9d.
READ BACK OF FORM BEFORE COMPLETING & SIGNING THIS FORM. 12. PATIENT'S OR AUTHORIZED PERSON'S SIGNATUREI authorize the release of any medical or other information necessary to process this claim. I also request payment of government benefits either to myself or to the party who accepts assignment below. SIGNED ______ DATE ______		13. INSURED'S OR AUTHORIZED PERSON'S SIGNATURE I authorize payment of medical benefits to the undersigned physician or supplier for services described below. SIGNED ______

2. Upon completion of blocks 1 through 13 of the claim form, double-check the following and explain why you completed the block in the manner that you did.

Block	How did you complete?	Explanation
Block 1a		
Block 2		
Block 7		
Block 8		
Block 10d		
Block 11d		

→ • Leave Ms. Anderson's chart open and continue to the next exercise.

Exercise 3

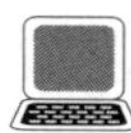

Online Activity—Completing the Physician/Supplier Section of the Claim Form

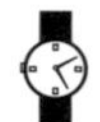

15 minutes

- Click on the **Patient Information** tab and select **1-Progress Notes** from the drop-down menu. (*Note:* If you have exited the program, sign in again to Mountain View Clinic, select Renee Anderson from the patient list, enter the Billing and Coding area, and open the Chart.)

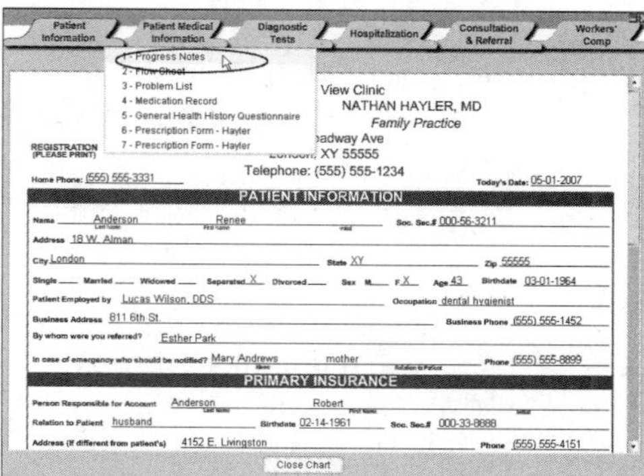

1. Using the information from Ms. Anderson's Progress Notes, complete blocks 14 through 20 of the claim form below. The NPI number is 0002223334 and should be placed in block 17b.

14. DATE OF CURRENT: ILLNESS, INJURY, or PREGNANCY(LMP) MM DD YY QUAL.	15. OTHER DATE QUAL. MM DD YY	16. DATES PATIENT UNABLE TO WORK IN CURRENT OCCUPATION FROM MM DD YY TO MM DD YY
17. NAME OF REFERRING PROVIDER OR OTHER SOURCE	17a. 17b. NPI	18. HOSPITALIZATION DATES RELATED TO CURRENT SERVICES FROM MM DD YY TO MM DD YY
19. ADDITIONAL CLAIM INFORMATION (Designated by NUCC)		20. OUTSIDE LAB? ☐ YES ☐ NO $ CHARGES

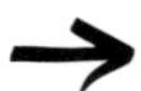

- Click **Close Chart** to return to the Billing and Coding area.
- Under the View heading, click on and review **Encounter Form** and **Fee Schedule** as needed to complete the following questions.

2. Continue filling in Ms. Anderson's claim form by recording the correct diagnosis codes in block 21 below. These codes are communicated by the physician to the health insurance specialist on the Encounter Form. You will learn how to perform diagnostic coding in Lesson 14. For this exercise, the diagnoses codes that you need are listed below:

V72.31: Annual GYN exam
611.72: Breast mass
054.12: Herpetic ulcer-vulva

21. DIAGNOSIS OR NATURE OF ILLNESS OR INJURY Relate A-L to service line below (24E)			ICD Ind.	22. RESUBMISSION CODE / ORIGINAL REF. NO.
A.	B.	C.	D.	
E.	F.	G.	H.	23. PRIOR AUTHORIZATION NUMBER
I.	J.	K.	L.	

3. Next, you will fill in block 24 of the claim form. To complete this section, you will need the correct procedural codes. These codes are communicated by the physician to the health insurance specialist on the Encounter Form. You will learn how to perform procedural coding in Lesson 15. For this exercise, the procedural codes are provided below:

   99396: Preventive care 40-64
   82270: Hemoccult
   88614: Pap smear
   81000: U/A dipstick
   99000: Handling/collection

Using Renee Anderson's Encounter Form and Fee Schedule, complete blocks 24A through 24J of the claim form for each service/procedure provided. (*Note:* Do not include services/procedures for which there is no charge. Also, since no provider NPI is provided in Mountain View Clinic's records, use NPI 0002223334 for the rendering provider ID # in column J, as you did in block 17b.)

	24. A. DATE(S) OF SERVICE From MM DD YY	To MM DD YY	B. PLACE OF SERVICE	C. EMG	D. PROCEDURES, SERVICES, OR SUPPLIES (Explain Unusual Circumstances) CPT/HCPCS	MODIFIER	E. DIAGNOSIS POINTER	F. $ CHARGES	G. DAYS OR UNITS	H. EPSDT Family Plan	I. ID. QUAL.	J. RENDERING PROVIDER ID. #
1											NPI	
2											NPI	
3											NPI	
4											NPI	
5											NPI	
6											NPI	

4. Complete blocks 25 through 33a of the claim form. (*Note:* Use the same date as shown on the Encounter Form. The Clinic NPI is 0001115670.)

25. FEDERAL TAX I.D. NUMBER SSN EIN	26. PATIENT'S ACCOUNT NO.	27. ACCEPT ASSIGNMENT? (For govt. claims, see back) YES NO	28. TOTAL CHARGE $	29. AMOUNT PAID $	30. Rsvd for NUCC Use $
31. SIGNATURE OF PHYSICIAN OR SUPPLIER INCLUDING DEGREES OR CREDENTIALS (I certify that the statements on the reverse apply to this bill and are made a part thereof.) SIGNED DATE	32. SERVICE FACILITY LOCATION INFORMATION a. NPI b.		33. BILLING PROVIDER INFO & PH # ( ) a. NPI b.		

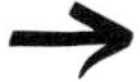

- Click **Finish** to close the Encounter Form or Fee Schedule and return to the Billing and Coding area.
- Click the exit arrow at the lower right corner of the screen to go to the Summary Menu.
- On the Summary Menu, click **Return to Map** to continue to the next lesson or click **Exit the Program**.

LESSON 7

Traditional Fee-for-Service (Indemnity) Insurance

Reading Assignment: Chapter 6—Traditional Fee-for-Service/Private Plans

Patients: Wilson Metcalf, Shaunti Begay, Jean Deere, Renee Anderson, Teresa Hernandez, Tristan Tsosie, Jose Imero, Louise Parlet, Jade Wong, John R. Simmons, Hu Huang

Learning Objectives:

- Identify insurance coverage.
- Determine primary/secondary carriers.
- Identify copayments for health services based on insurance card information.
- Determine the process for obtaining precertification for visits to specialists.

Overview:

In this lesson, you will learn about commercial insurance plans, specifically traditional indemnity (fee-for-service) and private plans. Blue Cross/Blue Shield is one of the most familiar carriers of commercial insurance. You will view various Mountain View Clinic patients' insurance information to identify type of insurance coverage and to recognize which policy is primary when patients are covered by more than one insurer. You will also review the Policy Manual to identify all policies that serve as a resource in understanding and collecting patient copayments. Finally, you will learn when a precertification is required and how to acquire it.

Exercise 1

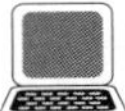

Online Activity—Identifying Insurance Coverage

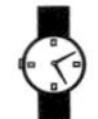

15 minutes

- Sign in to Mountain View Clinic.
- For this exercise, you will go through the same set of steps for each of the patients listed in the table in question 1. Begin by selecting **Wilson Metcalf** from the patient list. (*Note:* It is recommended that you select one patient and answer all questions in Exercise 1 that are pertinent to that patient before proceeding to the next patient.)

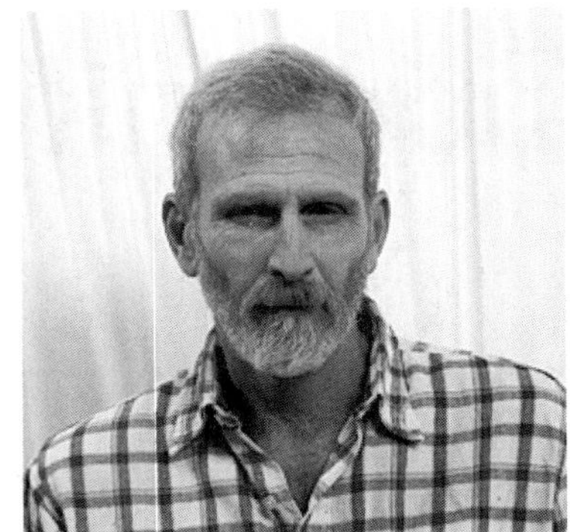

- On the office map, highlight and click on **Billing and Coding** to enter the Billing and Coding area.

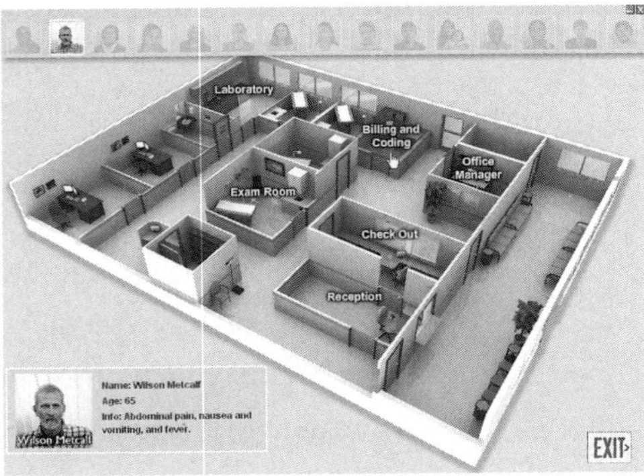

- Click on **Charts** to open Mr. Metcalf's medical record.

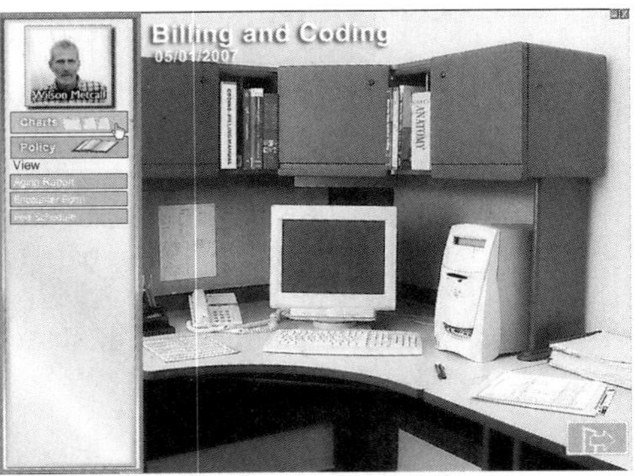

- Review the patient's insurance information as it appears on the Patient Information Form. (*Note:* If applicable you can also review the patient's insurance cards under the Patient Information tab.)

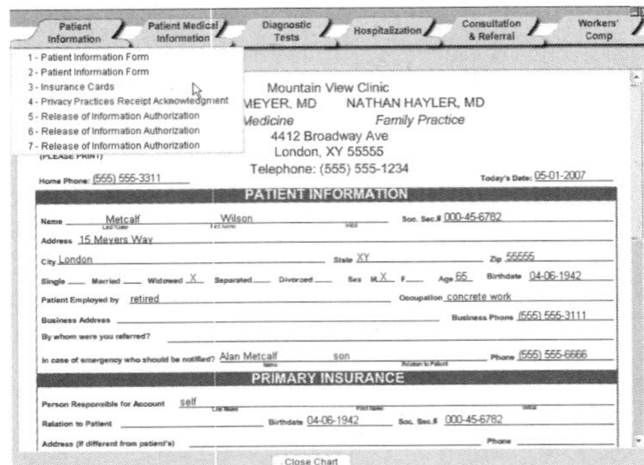

- Click **Close Chart** when finished with all the questions in this exercise pertaining to Mr. Metcalf and return to the Billing and Coding area.
- Click the exit arrow at the lower right corner of the screen to go to the Summary Menu.
- On the Summary Menu, click **Return to Map**.
- Repeat the previous steps with the remaining patients listed in the table in question 1.

1. For each patient listed below, place an X in the correct column to indicate the type of primary insurance (commercial or noncommercial health plan) the patient has.

Patient	Commercial Health Plan	Noncommercial Health Plan
Wilson Metcalf		
Shaunti Begay		
Jean Deere		
Renee Anderson		
Teresa Hernandez		
Louise Parlet		
Tristan Tsosie		
Jose Imero		
Jade Wong		
John Simmons		
Hu Huang		

2. Identify the name of the primary and secondary insurance company for each patient.

Patient	Primary	Secondary
Louise Parlet		
Tristan Tsosie		
Jose Imero		

3. What rule was used to determine the primary insurance coverage for Louise Parlet?
   a. The commercial health insurance rule
   b. The birthday rule
   c. The husband/wife rule
   d. No rule (however, when the patient is the subscriber, his or her insurance is usually primary)

4. What rule was used to determine the primary insurance coverage for Tristan Tsosie?
   a. The commercial health insurance rule
   b. The supplemental health insurance rule
   c. The birthday rule
   d. The coordination of benefits rule

5. For each patient below, identify the name of the subscriber for each plan the patient is enrolled with and note in parentheses the subscriber's relationship to the patient.

Patient	Primary Plan Subscriber (Relationship to Patient)	Secondary Plan Subscriber (Relationship to Patient)
Louise Parlet		
Tristan Tsosie		
Jose Imero		

6. Indicate the name of the group and the group number of each patient's primary insurance plan. (Refer to the Patient Information Form, under the Patient Information tab, for the Group Name).

Patient	Group Name	Group Number
Louise Parlet		
Tristan Tsosie		
Jose Imero		

7. What is the annual PPO or HMO deductible that must be paid out of pocket for these patients?

   Louise Parlet: $ __________

   Tristan Tsosie: $ __________

   Jose Imero: $ __________

8. Fill in the amount of copay these patients are responsible for when they see their primary care provider or a specialist under their primary insurance plan.

   Louise Parlet: primary care provider: $ __________ / specialist: $ __________

   Tristan Tsosie: primary care provider: $ __________ / specialist: $ __________

   Jose Imero: primary care provider: $ __________ / specialist: $ __________

9. Identify whether the following patients have a preferred provider organization (PPO) or a health maintenance organization (HMO) for their primary insurance plan by writing either PPO or HMO in the blank.

   Louise Parlet: ___________

   Tristan Tsosie: ___________

   Jose Imero: ___________

10. Which patients' *primary* insurance cards indicate that prior authorization is required before hospital admission? Place an X in the right column next to each patient this applies to.

Patient	Prior Authorization Required for Hospitalization
Louise Parlet	
Tristan Tsosie	
Jose Imero	

Exercise 2

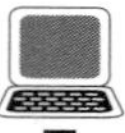

Online Activity—Clinic Copay Policy

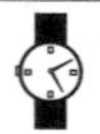

45 minutes

- Sign in to Mountain View Clinic.
- From the patient list, select **Renee Anderson**. (*Note:* If you have exited the program, sign in again to Mountain View Clinic and select Renee Anderson from the patient list.)

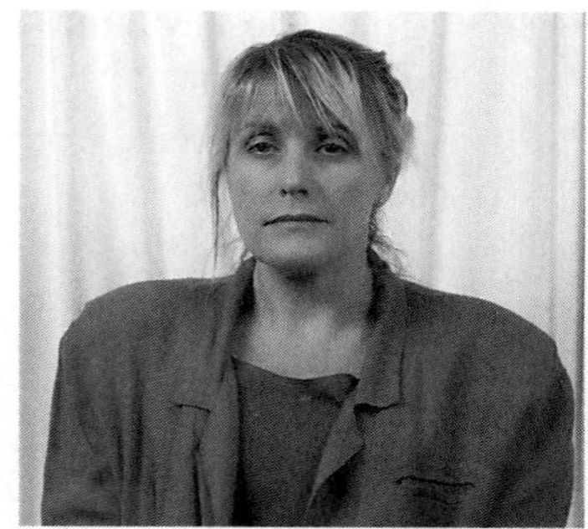

- On the office map, highlight and click on **Billing and Coding** to enter the Billing and Coding area.

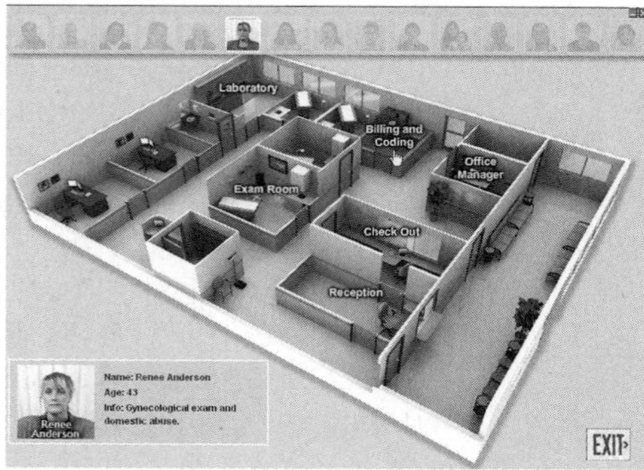

- Click on **Policy** to open the office Policy Manual.

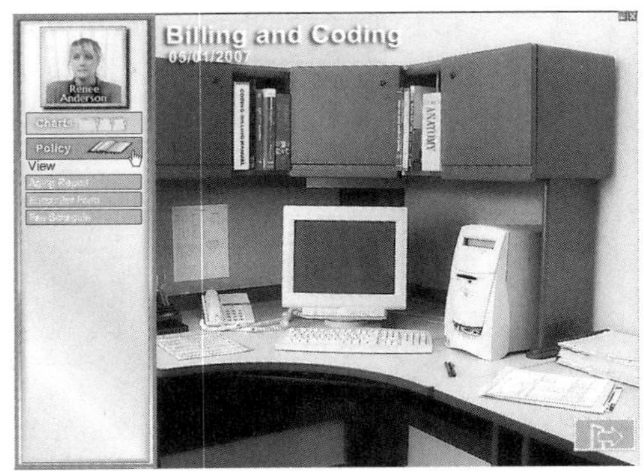

- Find answers to the following questions about copayments by using the Policy Manual Table of Contents or the search bar.

1. When should Mountain View Clinic patients be reminded that copayment is due at the time service is rendered?
   a. When they schedule their appointment
   b. When they check in
   c. When they check out
   d. When the clinic sends them a bill for the outstanding charge

2. According to the Mountain View Clinic Policy Manual, collection of copays at time of service is the responsibility of:
   a. scheduling staff.
   b. check-in staff.
   c. check-out staff.
   d. billing staff.

- Click **Close Manual** to return to the Billing and Coding area.
- For this exercise, you will go through the same set of steps for each of the patients listed in the table in question 3.
- Click on **Charts** to open Ms. Anderson's medical record.

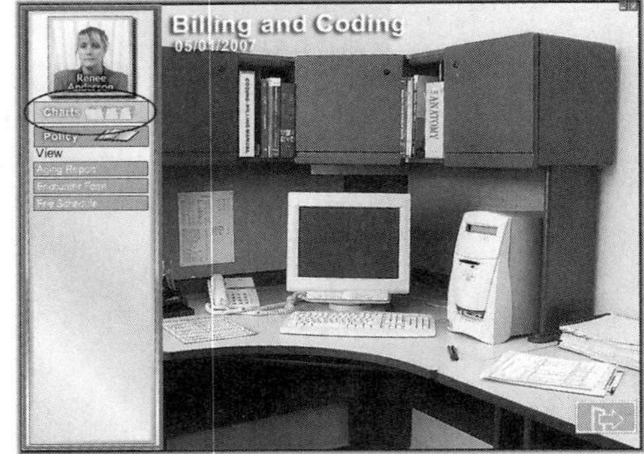

- Review the patient's insurance information as it appears on the Patient Information Form. (*Note:* If applicable you can also review the patient's insurance cards under the Patient Information tab.)
- Confirm the patient's copay for the primary insurance provider on the insurance card.
- Click **Close Chart** when finished to return to the Billing and Coding area.
- Click the exit arrow at the lower right corner of the screen to go to the Summary Menu.
- On the Summary Menu, click **Return to Map**.

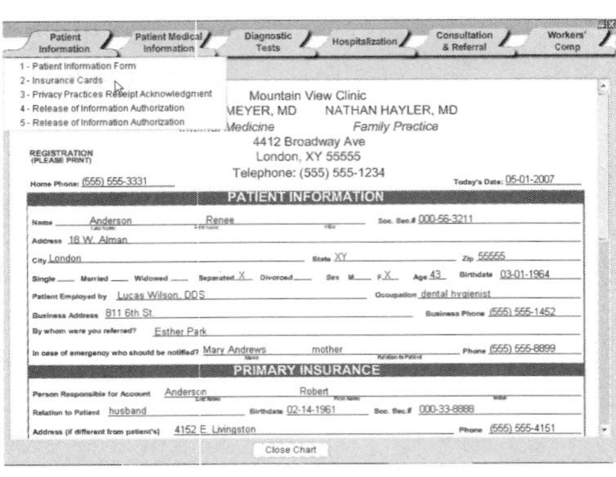

- Repeat the previous steps with the remaining patients listed in the table in question 3.

3. Using the same steps outlined above for Renee Anderson, confirm the amount of copay due from the following patients for their visit to see one of the primary care physicians at Mountain View Clinic. Indicate whether or not the copay was collected (and the amount collected) at the time of the visit. (*Note:* Find this information by reviewing the patient's Encounter Form for the day of the visit).

Patient	Amount of Copay for Patient's Primary Insurance	Amount Collected for Copay at Time of Visit
Renee Anderson		
Teresa Hernandez		
Louise Parlet		
Tristan Tsosie		
Jose Imero		
Jade Wong		
John R. Simmons		

→ • From the patient list, select **Jose Imero**. (*Note:* If you have exited the program, sign in again to Mountain View Clinic and select Jose Imero from the patient list.)

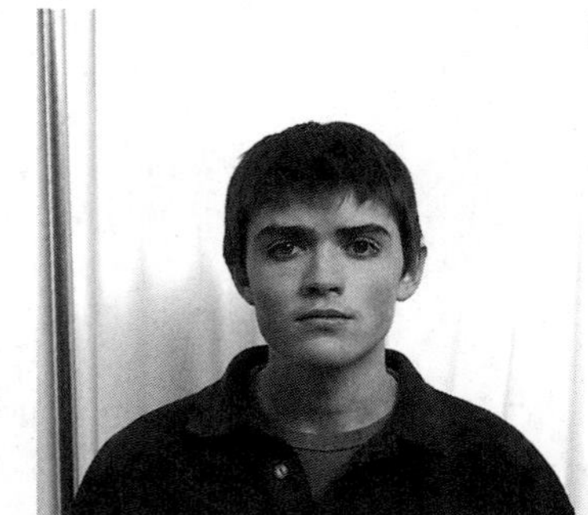

- On the office map, highlight and click on **Check Out** to enter the Check Out area.

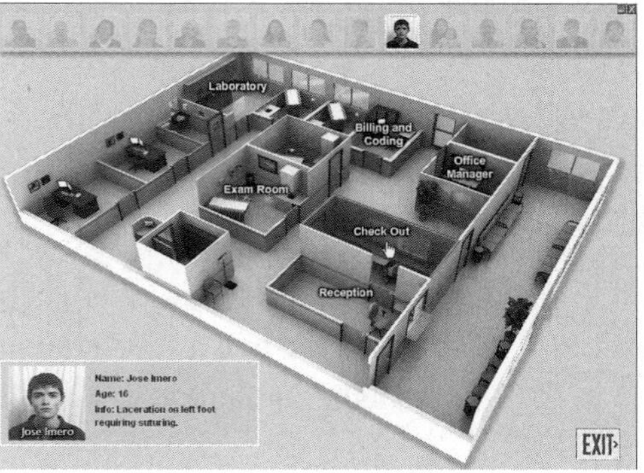

- Under the Watch heading, click on **Patient Check-Out** to view the video.

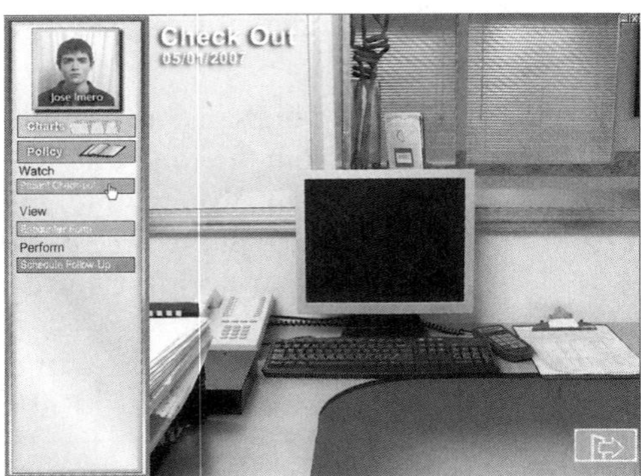

4. What concern does the receptionist voice to Jose's mother at check-out?

5. The receptionist at Mountain View Clinic offers an explanation for requesting collection of copayments by advising Jose's mother of the clinic's policy. What is the policy with regard to copayments?

6. What types of payment does Mountain View Clinic accept? Select all that apply.

   _____ Cash

   _____ Credit card

   _____ Small bank loan

   _____ Personal check

   _____ Credit union voucher

7. Did the receptionist at Mountain View Clinic handle collection of copayment from Jose's mother well? Explain.

→ • At the end of the video, click the **X** in the upper right corner to return to the Check Out area.
- Click the exit arrow at the lower right corner of the screen to go to the Summary Menu.
- On the Summary Menu, click **Return to Map** to continue to the next exercise.

Exercise 3

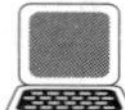

Online Activity—Precertifying a Visit to a Specialist

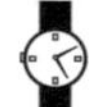

5 minutes

- Sign in to Mountain View Clinic.
- From the patient list, select **Louise Parlet**. (*Note:* If you have exited the program, sign in again to Mountain View Clinic and select Louise Parlet from the patient list.)

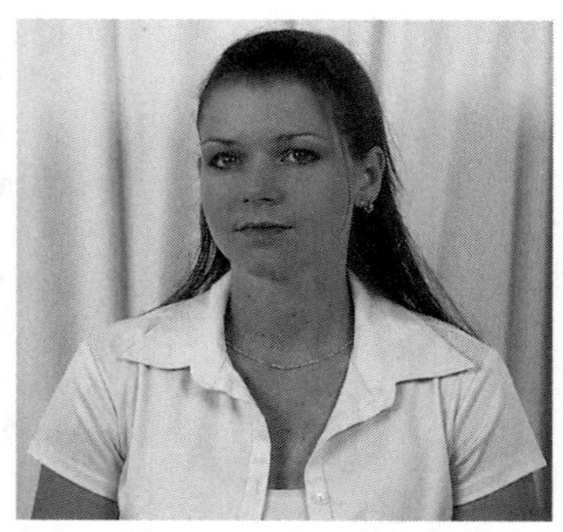

- On the office map, highlight and click on **Check-Out** to enter the Check Out area.

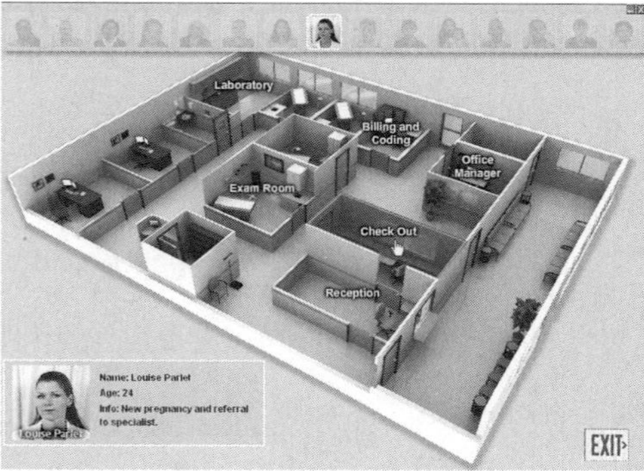

- Under the Watch heading, click on **Patient Check-Out** to view the video.

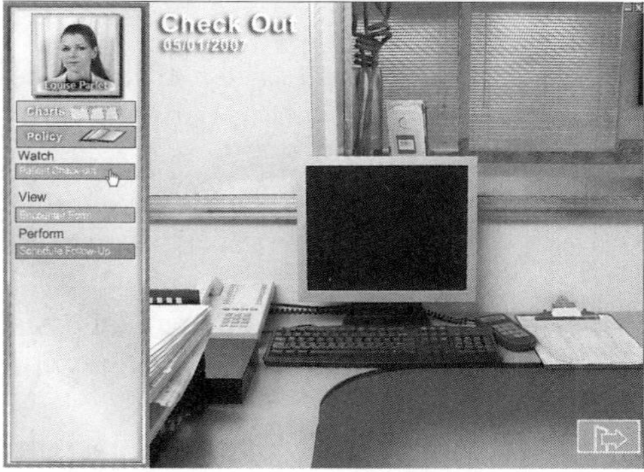

1. What indicator on Louise Parlet's primary insurance card would alert the check-out staff that precertification may be required for a referral to an obstetrician?
   a. Copay
   b. Group #
   c. Employer name
   d. PPO

2. What statement is on the back of Louise Parlet's insurance card with Teachers' Health Group that indicates precertification may be required for a referral to an obstetrician?
   a. "Certain services may require preauthorization"
   b. "To locate a preferred provider, call the phone number indicated"
   c. Neither a nor b
   d. Both a and b

3. Louise Parlet says that she assumes that both of her insurance providers will cover Dr. Lockett's services. Why should the check-out staff call her insurance providers to verify coverage of Dr. Lockett's services?
   a. Mountain View Clinic will not get paid for today's services if the insurance providers are not contacted.
   b. There is no need for her to verify coverage; it is safe to assume.
   c. There is no need for her to verify coverage; it is the responsibility of Dr. Lockett's office.
   d. Verifying this information complies with the practice's mission statement and the practice's Policy Manual to arrange referrals and to provide the highest professional care and patient satisfaction.

4. The office staff asks whether Dr. Lockett is an "in-network provider." If Dr. Lockett is an in-network provider, this means:
   a. Dr. Lockett is within driving distance from Mountain View Clinic.
   b. Dr. Lockett is a participating physician and out-of-pocket expenses will be less for the patient.
   c. Dr. Lockett is a participating physician and the provider will pay the patient directly.
   d. Dr. Lockett is employed by Teachers' Health Group so there will be an out-of-pocket discount for the patient.

5. Which steps are performed by the medical assistant to obtain authorization for a referral to a specialist? Select all that apply.

   _____ A telephone call is made to Teachers' Health Group.

   _____ A telephone call is made to Blue Cross/Blue Shield.

   _____ A fax is sent to Teachers' Health Group to obtain precertification.

   _____ A verification number is obtained from Teachers' Health Group.

   _____ The medical assistant asks Teachers' Health Group if Dr. Lockett is an "in-network" provider.

   _____ The medical assistant requests Teachers' Health Group to fax the completed precertification form.

   _____ The medical assistant asks Blue Cross/Blue Shield to schedule Ms. Parlet's appointment with Dr. Lockett.

6. If Dr. Lockett is not a participating provider with either Teachers' Health Group or Blue Cross/Blue Shield, which of the following is *not* an option open to Ms. Parlet?
   a. She can request the name(s) of participating obstetric providers in the area that do contract with either or both of her insurance plans.
   b. She can accept treatment from an out-of-network provider and pay a higher copay, according to the rules of her plan.
   c. She can accept treatment from an out-of-network provider and request a discount from the provider known as "insurance only" billing.
   d. She can opt to pay the charges herself.

→
- At the end of the video, click the **X** in the upper right corner to return to the Check Out area.
- Click the exit arrow at the lower right corner of the screen to go to the Summary Menu.
- On the Summary Menu, click **Return to Map** to continue to the next lesson or click **Exit the Program**.

LESSON 8

Blue Cross/Blue Shield Claims

Reading Assignment: Chapter 6—Traditional Fee-for-Service/Private Plans
- Blue Cross/Blue Shield Programs
- Submitting Blue Cross and Blue Shield and Commercial Claims

Patients: Renee Anderson, Louise Parlet

Learning Objectives:

- Complete a claim form for a patient with Blue Cross/Blue Shield as primary coverage.
- Complete a claim form for a patient with Blue Cross/Blue Shield as secondary coverage.
- Interpret the entries on an Explanation of Benefits (EOB) document.

Overview:

In this lesson you will learn about patients who have Blue Cross/Blue Shield insurance as their primary coverage and how to enter that information on a CMS-1500 form. You will also learn about completing the information the physician must provide for patients covered by Blue Cross/Blue Shield. The lesson demonstrates where to find the necessary information in the patient's chart and how to accurately transfer that information to the CMS-1500 form.

Exercise 1

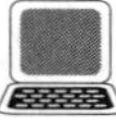

Online Activity—Completing the Patient/Insured Section of a CMS-1500 for Patient with Blue Cross/Blue Shield as Primary Coverage

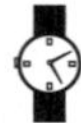

10 minutes

1. An open enrollment period means that employees can choose a health care plan:
   a. at a reduced rate of cost.
   b. without limitations regarding preexisting conditions.

2. Which of the following statements about the flexibility of a point-of-service plan are correct? Select all that apply.

_____ The insured may visit an HMO provider, where the service is covered in full.

_____ The insured may visit a provider in the PPO and make a copayment.

_____ The insured may see specialists without a referral and have full coverage with no copay.

_____ The insured must see the same provider, under all circumstances.

_____ The insured may visit a provider outside the network and pay a deductible; with this option, only a portion of the cost is paid by the plan.

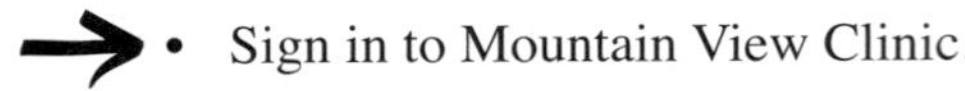

- Sign in to Mountain View Clinic.
- From the patient list, select **Renee Anderson**.

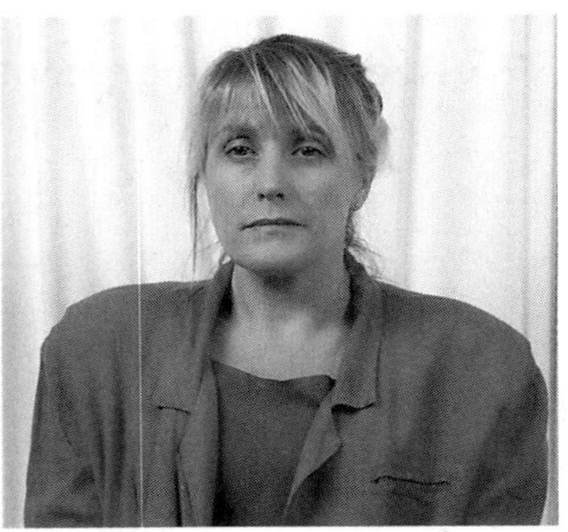

- On the office map, highlight and click on **Billing and Coding** to enter the Billing and Coding area.

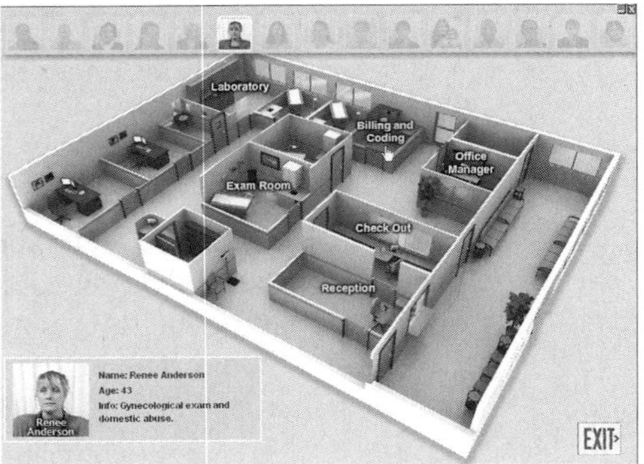

- Click on **Charts** to open Ms. Anderson's medical record.

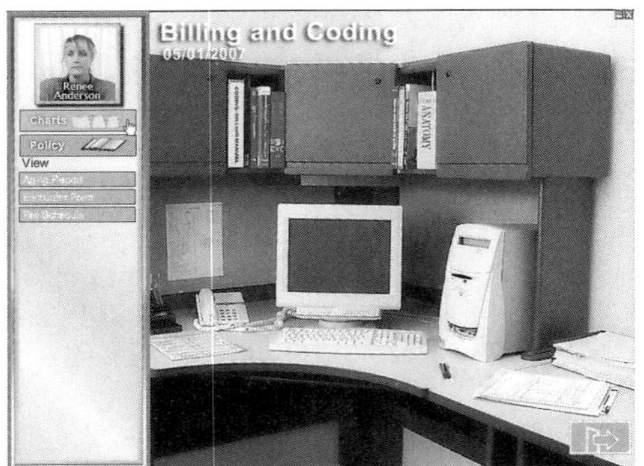

3. Using the Patient Information Form in Ms. Anderson's chart and referring to Figure 6-3 in the textbook, complete the CMS-1500 claim form below. Check the appropriate box(es) in block 1 and enter the patient's insurance ID number in block 1a of the form. Continue completing the form through block 13.

1. MEDICARE ☐ (Medicare#) MEDICAID ☐ (Medicaid#) TRICARE ☐ (ID#DoD#) CHAMPVA ☐ (Member ID#) GROUP HEALTH PLAN ☐ (ID#) FECA BLK LUNG ☐ (ID#) OTHER ☐ (ID#)		1a. INSURED'S I.D. NUMBER (For Program in Item 1)
2. PATIENT'S NAME (Last Name, First Name, Middle Initial)	3. PATIENT'S BIRTH DATE MM DD YY SEX M☐ F☐	4. INSURED'S NAME (Last Name, First Name, Middle Initial)
5. PATIENT'S ADDRESS (No., Street)	6. PATIENT RELATIONSHIP TO INSURED Self☐ Spouse☐ Child☐ Other☐	7. INSURED'S ADDRESS (No., Street)
CITY STATE	8. RESERVED FOR NUCC USE	CITY STATE
ZIP CODE TELEPHONE (Include Area Code) ( )		ZIP CODE TELEPHONE (Include Area Code) ( )
9. OTHER INSURED'S NAME (Last Name, First Name, Middle Initial)	10. IS PATIENT'S CONDITION RELATED TO:	11. INSURED'S POLICY GROUP OR FECA NUMBER
a. OTHER INSURED'S POLICY OR GROUP NUMBER	a. EMPLOYMENT? (Current or Previous) ☐YES ☐NO	a. INSURED'S DATE OF BIRTH MM DD YY SEX M☐ F☐
b. RESERVED FOR NUCC USE	b. AUTO ACCIDENT? ☐YES ☐NO PLACE (State)	b. OTHER CLAIM ID (Designated by NUCC)
c. RESERVED FOR NUCC USE	c. OTHER ACCIDENT? ☐YES ☐NO	c. INSURANCE PLAN NAME OR PROGRAM NAME
d. INSURANCE PLAN NAME OR PROGRAM NAME	10d. CLAIM CODES (Designated by NUCC)	d. IS THERE ANOTHER HEALTH BENEFIT PLAN? ☐YES ☐NO *If yes,* complete items 9, 9a, and 9d.
READ BACK OF FORM BEFORE COMPLETING & SIGNING THIS FORM. 12. PATIENT'S OR AUTHORIZED PERSON'S SIGNATURE I authorize the release of any medical or other information necessary to process this claim. I also request payment of government benefits either to myself or to the party who accepts assignment below. SIGNED ____	DATE ____	13. INSURED'S OR AUTHORIZED PERSON'S SIGNATURE I authorize payment of medical benefits to the undersigned physician or supplier for services described below. SIGNED ____

4. The insured's ID number in block 1a should have been listed as:
   a. 000-56-3211.
   b. 000338888.
   c. YLE250011333.
   d. YLE-250011333.

5. In block 4, the policy holder's name should be entered as:
   a. Anderson, Renee.
   b. Anderson Robert.
   c. Robert Anderson.
   d. SAME.

6. Was it necessary to complete blocks 9 through 9d?
   a. No, the patient did not have an additional insurance policy.
   b. Yes, the patient had an additional insurance policy.

7. If a current release of information is on file, block 12:
   a. does not need to be completed.
   b. should be entered as "SOF."

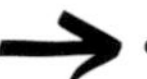

- Click on **Close Chart** to return to the Billing and Coding area.
- Remain in the Billing and Coding area with Renee Anderson as your patient and continue to the next exercise.

Exercise 2

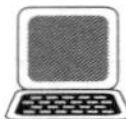

Online Activity—Completing the Physician/Supplier Section of the CMS-1500 for a Patient with Blue Cross/Blue Shield as Primary Coverage

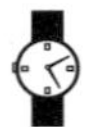

15 minutes

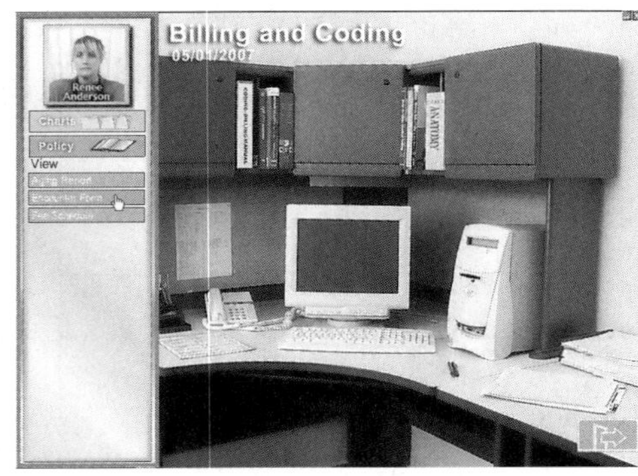

- Under the View heading, click on **Encounter Form** and **Fee Schedule** as needed to complete the following questions. (*Note:* If you have exited the program, sign in again to Mountain View Clinic, select Renee Anderson from the patient list, and go to the Billing and Coding area.)

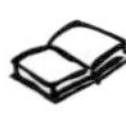

Throughout this exercise, you will need to refer to the Submitting BCBS and Commercial Claims section in your textbook and the Sample Completed Claim Form (Figure B-1) in Appendix B of the textbook. (*Hint:* Visit www.bcbs.com website for instructions.)

1. Using your resources, complete blocks 14 through 20 on the CMS-1500 claim form below. (*Note:* Dr. Hayler's NPI is 0002223334.)

14. DATE OF CURRENT: ILLNESS, INJURY, or PREGNANCY(LMP) MM DD YY QUAL.	15. OTHER DATE QUAL. MM DD YY	16. DATES PATIENT UNABLE TO WORK IN CURRENT OCCUPATION FROM MM DD YY TO MM DD YY
17. NAME OF REFERRING PROVIDER OR OTHER SOURCE	17a. 17b. NPI	18. HOSPITALIZATION DATES RELATED TO CURRENT SERVICES FROM MM DD YY TO MM DD YY
19. ADDITIONAL CLAIM INFORMATION (Designated by NUCC)		20. OUTSIDE LAB? $ CHARGES YES NO

2. The codes for Ms. Anderson's various diagnoses are as follows:

   V72.31: Annual GYN exam
   611.72: Breast mass
   054.12: Herpetic ulcer, vulva

   Enter these diagnosis codes in block 21 on the CMS-1500 claim form below.

21. DIAGNOSIS OR NATURE OF ILLNESS OR INJURY Relate A-L to service line below (24E)			ICD Ind.	22. RESUBMISSION CODE / ORIGINAL REF. NO.
A.	B.	C.	D.	
E.	F.	G.	H.	23. PRIOR AUTHORIZATION NUMBER
I.	J.	K.	L.	

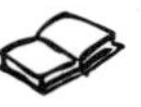

3. Using the information on Ms. Anderson's Encounter Form and the Fee Schedule, complete blocks 24A through 24J on the CMS-1500 claim form below for each service/procedure provided. (*Note:* Dr. Hayler's NPI is 0002223334. For the list of applicable service codes, log on to http://www.findacode.com/cms1500-claim-form/cms1500-place-of-service-codes.html.) The procedure codes (CPT) and associated diagnosis codes (ICD-9) are listed below:

CPT Code	Description	Associated ICD-9 Code
99396	Preventive care 40-64	V72.31
99000	Handling/collection	054.12
82270	Hemoccult	V72.31
88164	Pap smear	V72.31
81000	U/A dip	054.12

	24. A. DATE(S) OF SERVICE From MM DD YY To MM DD YY	B. PLACE OF SERVICE	C. EMG	D. PROCEDURES, SERVICES, OR SUPPLIES (Explain Unusual Circumstances) CPT/HCPCS MODIFIER	E. DIAGNOSIS POINTER	F. $ CHARGES	G. DAYS OR UNITS	H. EPSDT Family Plan	I. ID. QUAL.	J. RENDERING PROVIDER ID. #
1									NPI	
2									NPI	
3									NPI	
4									NPI	
5									NPI	
6									NPI	

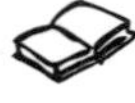

4. Complete blocks 25 through 33b on the CMS-1500 claim form below. (*Note:* The clinic NPI is 0001115670.) Use the same date as on the Encounter Form. Throughout this exercise, you will need to refer to the Sample Completed Claim Form (Figure B-1) in Appendix B of the textbook.

25. FEDERAL TAX I.D. NUMBER SSN EIN	26. PATIENT'S ACCOUNT NO.	27. ACCEPT ASSIGNMENT? (For govt. claims, see back) YES NO	28. TOTAL CHARGE $	29. AMOUNT PAID $	30. Rsvd for NUCC Use $
31. SIGNATURE OF PHYSICIAN OR SUPPLIER INCLUDING DEGREES OR CREDENTIALS (I certify that the statements on the reverse apply to this bill and are made a part thereof.) SIGNED DATE	32. SERVICE FACILITY LOCATION INFORMATION a. NPI b.		33. BILLING PROVIDER INFO & PH # ( ) a. NPI b.		

Based on your completion of the claim form, answer the following questions related to specific fields that insurance carriers frequently report as problematic areas.

5. Which of the following is true about block 15?
   a. This should be completed with the date of service for today's visit.
   b. This is not required for private plans.

6. Blocks 17 and 17a:
   a. do not need to be completed because the patient is not being referred to Dr. Hayler.
   b. must be completed with Dr. Hayler's name and NPI number.

7. For this claim, the code for block 24B (place of service) should be:
   a. 11.
   b. 21.
   c. 31.
   d. left blank.

8. For this particular claim, how many services/procedures are reported on the claim lines in field 24?
   a. One
   b. Two
   c. Four
   d. Five

9. In block 24E, the claim line to report the preventive care service (99396) provided would be linked to:
   a. V72.31, 611.72, 054.12.
   b. V72.31, 611.72.
   c. V72.31.

10. What should be recorded in block 24J?
    a. Dr. Hayler's name
    b. Dr. Hayler's NPI number

→ • Click **Finish** to close the Encounter Form or Fee Schedule and return to the Billing and Coding area.
- Click the exit arrow at the lower right corner of the screen to go to the Summary Menu.
- On the Summary Menu, click **Return to Map** and continue to the next exercise.

Exercise 3

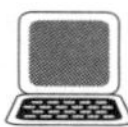

Online Activity—Completing an Insurance Claim for a Patient with Blue Cross/Blue Shield as Secondary Coverage

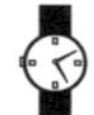

15 minutes

- From the patient list, select **Louise Parlet**. (*Note:* If you have exited the program, sign in again to Mountain View Clinic and select Louise Parlet from the patient list.)

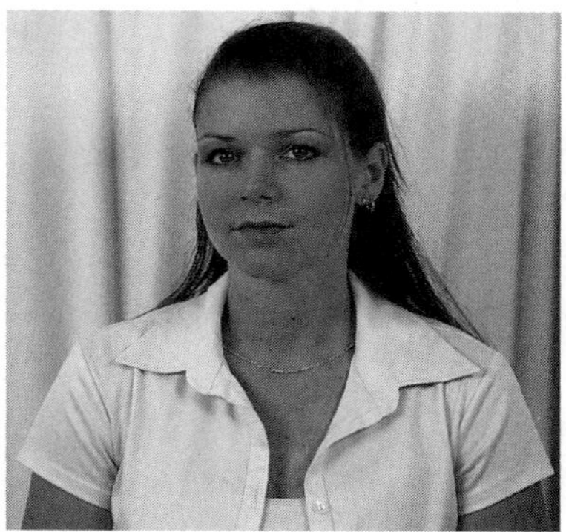

- On the office map, highlight and click on **Billing and Coding** to enter the Billing and Coding area.

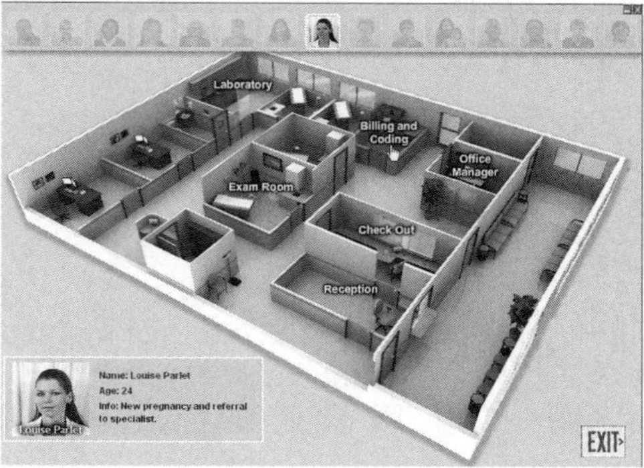

- Click on **Charts** to open Ms. Parlet's medical record.

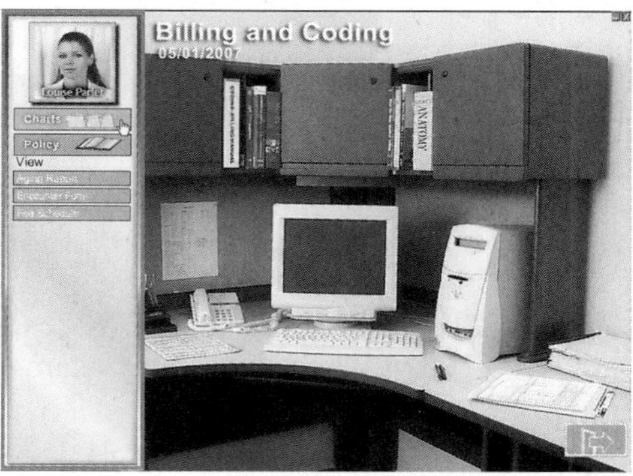

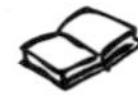

Throughout this exercise, you will need to refer to the Sample Completed Claim Form (Figure B-1) in Appendix B of the textbook.

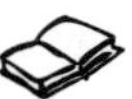

1. Using the Patient Information Form and referring to Figure 6-3 in the textbook, check the appropriate box(es) in block 1 and enter the patient's insurance ID number in block 1a on the CMS-1500 claim form below. Continue completing the form through block 13. (*Note:* Because this patient has an additional insurance policy, blocks 9 through 9d will need to be completed.)

1. MEDICARE ☐ (Medicare#) MEDICAID ☐ (Medicaid#) TRICARE ☐ (ID#DoD#) CHAMPVA ☐ (Member ID#) GROUP HEALTH PLAN ☐ (ID#) FECA BLK LUNG ☐ (ID#) OTHER ☐ (ID#)		1a. INSURED'S I.D. NUMBER (For Program in Item 1)
2. PATIENT'S NAME (Last Name, First Name, Middle Initial)	3. PATIENT'S BIRTH DATE MM DD YY SEX M ☐ F ☐	4. INSURED'S NAME (Last Name, First Name, Middle Initial)
5. PATIENT'S ADDRESS (No., Street)	6. PATIENT RELATIONSHIP TO INSURED Self ☐ Spouse ☐ Child ☐ Other ☐	7. INSURED'S ADDRESS (No., Street)
CITY / STATE	8. RESERVED FOR NUCC USE	CITY / STATE
ZIP CODE / TELEPHONE (Include Area Code) ( )		ZIP CODE / TELEPHONE (Include Area Code) ( )
9. OTHER INSURED'S NAME (Last Name, First Name, Middle Initial)	10. IS PATIENT'S CONDITION RELATED TO:	11. INSURED'S POLICY GROUP OR FECA NUMBER
a. OTHER INSURED'S POLICY OR GROUP NUMBER	a. EMPLOYMENT? (Current or Previous) ☐ YES ☐ NO	a. INSURED'S DATE OF BIRTH MM DD YY SEX M ☐ F ☐
b. RESERVED FOR NUCC USE	b. AUTO ACCIDENT? ☐ YES ☐ NO PLACE (State)	b. OTHER CLAIM ID (Designated by NUCC)
c. RESERVED FOR NUCC USE	c. OTHER ACCIDENT? ☐ YES ☐ NO	c. INSURANCE PLAN NAME OR PROGRAM NAME
d. INSURANCE PLAN NAME OR PROGRAM NAME	10d. CLAIM CODES (Designated by NUCC)	d. IS THERE ANOTHER HEALTH BENEFIT PLAN? ☐ YES ☐ NO *If yes,* complete items 9, 9a, and 9d.
READ BACK OF FORM BEFORE COMPLETING & SIGNING THIS FORM. 12. PATIENT'S OR AUTHORIZED PERSON'S SIGNATURE I authorize the release of any medical or other information necessary to process this claim. I also request payment of government benefits either to myself or to the party who accepts assignment below. SIGNED ____	DATE ____	13. INSURED'S OR AUTHORIZED PERSON'S SIGNATURE I authorize payment of medical benefits to the undersigned physician or supplier for services described below. SIGNED ____

2. Using the information on the patient's Encounter Form and referring to Figure 6-3 in the textbook, complete blocks 14 through 20 on the CMS-1500 claim form below. (*Note:* Dr. Hayler's NPI is 0002223334.)

14. DATE OF CURRENT: ILLNESS, INJURY, or PREGNANCY(LMP) MM DD YY QUAL.	15. OTHER DATE QUAL. MM DD YY	16. DATES PATIENT UNABLE TO WORK IN CURRENT OCCUPATION FROM MM DD YY TO MM DD YY
17. NAME OF REFERRING PROVIDER OR OTHER SOURCE	17a. / 17b. NPI	18. HOSPITALIZATION DATES RELATED TO CURRENT SERVICES FROM MM DD YY TO MM DD YY
19. ADDITIONAL CLAIM INFORMATION (Designated by NUCC)		20. OUTSIDE LAB? ☐ YES ☐ NO $ CHARGES

3. The codes for Ms. Parlet's various diagnoses are as follows:

V72.31: Routine GYN exam w/ Pap
V72.42: Pregnancy exam or test w/ positive result

Enter these diagnosis codes in block 21 on the CMS-1500 claim form below.

21. DIAGNOSIS OR NATURE OF ILLNESS OR INJURY Relate A-L to service line below (24E) ICD Ind. A. ___ B. ___ C. ___ D. ___ E. ___ F. ___ G. ___ H. ___ I. ___ J. ___ K. ___ L. ___	22. RESUBMISSION CODE / ORIGINAL REF. NO.
	23. PRIOR AUTHORIZATION NUMBER

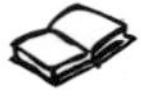

4. Using the information on the Encounter Form and the Fee Schedule, complete blocks 24A through 24J on the CMS-1500 claim form below for each service/procedure provided. The procedure codes are as follows:

   99212: Visit, level II, established patient
   99000: Handling/collection
   88164: Pap smear
   81025: Urine pregnancy test
   36415: Venipuncture

Throughout this exercise, you will need to refer to the Sample Completed Claim Form (Figure B-1) in Appendix B of the textbook.

	24. A. DATE(S) OF SERVICE From MM DD YY	To MM DD YY	B. PLACE OF SERVICE	C. EMG	D. PROCEDURES, SERVICES, OR SUPPLIES (Explain Unusual Circumstances) CPT/HCPCS	MODIFIER	E. DIAGNOSIS POINTER	F. $ CHARGES	G. DAYS OR UNITS	H. EPSDT Family Plan	I. ID. QUAL.	J. RENDERING PROVIDER ID. #
1											NPI	
2											NPI	
3											NPI	
4											NPI	
5											NPI	
6											NPI	

Based on your completion of the claim form, answer the following questions related to specific fields that insurance carriers frequently report as problematic areas.

5. In block 4, the policy holder's name should be entered as:
   a. Louise Parlet.
   b. Parlet Louise.
   c. Parlet Scott.
   d. Same.

6. Was it necessary to complete blocks 9 through 9d?
   a. No, the patient did not have an additional insurance policy.
   b. Yes, the patient had an additional insurance policy.

7. Block 14 reads, "ILLNESS (First symptom) OR INJURY (Accident) OR PREGNANCY (LMP)." Does this block need to be completed for Ms. Parlet's claim?
   a. Yes.
   b. No, this is not applicable to this case because there was no accident.

8. If it is necessary to enter information in block 14, where can you find the correct information to complete it?
   a. On the Encounter Form
   b. On the Patient Information Form
   c. In the Progress Notes
   d. In the Diagnostic Tests section of the chart
   e. By asking the patient directly

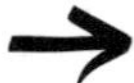

- Click **Close Chart** to return to the Billing and Coding area.
- Click the exit arrow at the lower right corner of the screen to go to the Summary Menu.
- On the Summary Menu, click **Return to Map** and continue to the next exercise.

Exercise 4

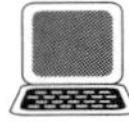

Online Activity—Interpreting an Explanation of Benefits (EOB)

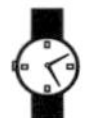

15 minutes

- Select any patient from the patient list.
- On the office map, highlight and click on **Reception** to enter the Reception area.

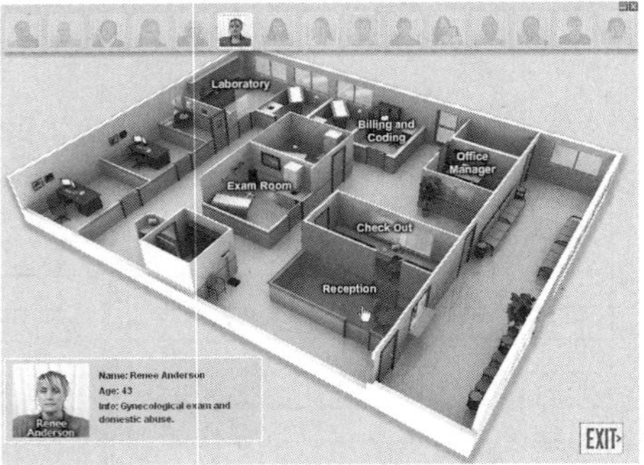

- Under the View heading, click on **Incoming Mail** to view the mail received by the clinic.

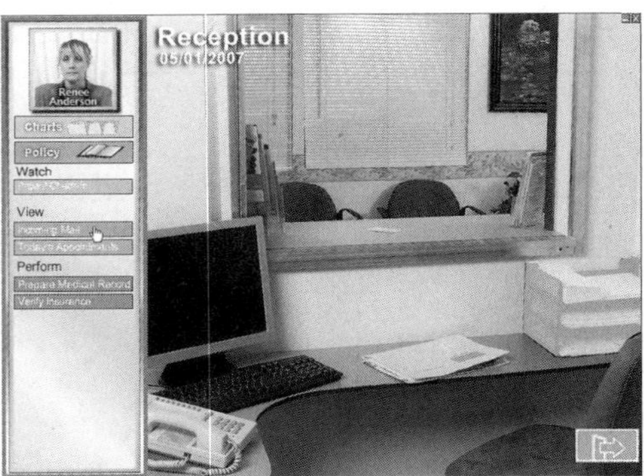

- Click the number **6** to examine that piece of mail.

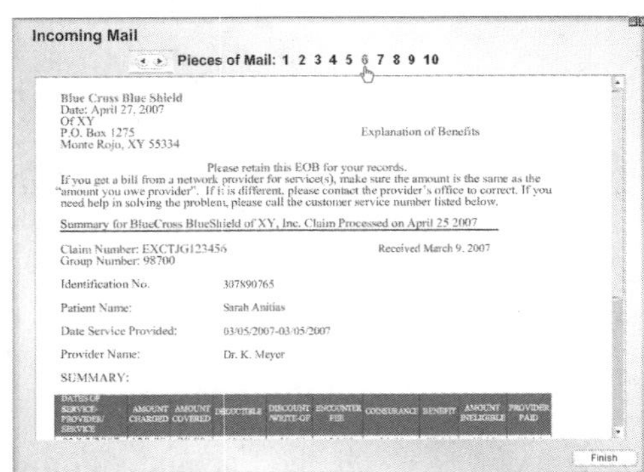

1. Indicate whether the following statement in true or false.

_________ The Explanation of Benefits (EOB) is also referred to as a bill.

2. Below, provide the requested information from the EOB document. If the information cannot be found on the EOB, write N/A.

Patient's name:

Policy holder's name:

Employer's name for group plan:

Date and type of service:

Amount charged for this service:

Amount applied to coinsurance:

Amount applied to deductible:

Amount of benefit:

Amount paid to patient:

Provider name:

Amount of patient's annual deductible:

Amount of patient's deductible met:

Amount of copayment:

Amount patient is responsible for:

Amount of benefits paid by the insurance carrier:

To whom benefits are being paid:

Customer service phone number to contact if questions:

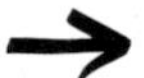

- Click **Finish** to return to the Reception area.
- Click the exit arrow at the lower right corner of the screen to go to the Summary Menu.
- On the Summary Menu, click **Return to Map** and continue to the next lesson or click **Exit the Program**.

LESSON 9

Managed Care

Reading Assignment: Chapter 7—Unraveling the Mysteries of Managed Care

Patients: Jade Wong, John R. Simmons, Kevin McKinzie, Hu Huang, Shaunti Begay

Learning Objectives:

- Identify the managed care patient.
- Identify characteristics of various types of managed care plans.
- Identify insurance information required to complete a managed care claim.
- Determine the need for preauthorization/precertification.
- Provide payment alternatives for a patient with noncontractual insurance coverage.

Overview:

This lesson addresses the diverse characteristics and functions of managed care plans, specifically HMOs and PPOs. You will learn that the goal of managed care is to maximize quality care while minimizing costs. You will identify the characteristics of managed care plans and learn how to identify the managed care patient. You will evaluate and verify information provided on the managed care insurance card. Finally, you will identify patients with noncontractual plans and take appropriate steps to properly advise them on related reimbursement issues.

Exercise 1

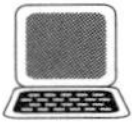

Online Activity—Managed Care Patients

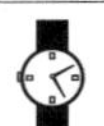

30 minutes

- Sign in to Mountain View Clinic.
- From the patient list, select **Jade Wong**.

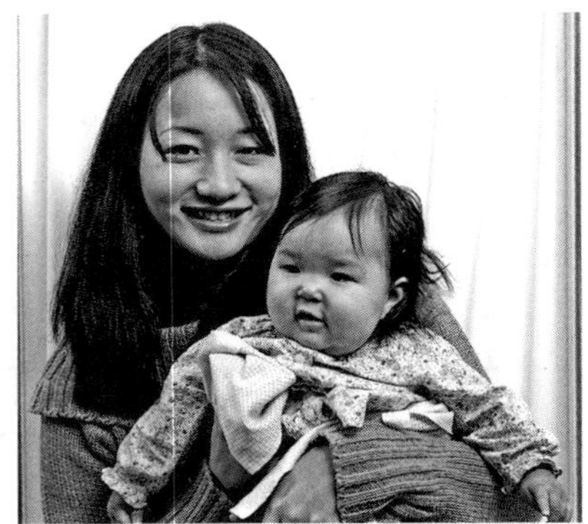

- On the office map, highlight and click on **Billing and Coding** to enter the Billing and Coding area.

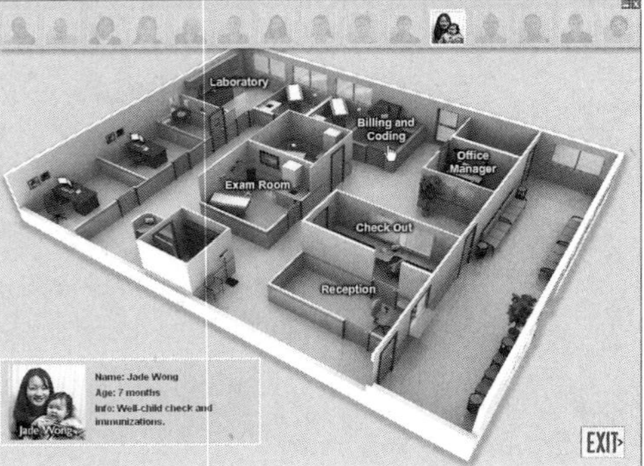

- Click on **Charts** to open Jade Wong's medical record.

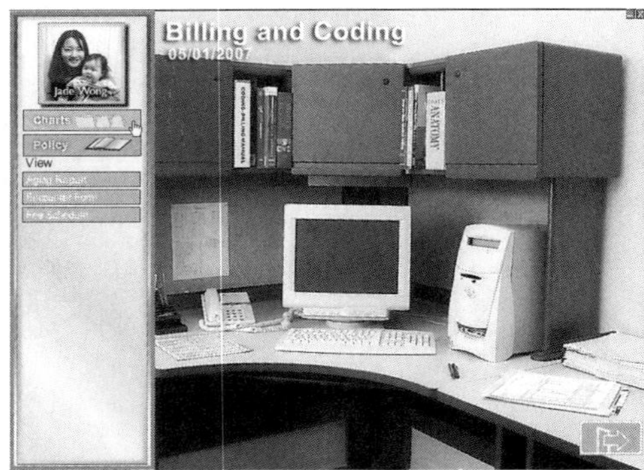

- Click on the **Patient Information** tab and select **2-Insurance Cards** from the drop-down menu.

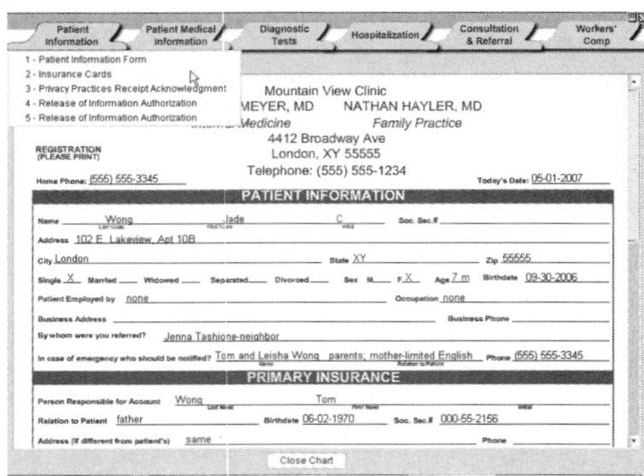

- After reviewing Jade Wong's insurance cards, click **Close Chart** to return to the Billing and Coding area.
- Click the exit arrow to return to the map.
- To answer the following questions, you will need to review the insurance cards for John R. Simmons, Kevin McKinzie, and Hu Huang, using the same steps you just completed for Jade Wong.

1. Which of the following is *not* a characteristic of an HMO?
   a. Patients who select providers out of network without approval will pay the entire bill.
   b. The PCP determines the need for a specialist.
   c. Patients may have to pay copayments.
   d. There are usually deductibles.

2. Which of the following patients is (are) enrolled in an HMO plan? Select all that apply.

   _____ Jade Wong

   _____ John R. Simmons

   _____ Hu Huang

   _____ Kevin McKinzie

3. Based on your review of the patients' insurance cards, provide the information requested in each column of the table below.

Patient	Type of Managed Care Plan (Primary Insurance)	Amount of Deductible	PCP Copayment	Specialist Copayment	Preauthorization/ Precertification May Be Required (Yes or No)
Jade Wong					
John R. Simmons					
Kevin McKinzie					

4. Based on your knowledge of managed care insurance plans and the information you recorded in question 3, which of the following statements typically apply to an HMO plan? Select all that apply.

   _____ There is no penalty for selecting out-of-network providers.

   _____ The patient is expected to pay an annual deductible.

   _____ Members have a copayment.

   _____ Patients do not have to choose a PCP.

5. Based on your knowledge of managed care insurance plans and the information you recorded in question 3, which of the following statements typically apply to a PPO plan? Select all that apply.

_____ There is no penalty for selecting out-of-network providers.

_____ The patient is expected to pay an annual deductible.

_____ Approval is not required before seeing a specialist.

_____ Patients do not have to choose a PCP.

6. Based on your knowledge of managed care insurance plans and the information you recorded in question 3, which of the following statements typically apply to a POS plan? Select all that apply.

_____ There is no penalty for selecting out-of-network providers.

_____ The patient is expected to pay an annual deductible.

_____ Approval is not required before seeing a specialist.

_____ Patients do not have to choose a PCP.

7. The office staff's most valuable source of information and most effective means of assisting patients with their managed care plans and any related costs or penalties is:
   a. the patient.
   b. the insurance plan.
   c. the insurance card.
   d. the patient registration form.

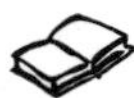

8. Assume that Dr. Hayler is referring Jade Wong to the WIC Program. Complete the form shown on the next page, using the information from the medical record. (*Note:* Some information can be found in the Progress Notes under the Patient Medical Information tab in Jade's chart. For complete instructions on how to fill out the form, see Figure 7-6 in your textbook.)

WIC Program Medical Referral Form 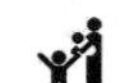

Shaded areas must be completed. **See instructions for completing this form on the reverse side.**

Is this client eligible for Healthy Start? ❑ Yes ❑ No

For WIC Office Use Only:
Date of WIC Certification Appointment ____________

Client's Name ________________________ **Birth Date** ____________ **Sex** M F

Address ________________________ **Phone Number** (______) ______-______

City ______________ **Zip Code** ________ **Social Security #** ______-_____-______

Parent's/Guardian's Name ________________________ (for infants and children only)

❑ *For Pregnant Women*

Height ________ **Weight** ________ **Date Taken** ________ (no older than 60 days)

Hemoglobin ________ **OR Hematocrit** ________ **Date Taken** ________ (must be taken during current pregnancy)

Expected Date of Delivery ________ **Date of First Prenatal Visit** ________ **Prepregnancy Weight** ________

❑ *For Breastfeeding and Postpartum (Non-Breastfeeding) Women*

Height ________ **Weight** ________ **Date Taken** ________ (no older than 60 days)

Hemoglobin ________ **OR Hematocrit** ________ **Date Taken** ________ (must be taken in postpartum period)

Date of Delivery ________ **Date of First Prenatal Visit** ________ **Weight at Last Prenatal Visit** ________

❑ *For Infants and Children less than 24 months of age*

Birth Weight ______ lb ______ oz **Birth Length** ________ inches

Current Height ______ **Current Weight** ______ **Date Taken** ________ (no older than 60 days)

Hemoglobin ________ **OR Hematocrit** ________ **Date Taken** ________ (required once between 6 to 12 months **AND** once between 12 to 24 months)

❑ *For Children 2 to 5 years of age*

Current Height ______ **Current Weight** ______ **Date Taken** ________ (no older than 60 days)

Hemoglobin ________ **OR Hematocrit** ________ **Date Taken** ________ (once a year unless value < 11.1 Hgb or < 33% Hct, then required in 6 months)

✓ **Check all that apply. Please refer your client to WIC, even if nothing is checked below.** This information assists the WIC nutritionist in determining eligibility, developing a nutrition care plan, and providing nutrition counseling. WIC staff may need to contact you or your staff to obtain more detailed medical information prior to providing WIC services.

❑ Medical condition (specify)
____

❑ High venous lead level (10 g/dl or more)
Lead level ______ Date taken ________

❑ Recent major surgery, trauma, burns (specify)
____

❑ Food allergy (specify) ________________

❑ Current or potential breastfeeding complications (specify) ________________

❑ Failure to Thrive

❑ **Special Formula Needed** (diagnosis/signature required)
Type of formula ________________
Number of months ________ (not to exceed 6 months)
Diagnosis ________________
Signature of physician, PA, or ARNP required for special formula ________________

❑ Other (specify) ________________

❑ **Nutrition Counseling Requested** – specify diet prescription/order ________________

WIC Local Agency Address:

I refer this client for WIC eligibility determination:
Signature/Title of Health Professional ________________
Date ________ **PLEASE PLACE OFFICE STAMP BELOW:**
Address:

Phone Number:

*****Parent or Guardian: Please bring a copy of your baby's/child's shot record to the WIC office.*****

DH Form 3075, 12/03 (Stock Number: 5744-000-3075-5) (Replaces 1/01 edition, which may be used.) *WIC is an equal opportunity provider.*

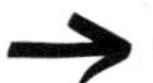

- Click **Close Chart** to return to the Billing and Coding area.
- Click the exit arrow at the lower right corner of the screen to go to the Summary Menu.
- On the Summary Menu, click **Return to Map** and continue to the next exercise.

Exercise 2

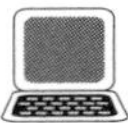

Online Activity—Noncontractual PPO Patient

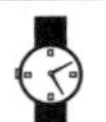

15 minutes

- From the patient list, select **Shaunti Begay**.

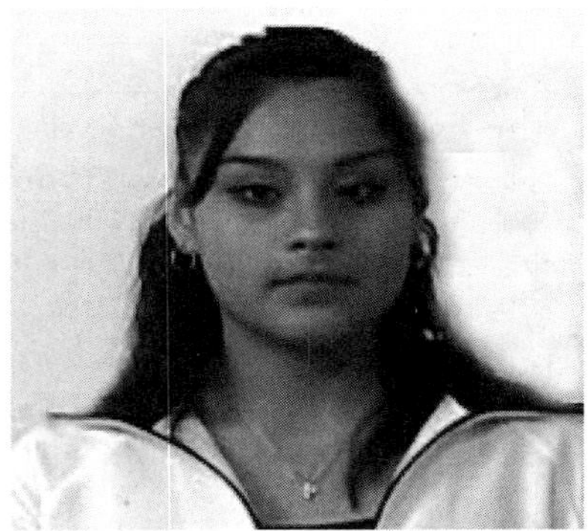

- On the office map, highlight and click on **Reception** to enter the Reception area.

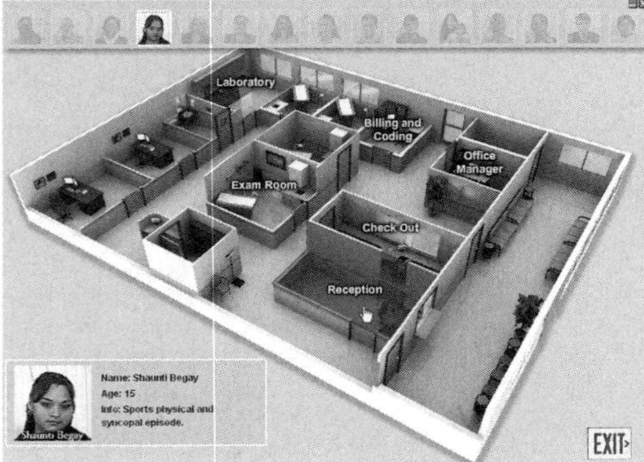

- Under the Watch heading, click on **Patient Check-In** to view the video.
- At the end of the video, click **Close** to return to the Reception area.

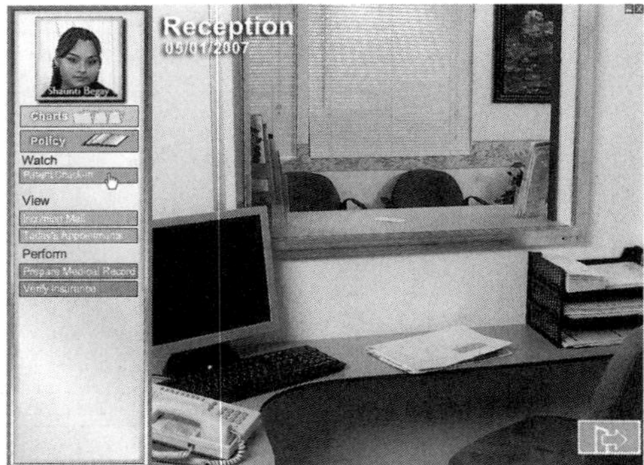

1. Shaunti Begay is covered by a PPO, Unity Health Care. In the video, Kristin advised Shaunti's parents that Mountain View Clinic does not participate with this plan. This means:
   a. Mountain View Clinic has a contract with Unity Health Care, but the contract has a stipulation that the clinic can pick and choose which patients to participate with.
   b. Mountain View Clinic has a contract with Unity Health Care but does not participate in coverage of sports physicals.
   c. Mountain View Clinic has no contract with Unity Health Care and would be considered an out-of-network provider.

2. As a result of Mountain View Clinic's nonparticipation with Shaunti's PPO:
   a. Mountain View Clinic must refuse to see the patient.
   b. Mountain View Clinic must refer the patient to an in-network provider.
   c. Mountain View Clinic may see the patient and offer a discount.
   d. Mountain View Clinic may see the patient but will expect full payment.

3. To avoid problems such as this in the future, Mountain View Clinic should:
   a. sign a contract to participate with Unity Health Care.
   b. advise the patient at the time the appointment is scheduled that the practice may not participate with the patient's insurance, which means the patient would be liable for the charges incurred on that day.
   c. offer the patient a discount to avoid any conflict with the patient and the family.
   d. implement an office policy refusing to see any patients who have managed care plans that the practice does not participate with.

- Click on **Policy** to open the office Policy Manual.

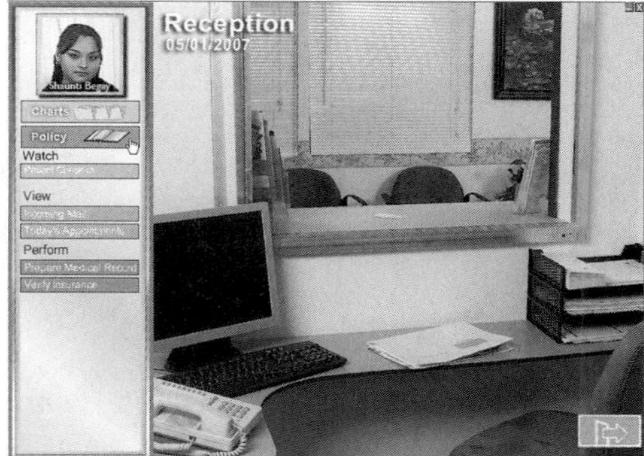

- Using the arrows at the top right of the page, navigate to page 17 and read the policy that applies when patients have insurance coverage that is not accepted by the clinic.

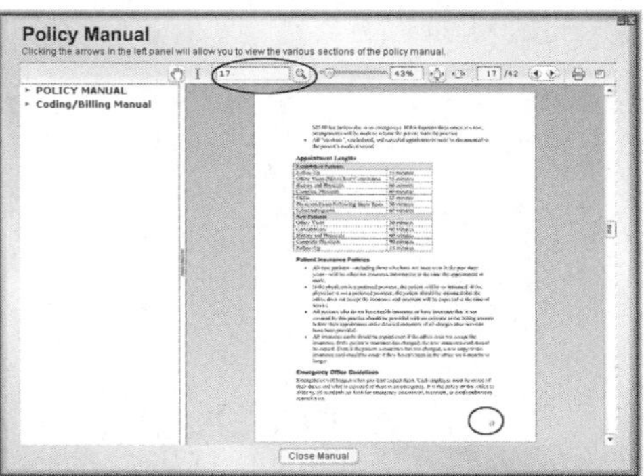

4. What is Mountain View Clinic's policy for patients who either do not have insurance or have insurance that is not accepted by the practice?

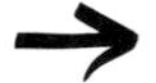

- Click on **Close Manual**.
- Under the Perform heading, click on **Verify Insurance** to obtain the required information for Shaunti's visit.

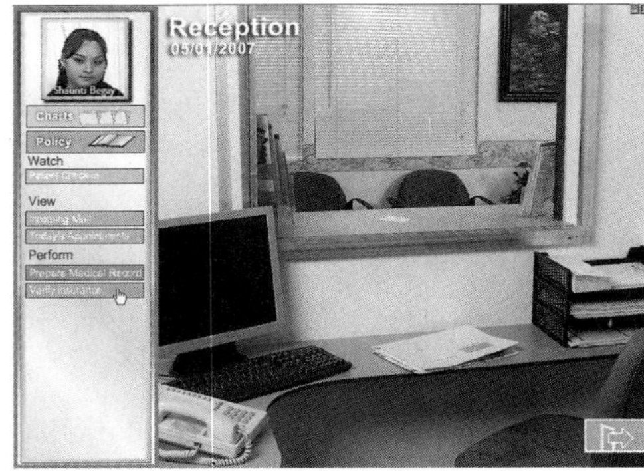

- Click on **Ask** next to the question "Do you have insurance?"

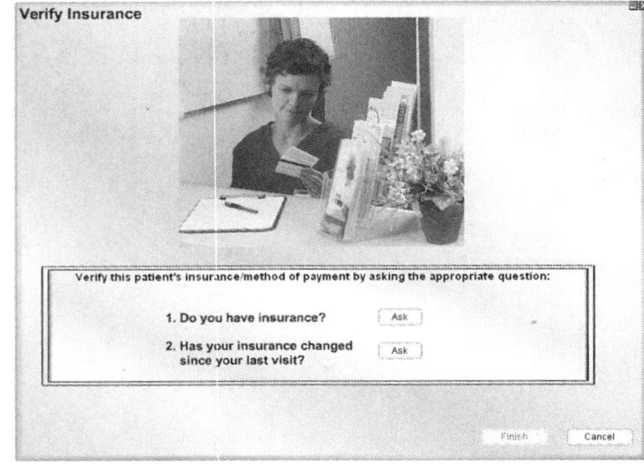

- Under View, click on **Insurance Card(s)**.

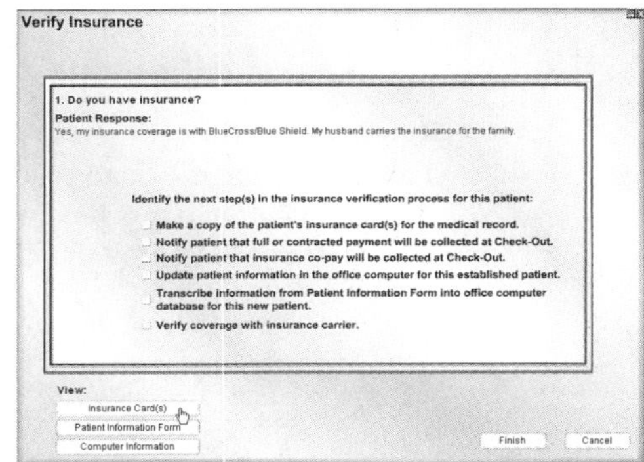

5. What type of plan is Unity Health Care?
   a. Fee-for-service
   b. Indemnity
   c. Preferred provider organization
   d. Health maintenance organization

6. What is the patient's copay for this encounter at Mountain View Clinic?
   a. None
   b. $15
   c. $25
   d. $40

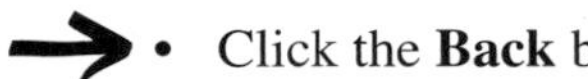

- Click the **Back** button.
- Click **Finish** to return to the Reception area.
- Click the exit arrow at the lower right corner of the screen to go to the Summary Menu.
- On the Summary Menu, click **Return to Map** to continue to the next lesson or click **Exit the Program**.

LESSON 10

Understanding Medicaid

Reading Assignment: Chapter 8—Understanding Medicaid

Patients: Rhea Davison, Wilson Metcalf

Learning Objectives:

- Determine Medicaid eligibility.
- Identify "mandated" Medicaid services.
- Verify patient eligibility for Medicaid.
- Complete a Medicaid claim.

Overview:

This lesson provides an opportunity to learn the basics of Medicaid, a medical assistance program jointly financed by state and federal governments for low-income, blind, or disabled individuals. Medicaid was enacted in 1965 as an amendment to the Social Security Act of 1935. It is a major social welfare program administered by the Centers for Medicare and Medicaid Services (CMS) under the direction of the U.S. Department of Health and Human Services (HHS).

You will view Mountain View Clinic's Policy Manual to familiarize yourself with office policies related to participation with the Medicaid program. You will identify the patient who qualifies for Medicaid assistance and verify Medicaid coverage. You will identify the payment process for Medicaid eligible patients. You will also complete a Medicaid claim form for Wilson Metcalf using the step-by-step claims completion guidelines for Medicaid claims.

Exercise 1

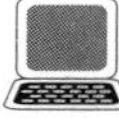

Online Activity—Determining Medicaid Eligibility

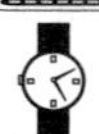

15 minutes

Answer the following questions, using Mountain View Clinic's Policy Manual and your knowledge of the Medicaid program based on information provided in the textbook.

1. Medicaid is a:
   a. commercial health insurance plan.
   b. managed care plan.
   c. federal and state health insurance plan.
   d. federal and state medical assistance program.

2. The Medicaid program covers patients:
   a. whose employers have selected the program as their insurance plan.
   b. over the age of 65 years old.
   c. whose income falls within the federal poverty guidelines.
   d. who have end-stage renal disease (ESRD).

3. Indicate whether each of the following statements is true or false.

   a. ________ Mountain View Clinic participates with the Medicaid program.

   b. ________ Based on federal and state guidelines, Mountain View Clinic must accept Medicaid patients.

4. The patient's Medicaid ID card should be verified at every visit or at least:
   a. once a week.
   b. once a month.
   c. once every 6 months.
   d. once a year.

5. When verifying eligibility of Medicaid coverage with the ID card, it is important to confirm:
   a. the eligibility period.
   b. the policy holder's name.
   c. the patient's PCP.
   d. the need for preauthorization or precertification.

6. Medi-Medi refers to patients who:
   a. are covered under both primary and secondary Medicaid plans.
   b. have Medicaid coverage for consecutive months.
   c. are covered under Medicare and Medicaid.
   d. are covered under managed care programs and Medicaid.

7. If the physicians at Mountain View Clinic decide to limit the number of Medicaid patients they see and therefore no longer accept new Medicaid patients, what procedure should the medical receptionist follow if a Medicaid patient insists on being seen anyway?
   a. Refuse to schedule any appointments for the patient.
   b. Inform the patient that the practice does not accept Medicaid patients and offer to schedule the appointment if the patient agrees to pay for the service.
   c. Keep a list of other local providers who are accepting new Medicaid patients and offer to provide that information to the patient.
   d. Confirm the patient's contact information and defer the final decision to the clinic physicians.

Exercise 2

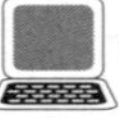

Online Activity—Identifying Medicaid Coverage

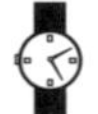

15 minutes

- Sign in to Mountain View Clinic.
- From the patient list, select **Rhea Davison**. (*Note:* If you have exited the program, sign in again to Mountain View Clinic and select Rhea Davison from the patient list.)

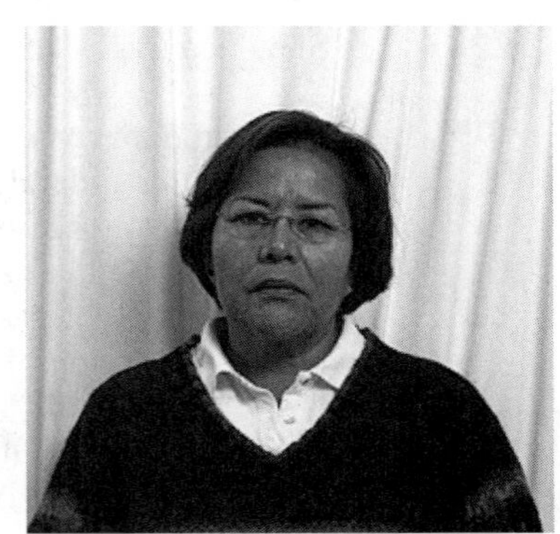

- On the office map, highlight and click on **Check Out** to enter the Check Out area.

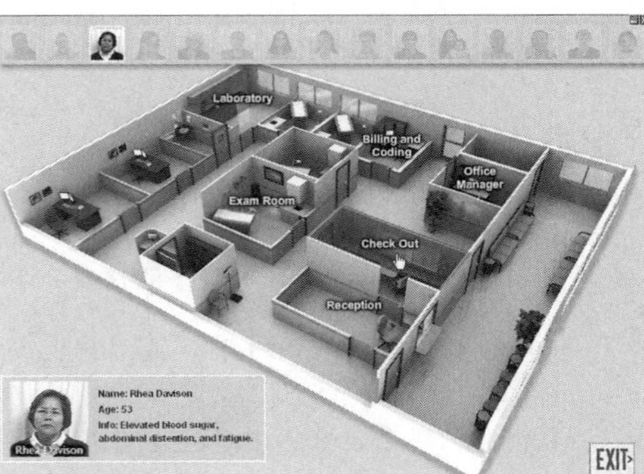

- Under the Watch heading, click on **Patient Check-Out** to view the video.

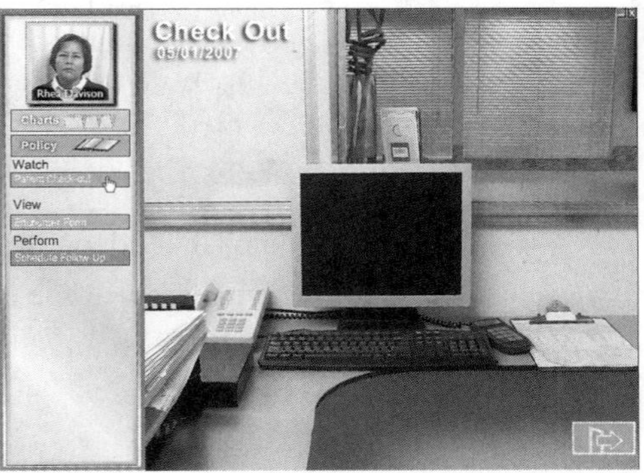

1. What type of health insurance does Rhea Davison have?
   a. Commercial insurance
   b. Managed care
   c. Medicaid
   d. None

2. How has Ms. Davison been paying for her medical services?
   a. By credit card
   b. Through her employer
   c. Through a payment plan set up by the clinic
   d. By providing child care for the physician's children

3. In the video, what does the medical assistant suggest to Ms. Davison to help her with paying for ongoing care?
   a. She offers to give Ms. Davison a discount.
   b. She offers to give Ms. Davison information on government-sponsored programs.
   c. She encourages her to enroll in Medicare.
   d. She encourages her to obtain a credit card so services can be charged.

4. Let's assume that Ms. Davison qualifies to receive Medicaid benefits because her income falls within the federal poverty guidelines. In what group would she be classified?
   a. The medically needy group
   b. The categorically needy group
   c. The medically necessary group
   d. The voluntary enrollee group

5. Title XIX of the Social Security Act requires that certain basic services (referred to as "mandated services") be offered to certain eligible groups. Which of the following services/procedures would qualify as mandated services and be available to Ms. Davison? (*Hint:* Use your textbook for assistance, if needed.) Select all that apply.

   _____ Physician services

   _____ Laboratory and x-ray services

   _____ Plastic surgery (face lifts, tummy tucks, etc.)

   _____ Home health care

   _____ Skilled Nursing facility services

   _____ Dental services (x-rays, cleaning, fillings)

   _____ Inpatient/outpatient hospital services

   _____ Prescription and over-the-counter drugs

→ • At the end of the video, click **Close** to return to the Check Out area.
• Click the exit arrow at the lower right corner of the screen to go to the Summary Menu.
• On the Summary Menu, click **Return to Map** and continue to the next exercise.

Exercise 3

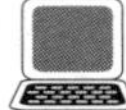

Online Activity—Payment for Medicaid Services

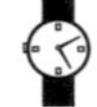

15 minutes

In this exercise, we will assume that Rhea Davison has met the criteria to receive Medicaid benefits and is eligible for coverage on this date of service.

- Keep **Rhea Davison** as your patient. (*Note:* If you have exited the program, sign in again to Mountain View Clinic and select Rhea Davison from the patient list.)
- On the office map, highlight and click on **Billing and Coding** to enter the Billing and Coding area.

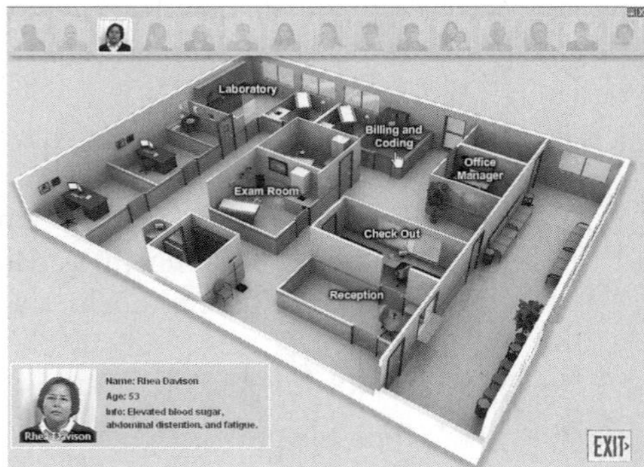

- Click on **Encounter Form** under the View heading.

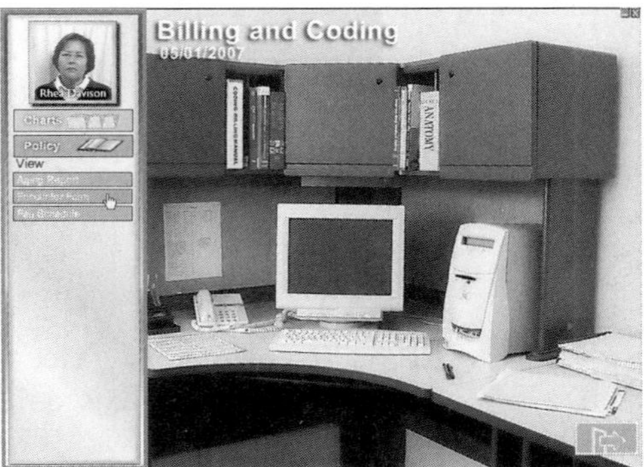

1. According to the Encounter Form, Ms. Davison received the following services during today's visit. Which of these procedures/services would qualify as "medically necessary" and be payable under Medicaid? Select all that apply.

   _____ Established patient visit, level IV

   _____ Blood sugar test

   _____ Pap smear

   _____ UA dipstick

   _____ Hemoccult

2. Indicate whether the following statement is true or false.

   _________ Under Medicaid regulations, Ms. Davison will never have to pay anything out of her pocket, as long she is eligible for Medicaid benefits.

3. Medicaid payments will be made directly to the:
   a. patient.
   b. provider.
   c. county health department.
   d. local state Medicaid office.

4. Providers participating in the Medicaid program:
   a. must accept Medicaid-approved amounts as payment in full.
   b. may balance-bill the patient.
   c. may balance-bill the patient for 20% of the approved amount.
   d. may balance-bill the county health department.

5. Medicaid reimbursements are calculated:
   a. by the provider.
   b. by the county health department.
   c. by the state health department.
   d. by the federal health department.

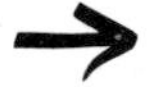

- Click **Finish** to close the Encounter Form and return to the Billing and Coding area.
- Click the exit arrow at the lower right corner of the screen to go to the Summary Menu.
- On the Summary Menu, click **Return to Map** and continue to the next exercise.

Exercise 4

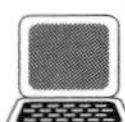

Online Activity—Completing a Medicaid Claim for the Medicare/Medicaid Patient

15 minutes

- From the patient list, select **Wilson Metcalf**. (*Note:* If you have exited the program, sign in again to Mountain View Clinic and select Wilson Metcalf from the patient list.)

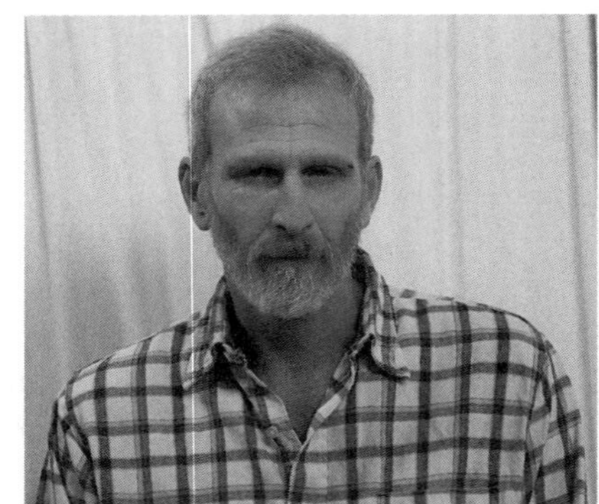

- On the office map, highlight and click on **Billing and Coding** to enter the Billing and Coding area.

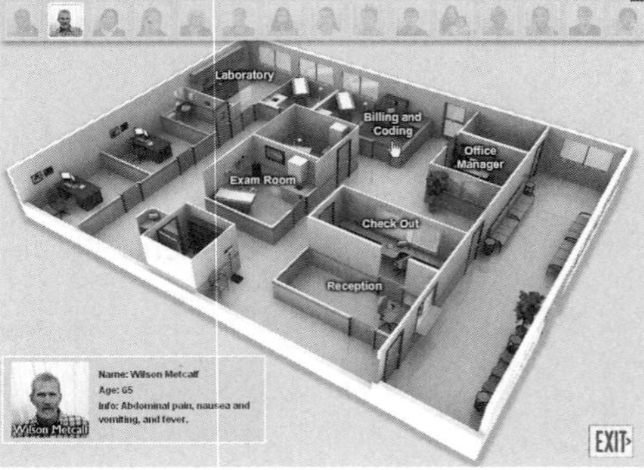

- Click on **Charts** to open Mr. Metcalf's medical record.

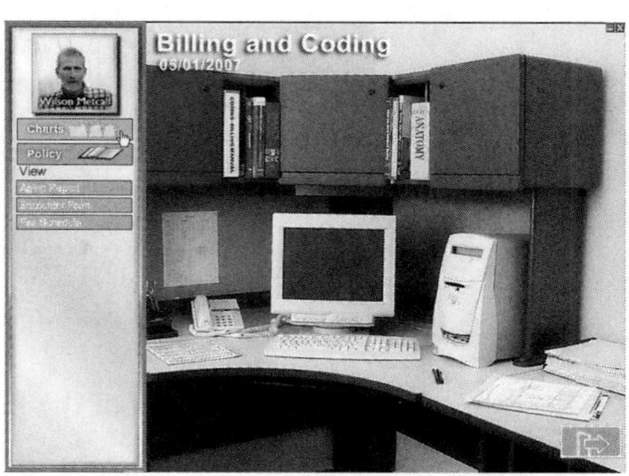

1. According to the Patient Information section of the chart, Mr. Metcalf now has Medicare Parts A and B. Let's also assume that he qualifies for Medicaid. A patient who is covered by both of these government programs is referred to as:
   a. dual eligible.
   b. categorically needy.
   c. medically needy.
   d. qualified.

2. To ensure that he qualified for Medicaid, Mr. Metcalf's total annual income and "countable" resources were reviewed and it was determined that they were less than 100% of the federal poverty level (FPL) guidelines. In light of this, and also considering his age, in what group would he be classified?
   a. Medically needy
   b. Categorically needy
   c. Medically necessary
   d. Qualified Medicare beneficiaries

3. Which methods can be used for verifying Mr. Metcalf's Medicaid eligibility? Select all that apply.

   _____ Asking the patient to produce his Medicaid identification (ID) card

   _____ Using an automated voice response (AVR) system

   _____ Using an electronic data interchange (EDI)

   _____ Asking the patient's son

   _____ Asking the physician

   _____ Using a point-of-sale device

   _____ Examining the patient's medical record

4. What other types of Medicare beneficiaries may receive some Medicaid assistance that would help pay for part or all of their health care expenses? Select all that apply.

   _____ Qualified disabled and working individuals

   _____ Qualified Medicare beneficiaries (QMBs)

   _____ Specified low-income Medicare beneficiaries (SLMBs)

   _____ Members of the Program of All-Inclusive Care for the Elderly (PACE)

   _____ Those with supplementary medical insurance (SMI)

5. If Mr. Metcalf has both Medicare and Medicaid coverage, a claim should be sent first to:
   a. Medicaid.
   b. Medicare.

6. If Mr. Metcalf's claim is not submitted to Medicaid within the time limit set by the state:
   a. the provider may bill the patient.
   b. the provider may not bill the patient.

→ • Click on the **Patient Information** tab and select **3-Insurance Cards** from the drop-down menu.

• Review Mr. Metcalf's Medicaid ID card.

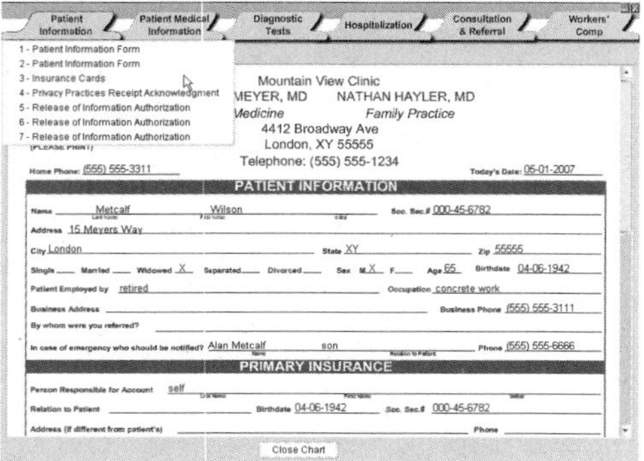

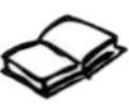

7. Using Mr. Metcalf's Medicaid ID card, along with Figure 8-3 in the textbook, complete the Patient/Insured section of the CMS-1500 form below for Mr. Metcalf. (*Remember:* He is now dual eligible. Refer to Figure B-4 in Appendix B of your textbook for a sample completed claim form for a patient who is dual eligible.)

1. MEDICARE ☐ (*Medicare#*) MEDICAID ☐ (Medicaid#) TRICARE ☐ (ID#DoD#) CHAMPVA ☐ (*Member ID#*) GROUP HEALTH PLAN ☐ (*ID#*) FECA BLK LUNG ☐ (ID#) OTHER ☐ (*ID#*)		1a. INSURED'S I.D. NUMBER (For Program in Item 1)
2. PATIENT'S NAME (Last Name, First Name, Middle Initial)	3. PATIENT'S BIRTH DATE MM | DD | YY SEX M☐ F☐	4. INSURED'S NAME (Last Name, First Name, Middle Initial)
5. PATIENT'S ADDRESS (No., Street)	6. PATIENT RELATIONSHIP TO INSURED Self☐ Spouse☐ Child☐ Other☐	7. INSURED'S ADDRESS (No., Street)
CITY / STATE	8. RESERVED FOR NUCC USE	CITY / STATE
ZIP CODE / TELEPHONE (Include Area Code) ( )		ZIP CODE / TELEPHONE (Include Area Code) ( )
9. OTHER INSURED'S NAME (Last Name, First Name, Middle Initial)	10. IS PATIENT'S CONDITION RELATED TO:	11. INSURED'S POLICY GROUP OR FECA NUMBER
a. OTHER INSURED'S POLICY OR GROUP NUMBER	a. EMPLOYMENT? (Current or Previous) ☐ YES ☐ NO	a. INSURED'S DATE OF BIRTH MM | DD | YY SEX M☐ F☐
b. RESERVED FOR NUCC USE	b. AUTO ACCIDENT? PLACE (State) ☐ YES ☐ NO	b. OTHER CLAIM ID (Designated by NUCC)
c. RESERVED FOR NUCC USE	c. OTHER ACCIDENT? ☐ YES ☐ NO	c. INSURANCE PLAN NAME OR PROGRAM NAME
d. INSURANCE PLAN NAME OR PROGRAM NAME	10d. CLAIM CODES (Designated by NUCC)	d. IS THERE ANOTHER HEALTH BENEFIT PLAN? ☐ YES ☐ NO ***If yes,*** complete items 9, 9a, and 9d.
READ BACK OF FORM BEFORE COMPLETING & SIGNING THIS FORM. 12. PATIENT'S OR AUTHORIZED PERSON'S SIGNATURE I authorize the release of any medical or other information necessary to process this claim. I also request payment of government benefits either to myself or to the party who accepts assignment below. SIGNED ______ DATE ______		13. INSURED'S OR AUTHORIZED PERSON'S SIGNATURE I authorize payment of medical benefits to the undersigned physician or supplier for services described below. SIGNED ______

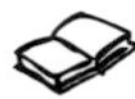

8. Compare your completed form above with the form in Appendix B of the textbook. Did you remember to mark both the Medicare and Medicaid box since the patient is dual enrolled?

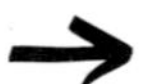

- Click **Close Chart** to return to the Billing and Coding area.
- Click the exit arrow at the lower right corner of the screen to go to the Summary Menu.
- On the Summary Menu, click **Return to Map** to continue to the next lesson or click **Exit the Program**.

LESSON 11

Medicare

Reading Assignment: Chapter 9—Conquering Medicare's Challenges
- Medicare Program
- Medicare Combination Coverages
- Preparing for the Medicare Patient
- Medicare Billing
- Using the CMS-1500 Form for Medicare Claims

Patients: Wilson Metcalf, Jean Deere, Hu Huang

Learning Objectives:

- Identify the Medicare beneficiary and determine eligibility.
- Extract important patient information from a Medicare ID card.
- Identify patient cost-sharing responsibilities under Medicare.
- Differentiate between Part A and Part B benefits.
- List the various Medicare combination coverages.
- Complete Medicare claim forms.

Overview:

This lesson addresses Medicare, which is an entitlement program for people age 65 or older, certain people under age 65 with disabilities, and people of any age who have permanent kidney failure or end-stage renal disease (ESRD). In this lesson you will view Mountain View Clinic's Policy Manual to familiarize yourself with office policies related to participation with the Medicare program, identify patients who qualify for Medicare coverage, and verify Medicare eligibility. You will view Wilson Metcalf's check-in video and identify the benefits available to him under the Medicare program and view Jean Deere's check-in video and identify her primary and secondary claim coverage. You will also view Hu Huang's insurance information to determine insurance coverage and benefits available to him under the Medicare program. Finally, you will complete a Medicare claim form for Wilson Metcalf, Jean Deere, and Hu Huang using the step-by-step claims completion guidelines for Medicare claims.

Exercise 1

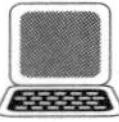

Online Activity—Identifying the Medicare Beneficiary

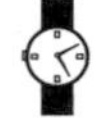

15 minutes

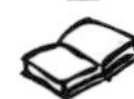

Answer the following questions, using Mountain View Clinic's Policy Manual and your knowledge of the Medicare program. Refer to Chapter 9 in your textbook for additional help.

1. Medicare is:
   a. a commercial health plan.
   b. a managed care plan.
   c. a comprehensive federal insurance program.
   d. a federal and state medical assistance program.

2. The Medicare program was established for:
   a. individuals whose incomes fall within the poverty or low-income guidelines.
   b. individuals over the age of 65.
   c. individuals who have been injured on the job.
   d. children whose parents do not have insurance coverage.

3. Since the origin of the Medicare program, it has been expanded to provide coverage to:
   a. patients with certain disabilities.
   b. patients with end-stage renal disease.
   c. patients with permanent kidney disorders.
   d. all of the above.

4. Indicate whether the following statement is true or false.

   _________ Mountain View Clinic participates with the Medicare program.

5. Medicare is composed of four parts (A, B, C, and D). Office visits provided by physicians at Mountain View Clinic would be billed to which of these parts?
   a. Part A
   b. Part B
   c. Part C
   d. Part D

Exercise 2

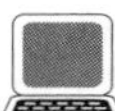

Online Activity—Determining Medicare Eligibility

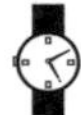

15 minutes

- Sign in to Mountain View Clinic.
- From the patient list, select **Wilson Metcalf**.

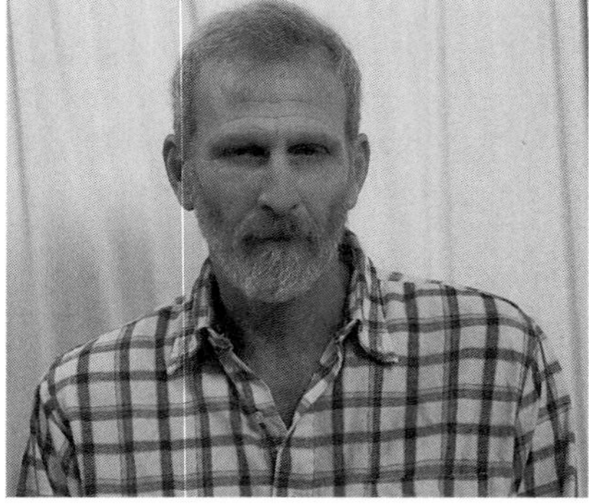

- On the office map, highlight and click on **Reception** to enter the Reception area.

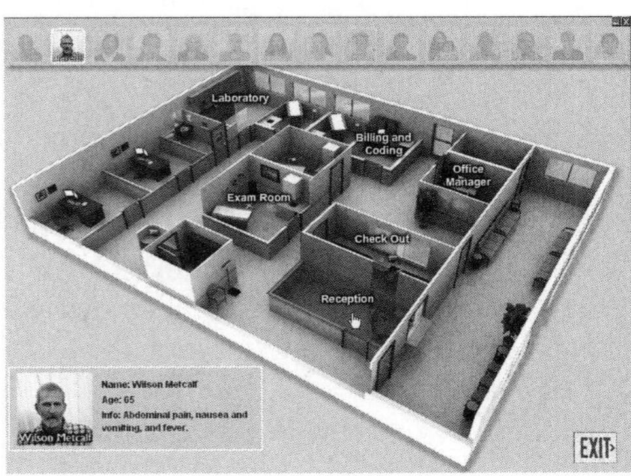

- Under the Watch heading, click on **Patient Check-In** to view the video.

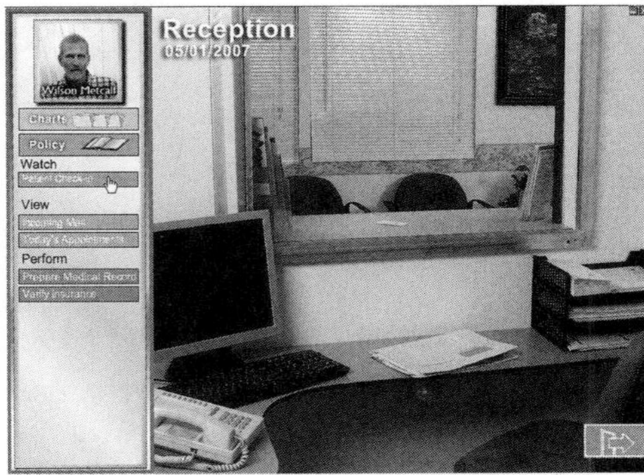

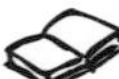 You may refer to Chapter 9 in your textbook as needed to answer the following questions.

1. How did Kristin know that Mr. Metcalf had Medicare?
   a. Kristin asked Mr. Metcalf whether his insurance had changed since his last visit.
   b. Kristin looked at his patient registration form.
   c. Kristin thought Mr. Metcalf looked like he was over 65.
   d. Kristin remembered that Mr. Metcalf had Medicare from his previous visit.

2. When Kristin asked Mr. Metcalf for his Medicare card, he asked her what the card looked like. Kristin described the card by saying which of the following?
   a. It says Medicare across the top of it.
   b. It has your name on it.
   c. It has a picture of an eagle on it.
   d. It is printed in red, white, and blue.

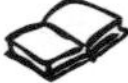

3. Which information is shown on the front of an authentic Medicare card? Select all that apply. (*Hint:* See Figure 9-7 in your textbook for help.)

_____ Name of beneficiary

_____ Beneficiary's address and phone number

_____ Medicare claim number

_____ Beneficiary's sex

_____ Beneficiary's telephone number

_____ Date(s) beneficiary became eligible for Parts A and/or B

_____ Medicare's toll-free phone number

_____ Signature of beneficiary

- At the end of the video, click **Close** to return to the Reception area.
- Click on **Verify Insurance** and select the appropriate question.
- Under the View heading on the next screen, click on **Insurance Cards** or on **Patient Information Form** as needed to answer the following questions.

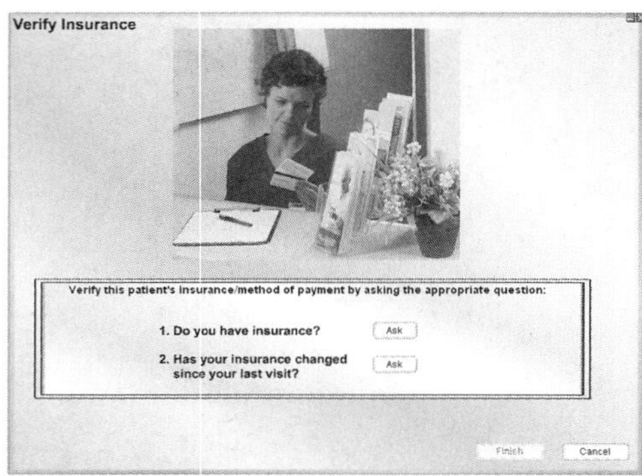

4. On what date did Mr. Metcalf become eligible for Medicare benefits?

5. The charges for Mr. Metcalf's office visit today would be eligible for payment under:
   a. Medicare Part A.
   b. Medicare Part B.
   c. Medicare Part C.
   d. Medicare Part D.

6. Mr. Metcalf's Medicare number is 000456782A. What does the "A" stand for at the end of the number?
   a. Nothing. All Medicare numbers end in A.
   b. It indicates that he is a retired wage earner.
   c. It indicates that he is a widower.
   d. It indicates that he is eligible for Part A benefits.

7. As a Medicare beneficiary with Part B benefits, how much will Mr. Metcalf have to pay for all covered services provided at Mountain View Clinic?
   a. Nothing. Medicare will pay for all covered services.
   b. He will pay a yearly deductible only.
   c. He will pay a 20% deductible only.
   d. He will pay a yearly deductible and a 20% copayment.

8. What is the most important reason for the health insurance professional to be able to answer the Medicare patients' questions about their cost-sharing responsibilities accurately?
   a. It is not important; the primary job of the health insurance professional is to complete CMS-1500 claim forms.
   b. It will help to avoid Medicare claim denial.
   c. It will help to ensure timely filing of Medicare claims.
   d. The Medicare program is confusing, and older adults will need assistance in understanding the program.

- Click **Finish** to return to the Reception area.
- Click the exit arrow at the lower right corner of the screen to go to the Summary Menu.
- On the Summary Menu, click **Return to Map** and continue to the next exercise.

Exercise 3

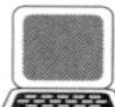

Online Activity—Patient with Medicare Combination Coverage

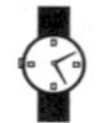

15 minutes

- From the patient list, select **Jean Deere**.

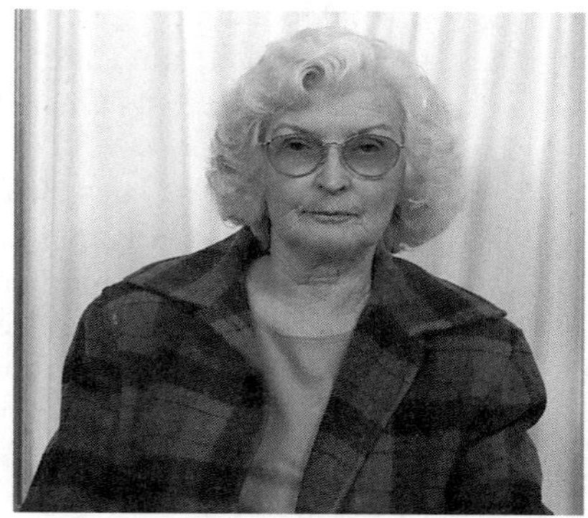

- On the office map, highlight and click on **Reception** to enter the Reception area.

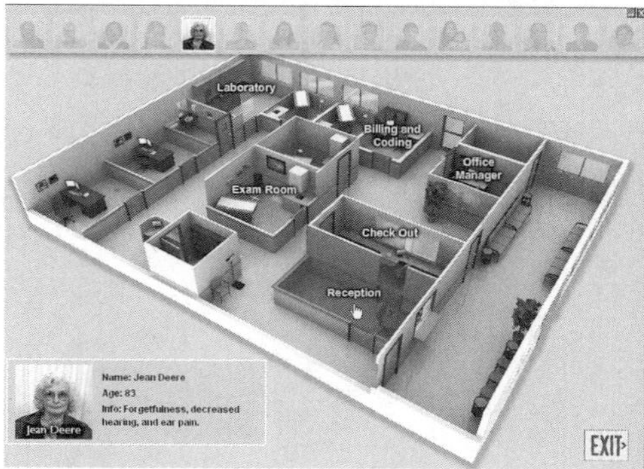

- Under the Watch heading, click on **Patient Check-In** to view the video.

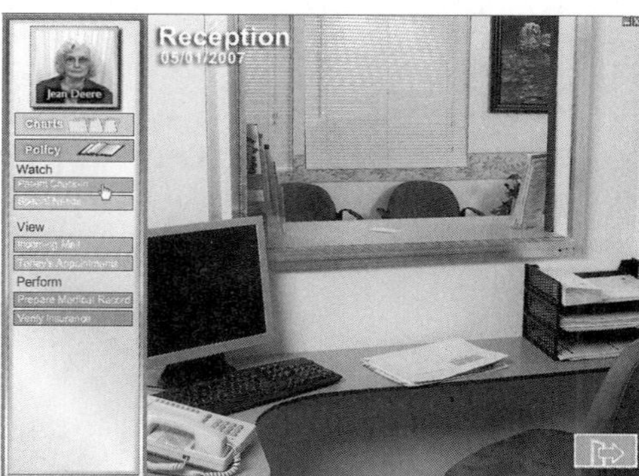

- At the end of the video, click **Finish** to return to the Reception area.
- Click on **Verify Insurance** and select the appropriate question.
- Under the "View" heading on the next screen, click on **Insurance Cards** and **Patient Information Form** to review Ms. Deere's insurance coverage information.
- Click **Finish** to return to the Reception area.
- Click on **Charts** to open Ms. Deere's medical record.

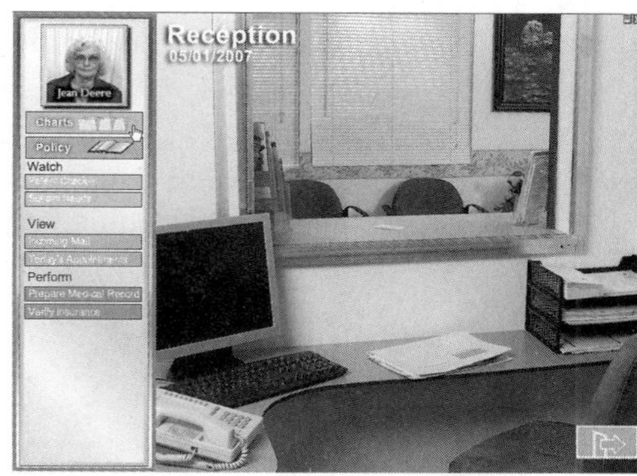

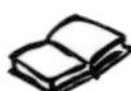 You may also refer to Chapter 9 in your textbook as needed to answer these questions.

1. The receptionist at Mountain View Clinic states that she will need to verify Jean Deere's Patient Information Form. Upon review of the form and the patient's insurance cards, the receptionist will confirm that Ms. Deere has coverage through:
   a. Medicaid.
   b. Medicare.
   c. Oasis Health Care.
   d. Medicare and Oasis Health Care.

2. Jean Deere's Oasis Health Care insurance card clearly states that this policy is a:
   a. Medicare Advantage Plan.
   b. Medicare Supplemental Insurance.
   c. Prescription Drug Benefit Plan.
   d. Dual Eligibility Plan.

3. Ms. Deere's Medigap Insurance will cover:
   a. physician services.
   b. hospital services.
   c. pharmacy charges.
   d. health care expenses not covered by Medicare (deductibles and coinsurance).

4. Explain why Jean Deere's insurance coverage under Oasis Health Care would not be considered a Medicare Secondary Payer (MSP).

5. What if Ms. Deere had Medicare as her primary insurance policy and Medicaid as her secondary insurance carrier? What would this be called?

6. If Jean Deere had no secondary coverage after Medicare, could Mountain View Clinic write off any unpaid balances after Medicare rather than bill her for them? (*Hint:* Refer to the Mountain View Clinic Policy Manual.)

7. If Ms. Deere chose to receive Medicare benefits through a managed care plan rather than through traditional Medicare, would she have the same coverage, the same premiums, and the same coinsurance? If not, explain.

8. The medical facility should maintain a current release of information that allows the health insurance professional to release information to the patient's insurance carriers. Does Mountain View Clinic have a release of information on file for Jean Deere? If so, who is listed as being authorized to receive information about her care?

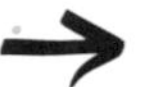

- Click **Close Chart** to return to the Reception area.
- Click the exit arrow at the lower right corner of the screen to go to the Summary Menu.
- On the Summary Menu, click **Return to Map** and continue to the next exercise.

Exercise 4

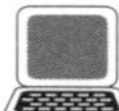

Online Activity—Billing the Medicare Patient

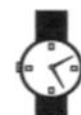

30 minutes

- From the patient list, select **Hu Huang**.

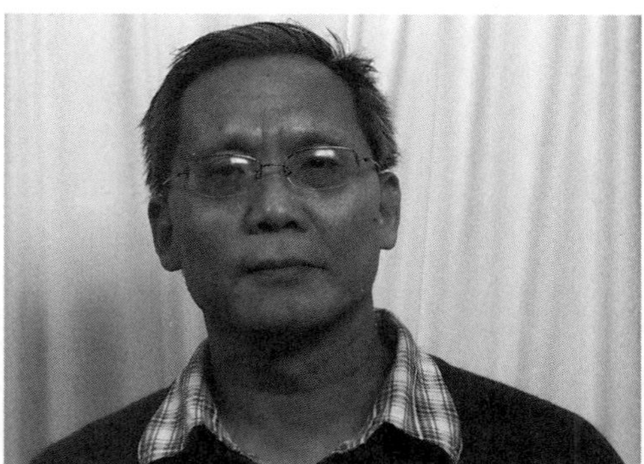

- On the office map, highlight and click on **Reception** to enter the Reception area.

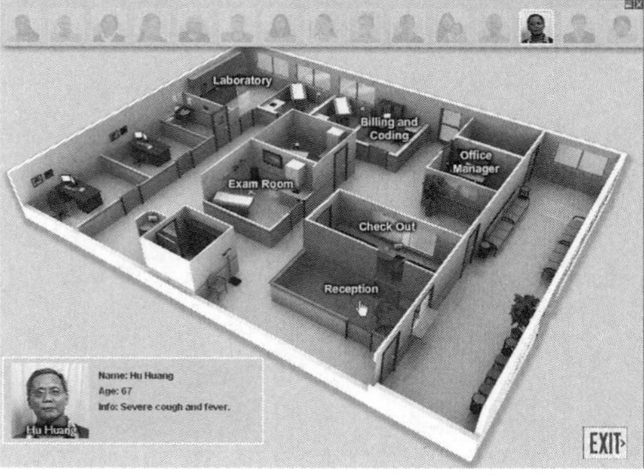

- Click on **Charts** to open Mr. Huang's medical record.

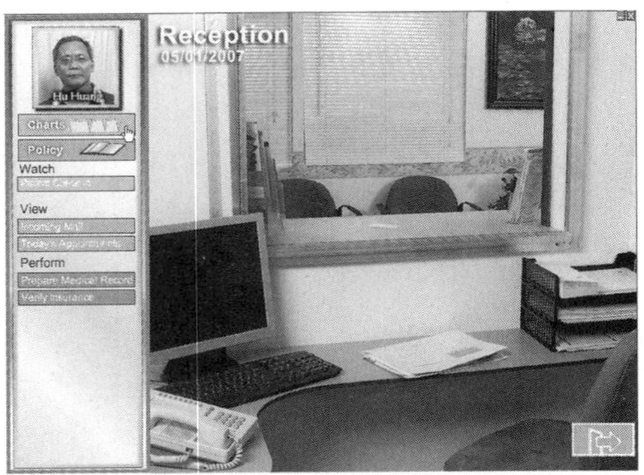

- Click on the **Patient Information** tab and select **2-Insurance Cards** from the drop-down menu.

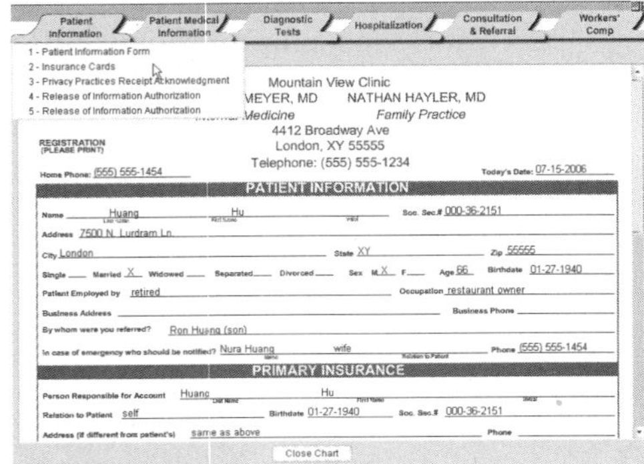

1. What type(s) of Medicare coverage does Mr. Huang have?

2. What type of policy is Oasis Health?

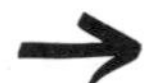

- Click **Close Chart** to return to the Reception area.
- Click the exit arrow at the lower right corner of the screen to go to the Summary Menu.
- On the Summary Menu, click **Return to Map**.
- On the office map, highlight and click on **Check Out** to enter the Check Out area.

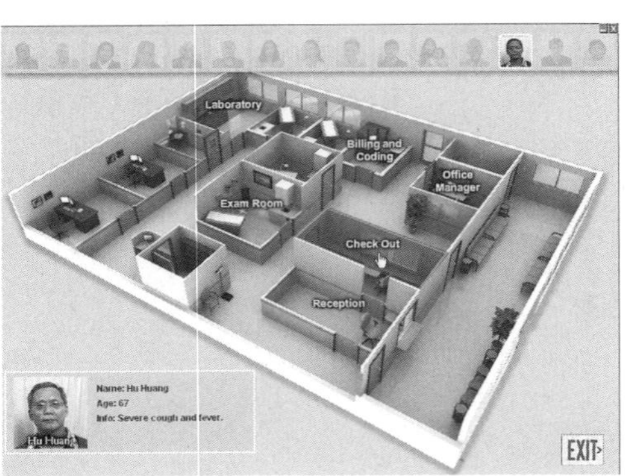

- Under the Watch heading, click on **Patient Check-Out** to view the video.

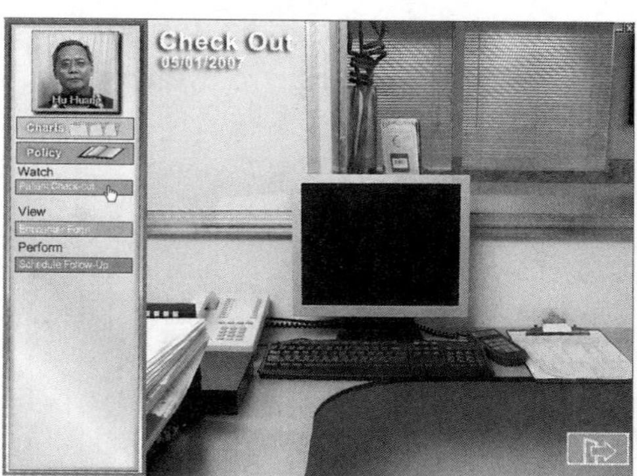

3. If Mr. Huang is ultimately admitted to the hospital as an inpatient, under which part of the Medicare program will the hospital charges fall?

4. For each service listed below, identify whether Medicare Part A or Part B would provide coverage.

	Type of Service	**Medicare Coverage**
_____	Inpatient hospital care	a. Medicare Part A
_____	Care in a skilled nursing facility	b. Medicare Part B
_____	Ambulance transport	
_____	Diagnostic tests/x-rays	
_____	Emergency Department services	
_____	Physician services	
_____	Hospice	
_____	Home health care	
_____	Ambulatory care services	
_____	Blood products	

5. Coverage requirements under Medicare state that for a service to be covered, it must be considered *medically necessary*. Explain what this means.

6. How would the health insurance professional determine whether the test the physician is ordering for Mr. Huang is considered medically necessary?

7. If the health insurance professional determines that the test the physician is ordering for Mr. Huang is not considered medically necessary, what action should be taken?

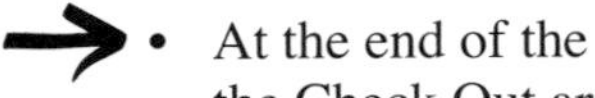

- At the end of the video, click **Close** to return to the Check Out area.
- Click the exit arrow at the lower right corner of the screen to go to the Summary Menu.
- On the Summary Menu, click **Return to Map**.
- On the office map, highlight and click on **Billing and Coding** to enter the Billing and Coding area.

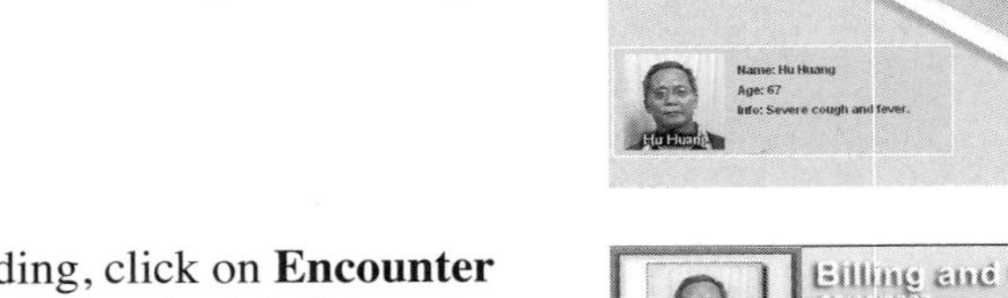

- Under the View heading, click on **Encounter Form** to review the charges for Mr. Huang's visit.

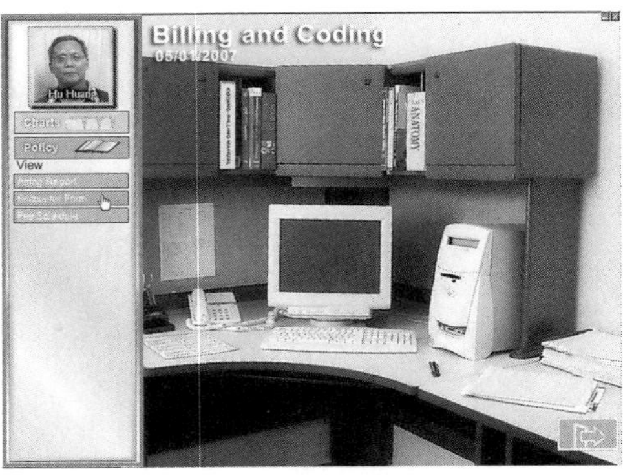

8. Mr. Huang's total fee for today's visit is ______________.

9. If Mr. Huang has not yet met his yearly Medicare Part B deductible of $155 (2010 figure), how much should be collected from him today? (*Hint:* $155 + 20% of the remaining balance.)

10. If Mr. Huang has met his yearly deductible of $155, how much should be collected from him today?

11. Indicate whether the following statement is true or false.

_________ Mountain View Clinic is a Medicare participating provider, which means it will accept Medicare's allowable fee as payment in full, after the beneficiary has paid his or her cost shares (deductible and coinsurance).

- Click **Finish** to close the Encounter Form and return to the Billing and Coding area.
- Remain in the Billing and Coding area with Hu Huang as your patient and continue to the next exercise.

Exercise 5

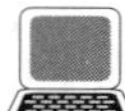

Online Activity—Completing a Medicare Claim

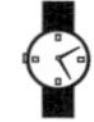

30 minutes

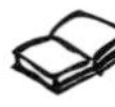

For help with this exercise, refer to Table 9-9 (CMS 1500 Claim Form Instructions for Medicare) in your textbook. You may also refer to sample completed claim forms in Appendix B (Figures B-3, B-4, B-5, and B-6) in your textbook.

- Click on **Charts** to open Mr. Huang's medical record. (*Note:* If you have exited the program, sign in again to Mountain View Clinic, select Hu Huang from the patient list, and enter the Billing and Coding area.)

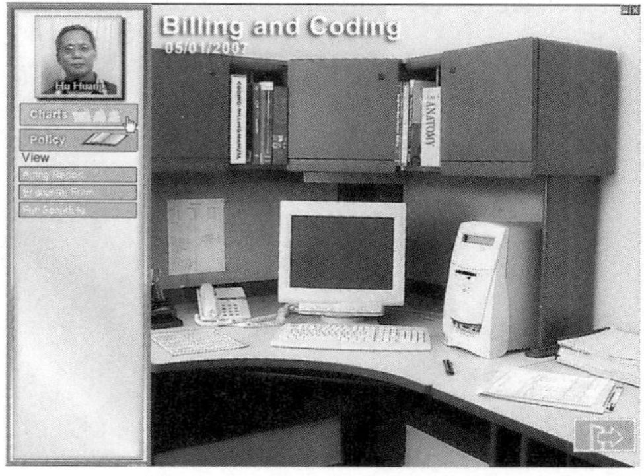

1. Using the information in Hu Huang's medical record, complete the CMS-1500 form on the next page for a Medicare claim. (*Note:* The clinic NPI is 0001115670, and the Rendering Provider ID # is 0011228890.)

   The procedure codes (CPT) and associated diagnosis codes (ICD-9) are listed below.

CPT Code	Description	Associated ICD-9 Code
99214	Office visit	465.9, 401.1
86580	Throat/sputum culture	780.6, 465.9
99000	Handling charge	780.6, 465.9
81000	Urinalysis	780.6
36415	Venipuncture	401.1
94760	Pulse oximetry	465.9

HEALTH INSURANCE CLAIM FORM

APPROVED BY NATIONAL UNIFOR MCLAIM COMMITTEE (NUCC) 02/12

PICA | PICA | CARR

1. MEDICARE (Medicare#) | MEDICAID (Medicaid#) | TRICARE (ID#DoD#) | CHAMPVA (Member ID#) | GROUP HEALTH PLAN (ID#) | FECA BLK LUNG (ID#) | OTHER (ID#)

1a. INSURED'S I.D. NUMBER (For Program in Item 1)

2. PATIENT'S NAME (Last Name, First Name, Middle Initial)

3. PATIENT'S BIRTH DATE MM DD YY SEX M F

4. INSURED'S NAME (Last Name, First Name, Middle Initial)

5. PATIENT'S ADDRESS (No., Street)

6. PATIENT RELATIONSHIP TO INSURED Self Spouse Child Other

7. INSURED'S ADDRESS (No., Street)

CITY STATE

8. RESERVED FOR NUCC USE

CITY STATE

ZIP CODE TELEPHONE (Include Area Code) ( )

ZIP CODE TELEPHONE (Include Area Code) ( )

9. OTHER INSURED'S NAME (Last Name, First Name, Middle Initial)

10. IS PATIENT'S CONDITION RELATED TO:

11. INSURED'S POLICY GROUP OR FECA NUMBER

a. OTHER INSURED'S POLICY OR GROUP NUMBER

a. EMPLOYMENT? (Current or Previous) YES NO

a. INSURED'S DATE OF BIRTH MM DD YY SEX M F

b. RESERVED FOR NUCC USE

b. AUTO ACCIDENT? YES NO PLACE (State)

b. OTHER CLAIM ID (Designated by NUCC)

c. RESERVED FOR NUCC USE

c. OTHER ACCIDENT? YES NO

c. INSURANCE PLAN NAME OR PROGRAM NAME

d. INSURANCE PLAN NAME OR PROGRAM NAME

10d. CLAIM CODES (Designated by NUCC)

d. IS THERE ANOTHER HEALTH BENEFIT PLAN? YES NO *If yes,* complete items 9, 9a, and 9d.

READ BACK OF FORM BEFORE COMPLETING & SIGNING THIS FORM.

12. PATIENT'S OR AUTHORIZED PERSON'S SIGNATUREI authorize the release of any medical or other information necessary to process this claim. I also request payment of government benefits either to myself or to the party who accepts assignment below.

SIGNED ______ DATE ______

13. INSURED'S OR AUTHORIZED PERSON'S SIGNATURE I authorize payment of medical benefits to the undersigned physician or supplier for services described below.

SIGNED ______

PATIENT AND INSURED INFORMATION

14. DATE OF CURRENT: ILLNESS, INJURY, or PREGNANCY(LMP) MM DD YY QUAL.

15. OTHER DATE QUAL. MM DD YY

16. DATES PATIENT UNABLE TO WORK IN CURRENT OCCUPATION FROM MM DD YY TO MM DD YY

17. NAME OF REFERRING PROVIDER OR OTHER SOURCE 17a. 17b. NPI

18. HOSPITALIZATION DATES RELATED TO CURRENT SERVICES FROM MM DD YY TO MM DD YY

19. ADDITIONAL CLAIM INFORMATION (Designated by NUCC)

20. OUTSIDE LAB? YES NO $ CHARGES

21. DIAGNOSIS OR NATURE OF ILLNESS OR INJURY Relate A-L to service line below (24E) ICD Ind.

A. B. C. D.
E. F. G. H.
I. J. K. L.

22. RESUBMISSION CODE ORIGINAL REF. NO.

23. PRIOR AUTHORIZATION NUMBER

24. A. DATE(S) OF SERVICE From MM DD YY To MM DD YY	B. PLACE OF SERVICE	C. EMG	D. PROCEDURES, SERVICES, OR SUPPLIES (Explain Unusual Circumstances) CPT/HCPCS MODIFIER	E. DIAGNOSIS POINTER	F. $ CHARGES	G. DAYS OR UNITS	H. EPSDT Family Plan	I. ID. QUAL.	J. RENDERING PROVIDER ID. #
1								NPI	
2								NPI	
3								NPI	
4								NPI	
5								NPI	
6								NPI	

25. FEDERAL TAX I.D. NUMBER SSN EIN

26. PATIENT'S ACCOUNT NO.

27. ACCEPT ASSIGNMENT? (For govt. claims, see back) YES NO

28. TOTAL CHARGE $

29. AMOUNT PAID $

30. Rsvd for NUCC Use $

31. SIGNATURE OF PHYSICIAN OR SUPPLIER INCLUDING DEGREES OR CREDENTIALS (I certify that the statements on the reverse apply to this bill and are made a part thereof.)

SIGNED DATE

32. SERVICE FACILITY LOCATION INFORMATION

a. NPI b.

33. BILLING PROVIDER INFO & PH # ( )

a. NPI b.

PHYSICIAN OR SUPPLIER INFORMATION

NUCC Instruction Manual available at: www.nucc.org *PLEASE PRINT OR TYPE* OMB APPROVAL PENDING

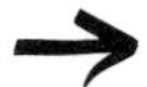

- Click **Close Chart** to return to the Billing and Coding area.
- Click the exit arrow at the lower right corner of the screen to go to the Summary Menu.
- On the Summary Menu, click **Return to Map**.
- From the patient list, select **Jean Deere**.

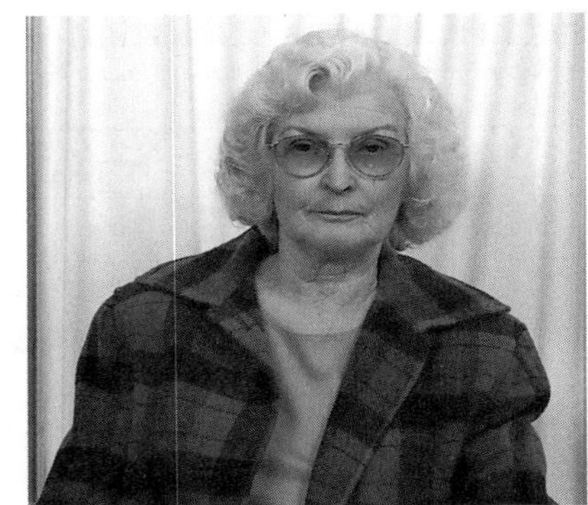

- On the office map, highlight and click on **Billing and Coding** to enter the Billing and Coding area.
- Click on **Charts** to open Jean Deere's medical record.

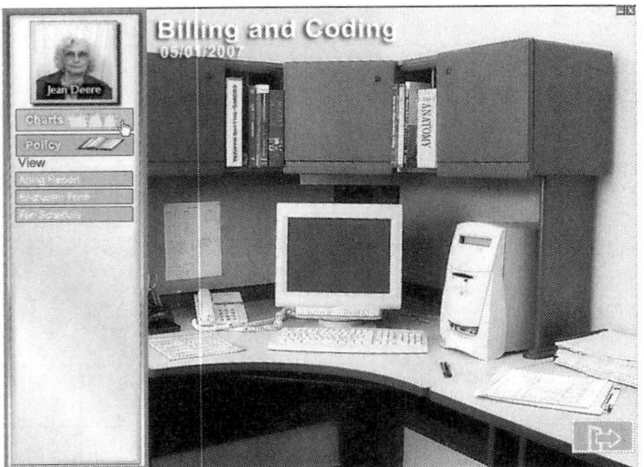

2. Using the information in Jean Deere's medical record, complete the CMS 1500 form on the next page for a Medicare claim. You will need to check the Progress Notes to locate the date of the first symptom, which should be reported in block 14. (*Note:* The clinic NPI is 0001115670, and the Rendering Provider ID # is 0011228890.) The procedure codes (CPT) and associated diagnosis codes (ICD-9) are listed below.

CPT Code	Description	Associated ICD-9 Code
99214	Office visit	380.4, 389.9, 388.70, 780.93
81000	Urinalysis	780.93
94760	Pulse oximetry	780.93

HEALTH INSURANCE CLAIM FORM

APPROVED BY NATIONAL UNIFOR MCLAIM COMMITTEE (NUCC) 02/12

PICA | PICA | CARRIER

1. MEDICARE (Medicare#) | MEDICAID (Medicaid#) | TRICARE (ID#DoD#) | CHAMPVA (Member ID#) | GROUP HEALTH PLAN (ID#) | FECA BLK LUNG (ID#) | OTHER (ID#)

1a. INSURED'S I.D. NUMBER (For Program in Item 1)

2. PATIENT'S NAME (Last Name, First Name, Middle Initial)

3. PATIENT'S BIRTH DATE MM DD YY SEX M F

4. INSURED'S NAME (Last Name, First Name, Middle Initial)

5. PATIENT'S ADDRESS (No., Street)

6. PATIENT RELATIONSHIP TO INSURED Self Spouse Child Other

7. INSURED'S ADDRESS (No., Street)

CITY STATE

8. RESERVED FOR NUCC USE

CITY STATE

ZIP CODE TELEPHONE (Include Area Code) ( )

ZIP CODE TELEPHONE (Include Area Code) ( )

9. OTHER INSURED'S NAME (Last Name, First Name, Middle Initial)

10. IS PATIENT'S CONDITION RELATED TO:

11. INSURED'S POLICY GROUP OR FECA NUMBER

a. OTHER INSURED'S POLICY OR GROUP NUMBER

a. EMPLOYMENT? (Current or Previous) YES NO

a. INSURED'S DATE OF BIRTH MM DD YY SEX M F

b. RESERVED FOR NUCC USE

b. AUTO ACCIDENT? YES NO PLACE (State)

b. OTHER CLAIM ID (Designated by NUCC)

c. RESERVED FOR NUCC USE

c. OTHER ACCIDENT? YES NO

c. INSURANCE PLAN NAME OR PROGRAM NAME

d. INSURANCE PLAN NAME OR PROGRAM NAME

10d. CLAIM CODES (Designated by NUCC)

d. IS THERE ANOTHER HEALTH BENEFIT PLAN? YES NO *If yes*, complete items 9, 9a, and 9d.

READ BACK OF FORM BEFORE COMPLETING & SIGNING THIS FORM.

12. PATIENT'S OR AUTHORIZED PERSON'S SIGNATUREI authorize the release of any medical or other information necessary to process this claim. I also request payment of government benefits either to myself or to the party who accepts assignment below.

SIGNED ______ DATE ______

13. INSURED'S OR AUTHORIZED PERSON'S SIGNATURE I authorize payment of medical benefits to the undersigned physician or supplier for services described below.

SIGNED ______

PATIENT AND INSURED INFORMATION

14. DATE OF CURRENT: ILLNESS, INJURY, or PREGNANCY(LMP) MM DD YY QUAL.

15. OTHER DATE QUAL. MM DD YY

16. DATES PATIENT UNABLE TO WORK IN CURRENT OCCUPATION MM DD YY FROM MM DD YY TO

17. NAME OF REFERRING PROVIDER OR OTHER SOURCE

17a. 17b. NPI

18. HOSPITALIZATION DATES RELATED TO CURRENT SERVICES MM DD YY FROM MM DD YY TO

19. ADDITIONAL CLAIM INFORMATION (Designated by NUCC)

20. OUTSIDE LAB? YES NO $ CHARGES

21. DIAGNOSIS OR NATURE OF ILLNESS OR INJURY Relate A-L to service line below (24E) ICD Ind.

A. B. C. D.
E. F. G. H.
I. J. K. L.

22. RESUBMISSION CODE ORIGINAL REF. NO.

23. PRIOR AUTHORIZATION NUMBER

	24. A. DATE(S) OF SERVICE From MM DD YY To MM DD YY	B. PLACE OF SERVICE	C. EMG	D. PROCEDURES, SERVICES, OR SUPPLIES (Explain Unusual Circumstances) CPT/HCPCS MODIFIER	E. DIAGNOSIS POINTER	F. $ CHARGES	G. DAYS OR UNITS	H. EPSDT Family Plan	I. ID. QUAL.	J. RENDERING PROVIDER ID. #
1									NPI	
2									NPI	
3									NPI	
4									NPI	
5									NPI	
6									NPI	

PHYSICIAN OR SUPPLIER INFORMATION

25. FEDERAL TAX I.D. NUMBER SSN EIN

26. PATIENT'S ACCOUNT NO.

27. ACCEPT ASSIGNMENT? (For govt. claims, see back) YES NO

28. TOTAL CHARGE $

29. AMOUNT PAID $

30. Rsvd for NUCC Use $

31. SIGNATURE OF PHYSICIAN OR SUPPLIER INCLUDING DEGREES OR CREDENTIALS (I certify that the statements on the reverse apply to this bill and are made a part thereof.)

SIGNED DATE

32. SERVICE FACILITY LOCATION INFORMATION

a. NPI b.

33. BILLING PROVIDER INFO & PH # ( )

a. NPI b.

NUCC Instruction Manual available at: www.nucc.org *PLEASE PRINT OR TYPE* OMB APPROVAL PENDING

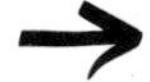

- Click **Close Chart** to return to the Billing and Coding area.
- Click the exit arrow at the lower right corner of the screen to go to the Summary Menu.
- On the Summary Menu, click **Return to Map**.
- From the patient list, select **Wilson Metcalf**.

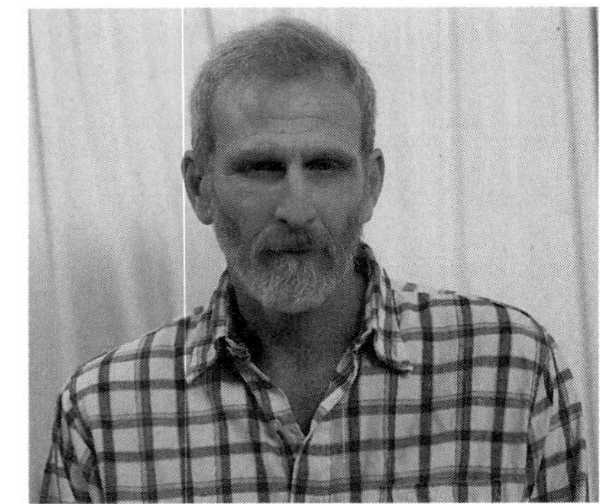

- On the office map, highlight and click on **Billing and Coding** to enter the Billing and Coding area.

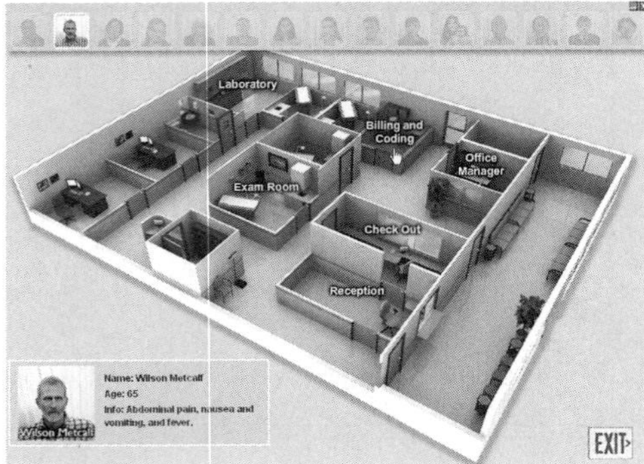

- Click on **Charts** to open Mr. Metcalf's medical record.

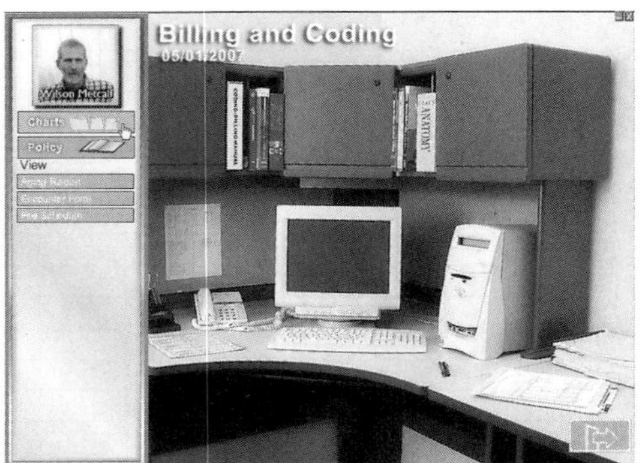

3. Using the information in Wilson Metcalf's medical record, complete the CMS 1500 form on the next page for a Medicare claim. (*Note:* The clinic NPI is 0001115670, and the Rendering Provider ID # is 0011228890.) The procedure codes (CPT) and associated diagnosis codes (ICD-9) are listed below.

CPT Code	Description	Associated ICD-9 Code
82948	Blood sugar	783.21, 788.1, 276.51
82272	Hemoccult	569.3, 789.01

HEALTH INSURANCE CLAIM FORM

APPROVED BY NATIONAL UNIFOR MCLAIM COMMITTEE (NUCC) 02/12

PICA PICA CARR

1. MEDICARE (Medicare#) MEDICAID (Medicaid#) TRICARE (ID#DoD#) CHAMPVA (Member ID#) GROUP HEALTH PLAN (ID#) FECA BLK LUNG (ID#) OTHER (ID#)

1a. INSURED'S I.D. NUMBER (For Program in Item 1)

2. PATIENT'S NAME (Last Name, First Name, Middle Initial)

3. PATIENT'S BIRTH DATE MM DD YY SEX M F

4. INSURED'S NAME (Last Name, First Name, Middle Initial)

5. PATIENT'S ADDRESS (No., Street)

6. PATIENT RELATIONSHIP TO INSURED Self Spouse Child Other

7. INSURED'S ADDRESS (No., Street)

CITY STATE

8. RESERVED FOR NUCC USE

CITY STATE

ZIP CODE TELEPHONE (Include Area Code) ( )

ZIP CODE TELEPHONE (Include Area Code) ( )

9. OTHER INSURED'S NAME (Last Name, First Name, Middle Initial)

10. IS PATIENT'S CONDITION RELATED TO:

11. INSURED'S POLICY GROUP OR FECA NUMBER

a. OTHER INSURED'S POLICY OR GROUP NUMBER

a. EMPLOYMENT? (Current or Previous) YES NO

a. INSURED'S DATE OF BIRTH MM DD YY SEX M F

b. RESERVED FOR NUCC USE

b. AUTO ACCIDENT? PLACE (State) YES NO

b. OTHER CLAIM ID (Designated by NUCC)

c. RESERVED FOR NUCC USE

c. OTHER ACCIDENT? YES NO

c. INSURANCE PLAN NAME OR PROGRAM NAME

d. INSURANCE PLAN NAME OR PROGRAM NAME

10d. CLAIM CODES (Designated by NUCC)

d. IS THERE ANOTHER HEALTH BENEFIT PLAN? YES NO *If yes,* complete items 9, 9a, and 9d.

READ BACK OF FORM BEFORE COMPLETING & SIGNING THIS FORM.

12. PATIENT'S OR AUTHORIZED PERSON'S SIGNATUREI authorize the release of any medical or other information necessary to process this claim. I also request payment of government benefits either to myself or to the party who accepts assignment below.

SIGNED ______ DATE ______

13. INSURED'S OR AUTHORIZED PERSON'S SIGNATURE I authorize payment of medical benefits to the undersigned physician or supplier for services described below.

SIGNED ______

PATIENT AND INSURED INFORMATION

14. DATE OF CURRENT: ILLNESS, INJURY, or PREGNANCY(LMP) MM DD YY QUAL.

15. OTHER DATE QUAL. MM DD YY

16. DATES PATIENT UNABLE TO WORK IN CURRENT OCCUPATION FROM MM DD YY TO MM DD YY

17. NAME OF REFERRING PROVIDER OR OTHER SOURCE

17a.

17b. NPI

18. HOSPITALIZATION DATES RELATED TO CURRENT SERVICES FROM MM DD YY TO MM DD YY

19. ADDITIONAL CLAIM INFORMATION (Designated by NUCC)

20. OUTSIDE LAB? YES NO $ CHARGES

21. DIAGNOSIS OR NATURE OF ILLNESS OR INJURY Relate A-L to service line below (24E) ICD Ind.

A. B. C. D.
E. F. G. H.
I. J K. L.

22. RESUBMISSION CODE ORIGINAL REF. NO.

23. PRIOR AUTHORIZATION NUMBER

	24. A. DATE(S) OF SERVICE From MM DD YY To MM DD YY	B. PLACE OF SERVICE	C. EMG	D. PROCEDURES, SERVICES, OR SUPPLIES (Explain Unusual Circumstances) CPT/HCPCS MODIFIER	E. DIAGNOSIS POINTER	F. $ CHARGES	G. DAYS OR UNITS	H. EPSDT Family Plan	I. ID. QUAL.	J. RENDERING PROVIDER ID. #
1									NPI	
2									NPI	
3									NPI	
4									NPI	
5									NPI	
6									NPI	

PHYSICIAN OR SUPPLIER INFORMATION

25. FEDERAL TAX I.D. NUMBER SSN EIN

26. PATIENT'S ACCOUNT NO.

27. ACCEPT ASSIGNMENT? (For govt. claims, see back) YES NO

28. TOTAL CHARGE $

29. AMOUNT PAID $

30. Rsvd for NUCC Use $

31. SIGNATURE OF PHYSICIAN OR SUPPLIER INCLUDING DEGREES OR CREDENTIALS (I certify that the statements on the reverse apply to this bill and are made a part thereof.)

SIGNED DATE

32. SERVICE FACILITY LOCATION INFORMATION

a. NPI b.

33. BILLING PROVIDER INFO & PH # ( )

a. NPI b.

NUCC Instruction Manual available at: www.nucc.org *PLEASE PRINT OR TYPE* OMB APPROVAL PENDING

- Click **Close Chart** to return to the Billing and Coding area.
- Click the exit arrow at the lower right corner of the screen to go to the Summary Menu.
- On the Summary Menu, click **Return to Map** to continue to the next lesson or click **Exit the Program**.

LESSON 12

TRICARE and CHAMPVA

Reading Assignment: Chapter 10—Military Carriers
- Military Health Programs
- TRICARE
- CHAMPVA
- Instructions for Completing TRICARE/CHAMPVA Claim Forms

Patients: Rhea Davison, Jesus Santo

Learning Objectives:

- Identify the TRICARE beneficiary and determine eligibility.
- Identify various TRICARE programs and payment types.
- Identify TRICARE claim submission and reimbursement policies.
- Identify the CHAMPVA beneficiary and determine eligibility.
- Determine CHAMPVA benefits, preauthorization, and reimbursement policies.
- Complete a claim for both a TRICARE and a CHAMPVA patient.

Overview:

This lesson addresses the two basic military programs—TRICARE and CHAMPVA—offered by the federal government for qualifying military personnel and their eligible dependents. You will identify the patient who qualifies for TRICARE and CHAMPVA coverage and verify eligibility. Next, you will complete a TRICARE claim form for Rhea Davison using the step-by-step claims completion guidelines for TRICARE. Then you will complete a CHAMPVA claim form for Jesus Santo using the step-by-step claims completion guidelines for CHAMPVA.

Exercise 1

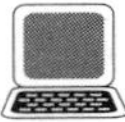

Online Activity—The TRICARE Patient

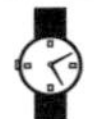

30 minutes

1. Who is eligible for TRICARE benefits?

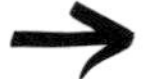

- Sign in to Mountain View Clinic.
- From the patient list, select **Rhea Davison**.

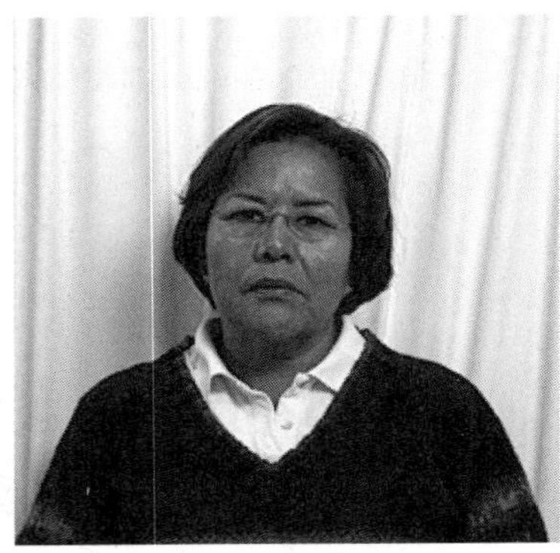

- On the office map, highlight and click on **Check Out** to enter the Check Out area.

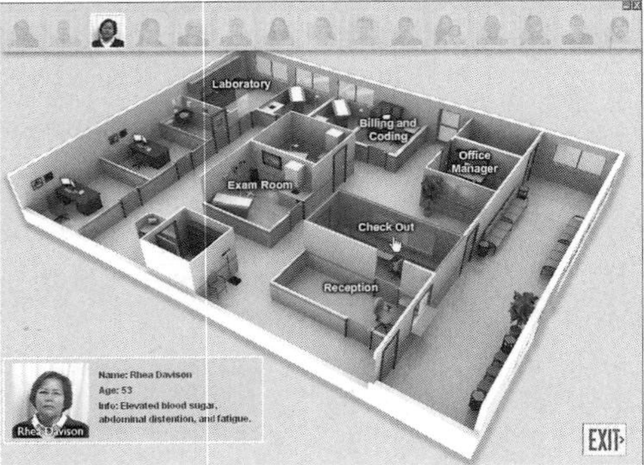

- Click on **Charts** to open Ms. Davison's medical record.

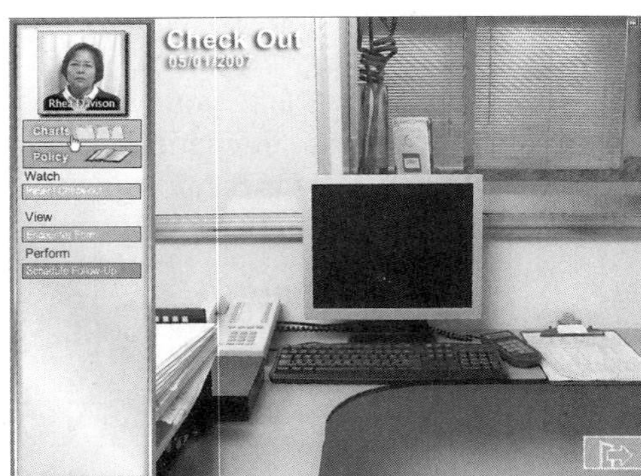

- Click on the **Patient Medical Information** tab and select **1-Progress Notes** from the drop-down menu to review Ms. Davison's information for this encounter.

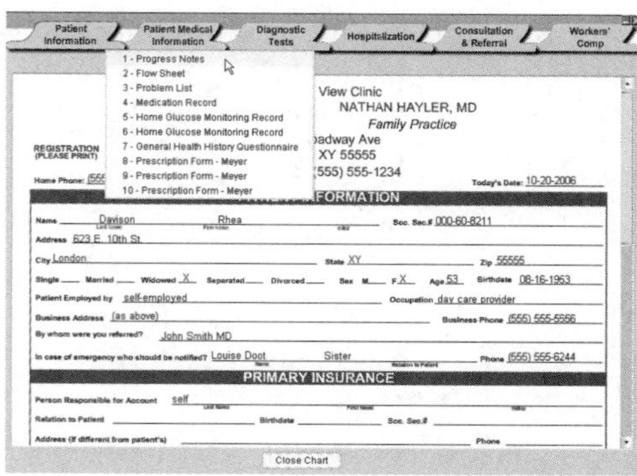

2. What type of insurance coverage does Ms. Davison have, if any?
   a. She has no insurance coverage; she is a self-pay patient.
   b. She has TRICARE.
   c. She has CHAMPUS.
   d. She has CHAMPVA.

3. Assume that Ms. Davison recently married. Below, complete the primary insurance section of Ms. Davison's Patient Information Form using the following information:

   Sponsor: Arthur T. Bentler, U.S. Army Reservist
   SSN: 000123456
   Birth date: 03/10/1959
   Address: Use patient's address for the sponsor as well (same address)

   (*Note:* Rhea Davison now goes by the name of Rhea Davison-Bentler.)

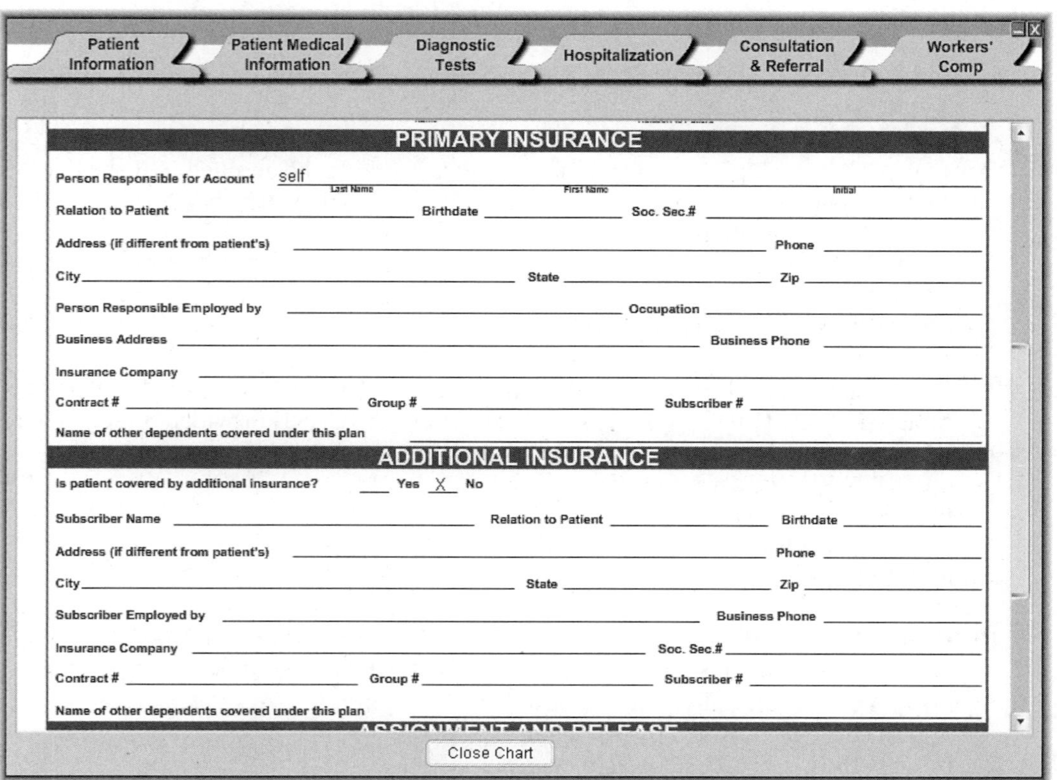

Patient Information | Patient Medical Information | Diagnostic Tests | Hospitalization | Consultation & Referral | Workers' Comp

PRIMARY INSURANCE

Person Responsible for Account self ________ (Last Name) ________ (First Name) ________ (Initial)

Relation to Patient ________ Birthdate ________ Soc. Sec.# ________

Address (if different from patient's) ________ Phone ________

City ________ State ________ Zip ________

Person Responsible Employed by ________ Occupation ________

Business Address ________ Business Phone ________

Insurance Company ________

Contract # ________ Group # ________ Subscriber # ________

Name of other dependents covered under this plan ________

ADDITIONAL INSURANCE

Is patient covered by additional insurance? ___ Yes _X_ No

Subscriber Name ________ Relation to Patient ________ Birthdate ________

Address (if different from patient's) ________ Phone ________

City ________ State ________ Zip ________

Subscriber Employed by ________ Business Phone ________

Insurance Company ________ Soc. Sec.# ________

Contract # ________ Group # ________ Subscriber # ________

Name of other dependents covered under this plan ________

Close Chart

4. Ms. Davison-Bentler is eligible for coverage under which of the following military programs?
   a. MHP
   b. TRICARE
   c. CHAMPVA
   d. DEERS

5. In which of the following programs, if any, is Ms. Davison-Bentler eligible to enroll? Select all that apply.

   _____ TRICARE Standard

   _____ TRICARE Extra

   _____ TRICARE Prime

   _____ CHAMPVA

   _____ TRICARE-for-Life

6. Who would be considered the sponsor for her coverage under this military program?
   a. The patient, Rhea Davison-Bentler
   b. Her husband, Arthur Bentler
   c. The U.S. Army Reserve
   d. The federal government

7. Immediately after her enrollment, Rhea Davison-Bentler's information is entered into the national computerized military database. What is the acronym for this database?
   a. MHS
   b. MTF
   c. DEERS
   d. TAMP

8. Which TRICARE program would Rhea Davison-Bentler be enrolled in if she does not pay an enrollment fee and a fee-for-service option is available worldwide?
   a. TRICARE Standard
   b. TRICARE Extra
   c. TRICARE Prime
   d. TRICARE Standard Supplemental

9. Let's assume that Rhea Davison-Bentler enrolls in TRICARE Standard and that the Mountain View Clinic physicians are listed in the TRICARE Provider Directory. Under which TRICARE program would she essentially be receiving benefits?
   a. TRICARE Standard
   b. TRICARE Extra
   c. TRICARE Prime
   d. TRICARE for Life

10. If Rhea Davison-Bentler enrolls in TRICARE Standard and receives treatment from a physician at Mountain View Clinic who is *not* a participating physician with TRICARE, how much will the patient be responsible for?
   a. The entire fee charged by Mountain View Clinic
   b. Only the TRICARE allowable charge
   c. 15% above the TRICARE allowable charge
   d. Only the cost share and deductible, if any

11. The health insurance professional at Mountain View Clinic should be aware that the deadline for submitting claims to TRICARE is:
    a. 30 days from the date services were rendered.
    b. 90 days from the date services were rendered.
    c. 1 year from the date services were rendered.
    d. 2 years from the date services were rendered.

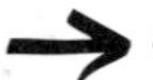

- Click **Close Chart** to return to the Check Out area.
- Click the exit arrow at the lower right corner of the screen to go to the Summary Menu.
- On the Summary Menu, click **Return to Map**.

Exercise 2

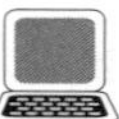

Online Activity—The CHAMPVA Patient

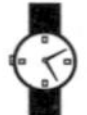

15 minutes

1. CHAMPVA is:
    a. the same as TRICARE.
    b. for active-duty members of the military services and their families.
    c. for retired members of the military services and their dependents.
    d. for veterans with permanent service-related disabilities and their spouses, dependents, or survivors.

- From the patient list, select **Jesus Santo**.

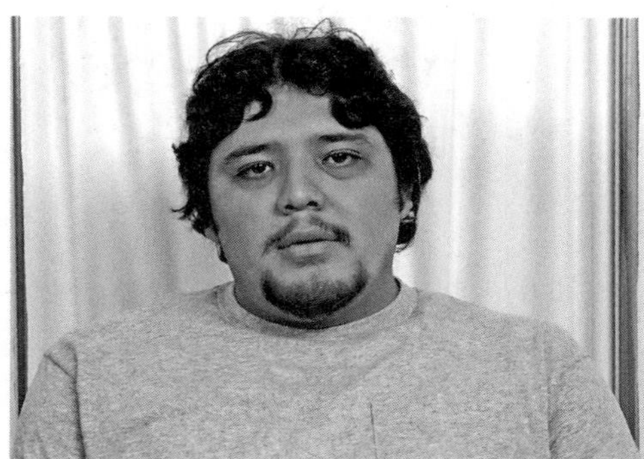

- On the office map, highlight and click on **Reception** to enter the Reception area.

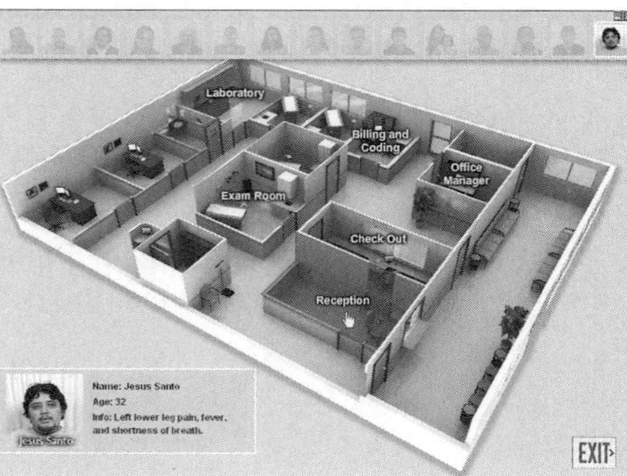

- Under the Watch heading, click on **Patient Check-In** to view the video.

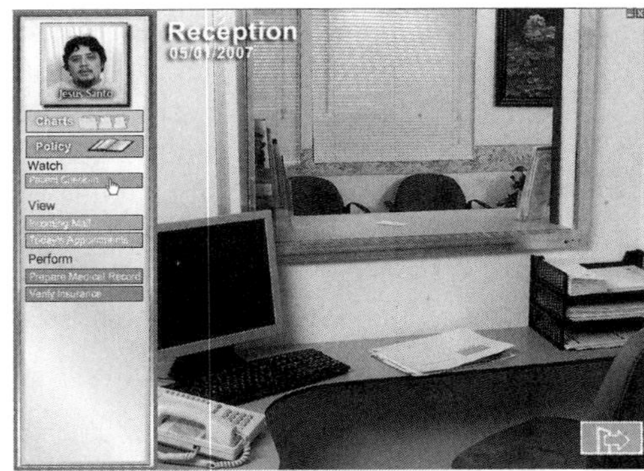

- At the end of the video, click **Close** to return to the Reception area.
- Click the exit arrow at the lower right corner of the screen to go to the Summary Menu.
- On the Summary Menu, click **Return to Map**.
- On the office map, highlight and click on **Check Out** to enter the Check Out area.

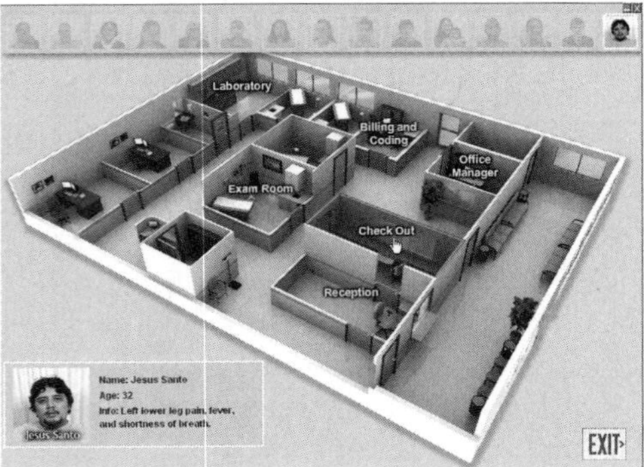

- Under the Watch heading, click on **Patient Check-Out** to view the video.

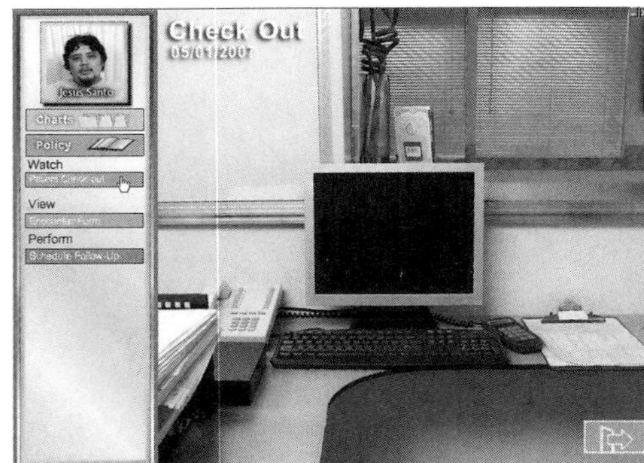

- At the end of the video, click **Close** to return to the Check Out area.
- Click the exit arrow at the lower right corner of the screen to go to the Summary Menu.
- On the Summary Menu, click **Return to Map**.
- On the office map, highlight and click on **Billing and Coding** to enter the Billing and Coding area.

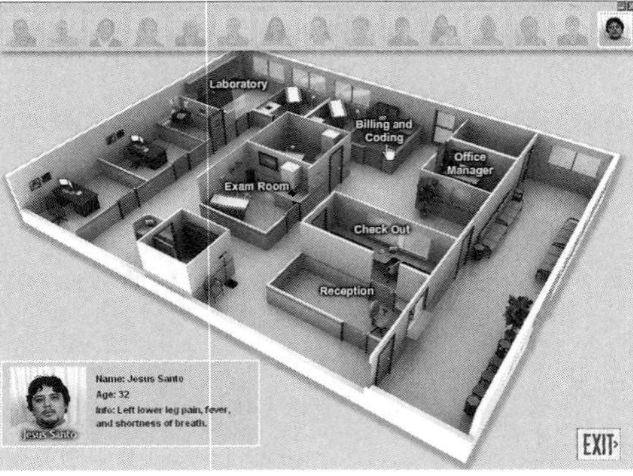

- Click on **Charts** to open Mr. Santo's medical record.

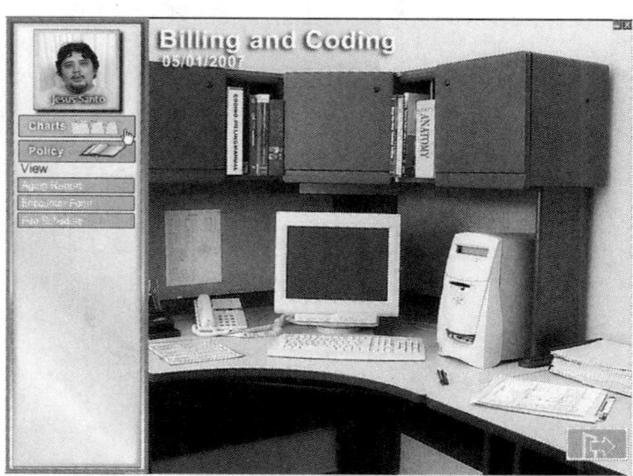

For this exercise, assume that while taking a detailed history of Mr. Santo, a member of the health care team discovers that the patient is the surviving spouse of Anita L. Santo, a veteran of Desert Storm who died from service-related injuries.

2. In this case, is Mr. Santo eligible to receive CHAMPVA health care benefits? Which statement most accurately explains why or why not?
   a. No, only the dependent children of Ms. Santo would be eligible for coverage.
   b. No, Mr. Santo would be eligible for benefits under CHAMPUS.
   c. Yes, Mr. Santo is eligible for benefits under CHAMPVA since his wife served in the military.
   d. Yes, Mr. Santo is eligible for benefits under CHAMPVA since he is the surviving spouse of a person who died of service-related injuries.

3. Mr. Santo will no longer be eligible for CHAMPVA health care benefits:
   a. if he remarries.
   b. if he becomes eligible for TRICARE.
   c. if he becomes eligible for Medicare.
   d. if any of the above occur.

4. Below, complete the primary insurance section of Mr. Santo's Patient Information Form using the following information:

   Sponsor's name: Anita L. Santo (deceased)
   SSN: 000121234
   Date of birth: 12/06/1979
   Relationship to patient: spouse

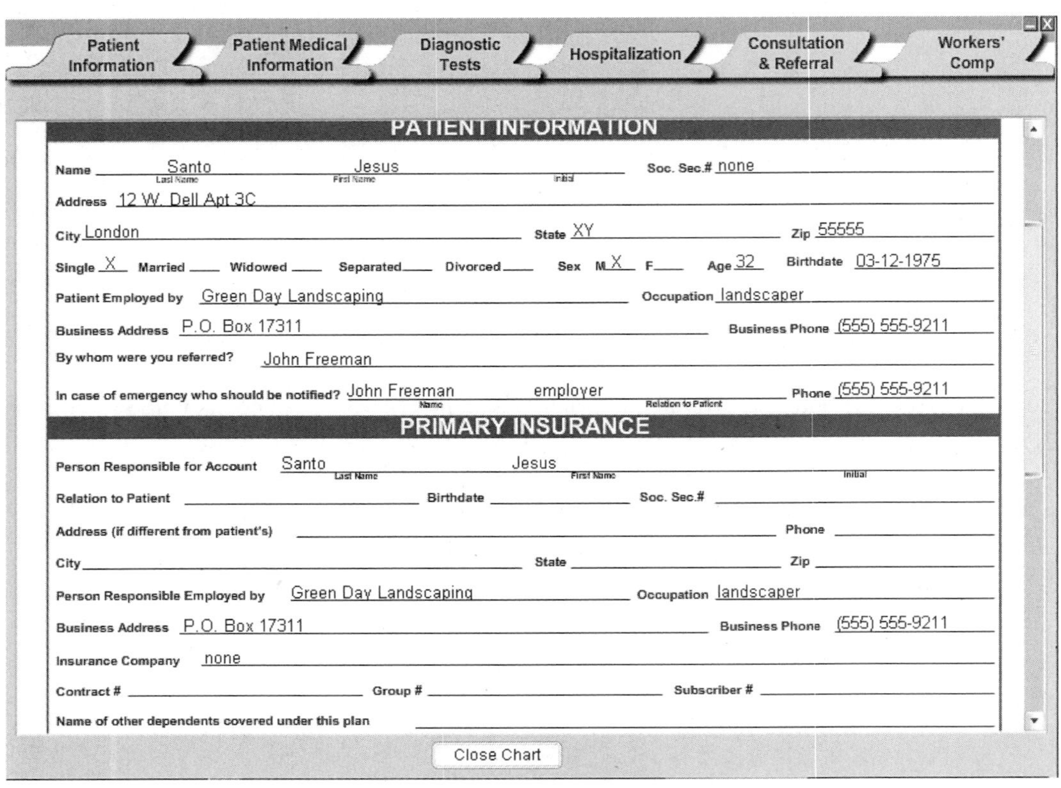

Patient Information | Patient Medical Information | Diagnostic Tests | Hospitalization | Consultation & Referral | Workers' Comp

PATIENT INFORMATION

Name: Santo (Last Name) Jesus (First Name) (Initial) Soc. Sec.# none
Address: 12 W. Dell Apt 3C
City: London State: XY Zip: 55555
Single: X Married: ___ Widowed: ___ Separated: ___ Divorced: ___ Sex M: X F: ___ Age: 32 Birthdate: 03-12-1975
Patient Employed by: Green Day Landscaping Occupation: landscaper
Business Address: P.O. Box 17311 Business Phone: (555) 555-9211
By whom were you referred? John Freeman
In case of emergency who should be notified? John Freeman (Name) employer (Relation to Patient) Phone: (555) 555-9211

PRIMARY INSURANCE

Person Responsible for Account: Santo (Last Name) Jesus (First Name) (Initial)
Relation to Patient ___ Birthdate ___ Soc. Sec.# ___
Address (if different from patient's) ___ Phone ___
City ___ State ___ Zip ___
Person Responsible Employed by: Green Day Landscaping Occupation: landscaper
Business Address: P.O. Box 17311 Business Phone: (555) 555-9211
Insurance Company: none
Contract # ___ Group # ___ Subscriber # ___
Name of other dependents covered under this plan ___

Close Chart

5. Indicate whether each of the following statements is true or false.

   a. _________ The physicians at Mountain View Clinic do not list CHAMPVA as an insurance that they participate with. Therefore they will not be able to treat Mr. Santos.

   b. _________ CHAMPVA will cover 75% of all health care services that Mr. Santo will receive.

6. The staff at Mountain View Clinic should confirm CHAMPVA eligibility by doing which of the following? Select all that apply.

   _____ Using the DEERS system

   _____ Using the IVR system

   _____ Making EDI requests through the EDI clearinghouse

   _____ Examining and copying the patient's CHAMPVA card

7. CHAMPVA benefits include which of the following? Select all that apply.

   _____ Prescription medication by mail

   _____ Over-the-counter medications

   _____ Dental care

   _____ Eye care

8. Under CHAMPVA, preauthorization is required for:
   a. visits to specialists.
   b. diagnostic radiology services.
   c. mental health.
   d. laboratory services.

9. The CHAMPVA fee schedule is based on:
   a. the fee charged by the provider at Mountain View Clinic.
   b. the Medicare rate.
   c. 15% of the TRICARE fee schedule.
   d. the usual, reasonable, and customary rates.

10. If a patient has coverage with Medicare and CHAMPVA, which insurance is considered primary?
   a. CHAMPVA
   b. Medicare

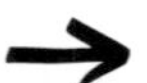

- Click **Close Chart** to return to the Billing and Coding area.
- Click the exit arrow at the lower right corner of the screen to go to the Summary Menu.
- On the Summary Menu, click **Return to Map** and continue to the next exercise.

Exercise 3

Writing Activity—Completing Claims for TRICARE/CHAMPVA-Eligible Patients

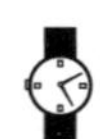

15 minutes

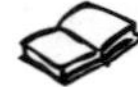

In this exercise, you will complete a TRICARE claim form for Rhea Davison-Bentler and a CHAMPVA claim form for Jesus Santos. For help, use Table 10-4 in your textbook, along with the Patient Information Forms you completed in Exercises 1 and 2 of this lesson. You may also refer to the sample completed claim forms in Appendix B (Figures B-7 and B-8) in your textbook.

1. Below, complete blocks 1 through 33 for patient Rhea Davison-Bentler.

HEALTH INSURANCE CLAIM FORM

APPROVED BY NATIONAL UNIFOR MCLAIM COMMITTEE (NUCC) 02/12

PICA | PICA | CARR

1. MEDICARE (Medicare#) MEDICAID (Medicaid#) TRICARE (ID#DoD#) CHAMPVA (Member ID#) GROUP HEALTH PLAN (ID#) FECA BLK LUNG (ID#) OTHER (ID#)
1a. INSURED'S I.D. NUMBER (For Program in Item 1)

2. PATIENT'S NAME (Last Name, First Name, Middle Initial)
3. PATIENT'S BIRTH DATE MM DD YY SEX M F
4. INSURED'S NAME (Last Name, First Name, Middle Initial)

5. PATIENT'S ADDRESS (No., Street)
6. PATIENT RELATIONSHIP TO INSURED Self Spouse Child Other
7. INSURED'S ADDRESS (No., Street)

CITY STATE
8. RESERVED FOR NUCC USE
CITY STATE

ZIP CODE TELEPHONE (Include Area Code) ( )
ZIP CODE TELEPHONE (Include Area Code) ( )

9. OTHER INSURED'S NAME (Last Name, First Name, Middle Initial)
10. IS PATIENT'S CONDITION RELATED TO:
11. INSURED'S POLICY GROUP OR FECA NUMBER

a. OTHER INSURED'S POLICY OR GROUP NUMBER
a. EMPLOYMENT? (Current or Previous) YES NO
a. INSURED'S DATE OF BIRTH MM DD YY SEX M F

b. RESERVED FOR NUCC USE
b. AUTO ACCIDENT? YES NO PLACE (State)
b. OTHER CLAIM ID (Designated by NUCC)

c. RESERVED FOR NUCC USE
c. OTHER ACCIDENT? YES NO
c. INSURANCE PLAN NAME OR PROGRAM NAME

d. INSURANCE PLAN NAME OR PROGRAM NAME
10d. CLAIM CODES (Designated by NUCC)
d. IS THERE ANOTHER HEALTH BENEFIT PLAN? YES NO *If yes*, complete items 9, 9a, and 9d.

READ BACK OF FORM BEFORE COMPLETING & SIGNING THIS FORM.

12. PATIENT'S OR AUTHORIZED PERSON'S SIGNATUREI authorize the release of any medical or other information necessary to process this claim. I also request payment of government benefits either to myself or to the party who accepts assignment below.

SIGNED DATE

13. INSURED'S OR AUTHORIZED PERSON'S SIGNATURE I authorize payment of medical benefits to the undersigned physician or supplier for services described below.

SIGNED

PATIENT AND INSURED INFORMATION

14. DATE OF CURRENT: ILLNESS, INJURY, or PREGNANCY(LMP) MM DD YY QUAL.
15. OTHER DATE QUAL. MM DD YY
16. DATES PATIENT UNABLE TO WORK IN CURRENT OCCUPATION MM DD YY FROM TO

17. NAME OF REFERRING PROVIDER OR OTHER SOURCE 17a. 17b. NPI
18. HOSPITALIZATION DATES RELATED TO CURRENT SERVICES MM DD YY FROM TO

19. ADDITIONAL CLAIM INFORMATION (Designated by NUCC)
20. OUTSIDE LAB? YES NO $ CHARGES

21. DIAGNOSIS OR NATURE OF ILLNESS OR INJURY Relate A-L to service line below (24E) ICD Ind.
A. B. C. D.
E. F. G. H.
I. J. K. L.
22. RESUBMISSION CODE ORIGINAL REF. NO.
23. PRIOR AUTHORIZATION NUMBER

	24. A. DATE(S) OF SERVICE From MM DD YY	To MM DD YY	B. PLACE OF SERVICE	C. EMG	D. PROCEDURES, SERVICES, OR SUPPLIES (Explain Unusual Circumstances) CPT/HCPCS	MODIFIER	E. DIAGNOSIS POINTER	F. $ CHARGES	G. DAYS OR UNITS	H. EPSDT Family Plan	I. ID. QUAL.	J. RENDERING PROVIDER ID. #
1											NPI	
2											NPI	
3											NPI	
4											NPI	
5											NPI	
6											NPI	

PHYSICIAN OR SUPPLIER INFORMATION

25. FEDERAL TAX I.D. NUMBER SSN EIN
26. PATIENT'S ACCOUNT NO.
27. ACCEPT ASSIGNMENT? (For govt. claims, see back) YES NO
28. TOTAL CHARGE $
29. AMOUNT PAID $
30. Rsvd for NUCC Use $

31. SIGNATURE OF PHYSICIAN OR SUPPLIER INCLUDING DEGREES OR CREDENTIALS (I certify that the statements on the reverse apply to this bill and are made a part thereof.)

SIGNED DATE

32. SERVICE FACILITY LOCATION INFORMATION
a. NPI b.

33. BILLING PROVIDER INFO & PH # ( )
a. NPI b.

NUCC Instruction Manual available at: www.nucc.org *PLEASE PRINT OR TYPE* OMB APPROVAL PENDING

2. Below, complete blocks 1 through 33 for patient Jesus Santos.

HEALTH INSURANCE CLAIM FORM

APPROVED BY NATIONAL UNIFOR MCLAIM COMMITTEE (NUCC) 02/12

PICA | PICA | CARRIER

1. MEDICARE (Medicare#) | MEDICAID (Medicaid#) | TRICARE (ID#DoD#) | CHAMPVA (Member ID#) | GROUP HEALTH PLAN (ID#) | FECA BLK LUNG (ID#) | OTHER (ID#)

1a. INSURED'S I.D. NUMBER (For Program in Item 1)

2. PATIENT'S NAME (Last Name, First Name, Middle Initial)

3. PATIENT'S BIRTH DATE MM | DD | YY SEX M F

4. INSURED'S NAME (Last Name, First Name, Middle Initial)

5. PATIENT'S ADDRESS (No., Street)

6. PATIENT RELATIONSHIP TO INSURED Self Spouse Child Other

7. INSURED'S ADDRESS (No., Street)

CITY STATE

8. RESERVED FOR NUCC USE

CITY STATE

ZIP CODE TELEPHONE (Include Area Code) ( )

ZIP CODE TELEPHONE (Include Area Code) ( )

9. OTHER INSURED'S NAME (Last Name, First Name, Middle Initial)

10. IS PATIENT'S CONDITION RELATED TO:

11. INSURED'S POLICY GROUP OR FECA NUMBER

a. OTHER INSURED'S POLICY OR GROUP NUMBER

a. EMPLOYMENT? (Current or Previous) YES NO

a. INSURED'S DATE OF BIRTH MM | DD | YY SEX M F

b. RESERVED FOR NUCC USE

b. AUTO ACCIDENT? YES NO PLACE (State)

b. OTHER CLAIM ID (Designated by NUCC)

c. RESERVED FOR NUCC USE

c. OTHER ACCIDENT? YES NO

c. INSURANCE PLAN NAME OR PROGRAM NAME

d. INSURANCE PLAN NAME OR PROGRAM NAME

10d. CLAIM CODES (Designated by NUCC)

d. IS THERE ANOTHER HEALTH BENEFIT PLAN? YES NO *If yes,* complete items 9, 9a, and 9d.

READ BACK OF FORM BEFORE COMPLETING & SIGNING THIS FORM.

12. PATIENT'S OR AUTHORIZED PERSON'S SIGNATUREI authorize the release of any medical or other information necessary to process this claim. I also request payment of government benefits either to myself or to the party who accepts assignment below.

SIGNED ____ DATE ____

13. INSURED'S OR AUTHORIZED PERSON'S SIGNATURE I authorize payment of medical benefits to the undersigned physician or supplier for services described below.

SIGNED ____

PATIENT AND INSURED INFORMATION

14. DATE OF CURRENT: ILLNESS, INJURY, or PREGNANCY(LMP) MM | DD | YY QUAL.

15. OTHER DATE QUAL. MM | DD | YY

16. DATES PATIENT UNABLE TO WORK IN CURRENT OCCUPATION FROM MM | DD | YY TO MM | DD | YY

17. NAME OF REFERRING PROVIDER OR OTHER SOURCE

17a. 17b. NPI

18. HOSPITALIZATION DATES RELATED TO CURRENT SERVICES FROM MM | DD | YY TO MM | DD | YY

19. ADDITIONAL CLAIM INFORMATION (Designated by NUCC)

20. OUTSIDE LAB? YES NO $ CHARGES

21. DIAGNOSIS OR NATURE OF ILLNESS OR INJURY Relate A-L to service line below (24E) ICD Ind.

A. B. C. D.

E. F. G. H.

I. J K. L.

22. RESUBMISSION CODE ORIGINAL REF. NO.

23. PRIOR AUTHORIZATION NUMBER

24. A. DATE(S) OF SERVICE From MM DD YY To MM DD YY	B. PLACE OF SERVICE	C. EMG	D. PROCEDURES, SERVICES, OR SUPPLIES (Explain Unusual Circumstances) CPT/HCPCS MODIFIER	E. DIAGNOSIS POINTER	F. $ CHARGES	G. DAYS OR UNITS	H. EPSDT Family Plan	I. ID. QUAL.	J. RENDERING PROVIDER ID. #
1								NPI	
2								NPI	
3								NPI	
4								NPI	
5								NPI	
6								NPI	

25. FEDERAL TAX I.D. NUMBER SSN EIN

26. PATIENT'S ACCOUNT NO.

27. ACCEPT ASSIGNMENT? (For govt. claims, see back) YES NO

28. TOTAL CHARGE $

29. AMOUNT PAID $

30. Rsvd for NUCC Use $

31. SIGNATURE OF PHYSICIAN OR SUPPLIER INCLUDING DEGREES OR CREDENTIALS (I certify that the statements on the reverse apply to this bill and are made a part thereof.)

SIGNED DATE

32. SERVICE FACILITY LOCATION INFORMATION

a. NPI b.

33. BILLING PROVIDER INFO & PH # ( )

a. NPI b.

PHYSICIAN OR SUPPLIER INFORMATION

NUCC Instruction Manual available at: www.nucc.org *PLEASE PRINT OR TYPE* OMB APPROVAL PENDING

LESSON 13

Workers' Compensation

Reading Assignment: Chapter 11—Miscellaneous Carriers: Workers' Compensation and Disability Insurance

Patient: Janet Jones

Learning Objectives:

- Discuss the purpose of workers' compensation insurance.
- Identify workers' compensation eligibility requirements.
- Determine the physician's role in workers' compensation cases.
- Identify key terms associated with disability claims.
- Complete a workers' compensation claim.

Overview:

This lesson addresses the concept of workers' compensation (W/C) insurance and the fact that most workers in the United States are covered by workers' compensation laws. The employer, rather than the employee, pays the premiums, and the legal contract is between the employer and the health care provider.

In this lesson you will identify the patient who qualifies for workers' compensation benefits, verify eligibility, complete the required documents for filing a workers' compensation claim, and identify the appropriate parties who must receive the documents. You will become familiar with terms related to disability benefits and how it is differentiated from workers' compensation benefits. You will also complete a workers' compensation claim for Janet Jones using the step-by-step claims completion guidelines for workers' compensation.

Exercise 1

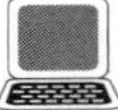

Online Activity—Understanding Workers' Compensation

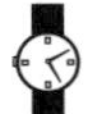

60 minutes

1. Workers' compensation is:
   a. insurance that pays medical expenses for individuals who are injured or become ill as a result of job-related circumstances.
   b. insurance that pays an individual's wages or salary if he or she becomes permanently disabled.
   c. an insurance program that protects workers from loss of income as a result of disability.
   d. a program that provides monthly cash payments to disabled individuals.

2. Workers' compensation insurance is regulated by:
   a. county laws.
   b. state laws.
   c. federal laws.
   d. none of the above.

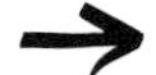

- Sign in to Mountain View Clinic.
- From the patient list, select **Janet Jones**.

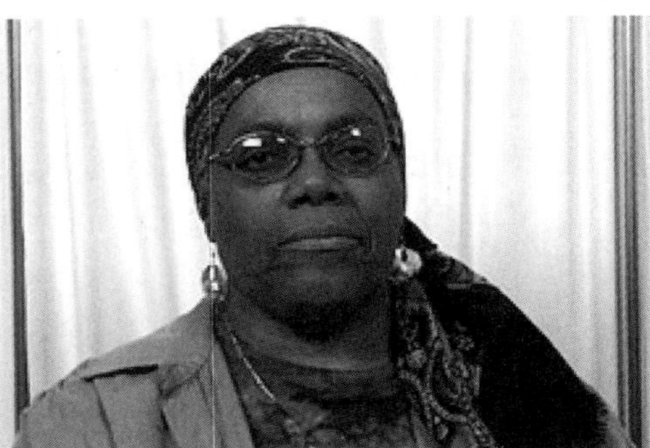

- On the office map, highlight and click on **Reception** to enter the Reception area.

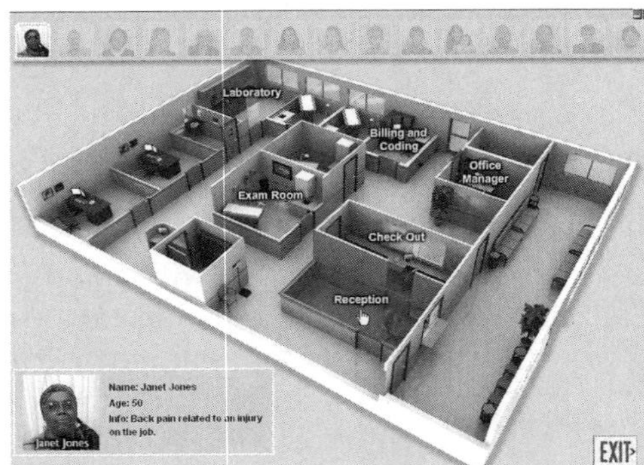

- Under the Watch heading, click on **Patient Check-In** to view the video.

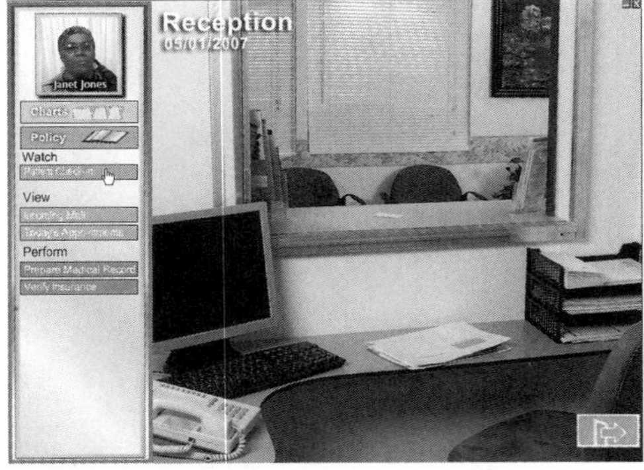

3. Indicate whether the following statement is true or false.

_________ If any "horseplay," drunkenness, or illegal drugs are involved, workers' compensation usually does not pay. The same applies for self-inflicted injuries.

4. If it is determined that Ms. Jones is a casual employee, she will more than likely not be eligible for workers' compensation benefits. A casual employee is an employee who:
   a. is allowed to wear jeans to work.
   b. does not have a desk job.
   c. works part-time.
   d. is not entitled to paid holiday or sick leave and has no expectation of ongoing employment.

5. If it is determined that Ms. Jones' fall occurred because she was not wearing appropriate footwear despite the recommendations in the employee handbook to wear sturdy shoes, will she be eligible for workers' compensation benefits?
   a. No, Ms. Jones was warned about appropriate footwear and precautions to prevent injury, so use of improper footwear would make her ineligible.
   b. Yes, workers' compensation insurance is no-fault insurance.

6. If it is determined that Ms. Jones' fall occurred at a local fast-food restaurant during her lunch period, will she be eligible for workers' compensation benefits?
   a. No, this is usually considered outside the scope of the employment relationship.
   b. Yes, the employer is responsible for the employee for the entire work day.

7. If it is determined that Ms. Jones' fall occurred during her lunch hour, but while she was at the bank making a deposit for her employer, will she be eligible for workers' compensation benefits?
   a. No, because this is on her lunch hour, it is out of the scope of the employment relationship.
   b. Yes, workers' compensation insurance should provide benefits because the employee is running a work-related errand during her lunch hour.

8. If Ms. Jones' fall occurred under the circumstances described in question 7, but the insurance carrier denies eligibility for workers' compensation benefits:
   a. Ms. Jones will have to pay for all medical bills.
   b. Ms. Jones can bill the employer directly for her medical services.
   c. Ms. Jones can request an appeal by the insurance carrier.
   d. Ms. Jones should sue the insurance carrier.

9. During check-in, what "paperwork" was Kristin referring to when she asked for documents from Ms. Jones' employer?
   a. Ms. Jones' insurance identification card
   b. The employer's workers' compensation identification card
   c. The patient information and problem forms
   d. The employer's written authorization for the visit and the "first report of injury"

10. Kristin did not ask Janet Jones for her insurance ID card. Was this an oversight on Kristin's part?
   a. Yes
   b. No

11. Who is considered the responsible party in Ms. Jones' case?
    a. The patient, Janet Jones
    b. The patient's employer
    c. State health insurance
    d. Elaine Meere

- At the end of the video, click **Close** to return to the Reception area.
- Click the exit arrow at the lower right corner of the screen to go to the Summary Menu.
- On the Summary Menu, click **Return to Map**.
- On the office map, highlight and click on **Billing and Coding** to enter the Billing and Coding area.

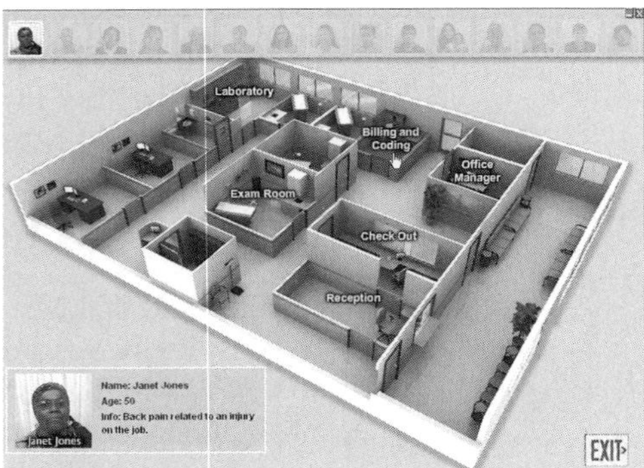

- Click on **Charts** to open Ms. Jones' medical record. View the information under the **Workers' Compensation** tab.

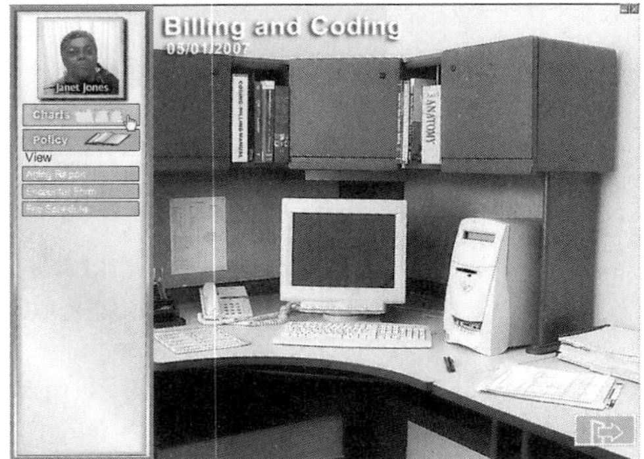

12. Did Ms. Jones correctly fill out the Primary Insurance section of her Patient Information Form? Explain.

13. Most state workers' compensation laws exclude coverage for injuries sustained while an employee is commuting to and from work, which is commonly referred to as the:
    a. commuter rule.
    b. to and from work rule.
    c. coming and going rule.
    d. travel rule.

14. Indicate whether the following statement is true or false.

    _________ Each state has rules establishing a time limit for the employee to file a workers' compensation claim. The procedure for reporting injuries and filing claims varies from state to state.

15. What is the physician's role in workers' compensation cases? Select all that apply.

_____ To diagnose and treat work-related injuries/illnesses

_____ To provide opinions in response to specific medical and/or legal questions from claims administrators about work-related illness or injury

_____ To ensure that the cause of the injury/illness is remedied

_____ To help the injured person find alternative work

_____ To determine the degree of disability

_____ To make recommendations concerning when the patient can return to work

16. Once the physician at Mountain View Clinic is advised that Ms. Jones' injury is work-related, he or she must complete a(n):
    a. first report of injury or illness.
    b. attending physician statement.
    c. temporary disability form.
    d. workers' compensation medical progress report form.

17. The physician at Mountain View Clinic must complete all workers' compensation paperwork promptly to avoid:
    a. claim denial.
    b. any delay in income to the patient.
    c. duplicate claim submissions.
    d. penalties imposed by the Workers' Compensation Board.

18. What is the health insurance professional's role in the claims process?

19. If Janet Jones' work-related injury keeps her out of work after her initial visit to Mountain View Clinic, periodic reports must be filed to apprise the insurance carrier as to the patient's treatment plan, progress, and status. These reports are referred to as:
    a. follow-up reports.
    b. progress reports.
    c. claims for compensation.
    d. second report of injury or illness.

20. Upon Ms. Jones' return to work, the physician at Mountain View Clinic must submit a:
    a. final report.
    b. last report.
    c. summary report.
    d. final claim for compensation.

21. The charge for Janet Jones' encounter for 5/1/2007 is $160. If the workers' compensation insurer pays $135, how much can be billed to the patient?
    a. $160
    b. $25
    c. Nothing

22. If Ms. Jones' workers' compensation insurer does not reimburse Mountain View Clinic in a timely manner because the claim is pending, the health insurance professional:
    a. may bill the patient.
    b. may not bill the patient.

23. If Ms. Jones' workers' compensation claim is denied and all efforts for appeal have been exhausted, the health insurance professional should:
    a. write off the bill.
    b. bill the patient.
    c. bill the patient or her private insurance company.

24. Because this is a job-related illness/injury, the patient will not be billed. Therefore the possibility of fraud and/or abuse is eliminated.
    a. Yes
    b. No

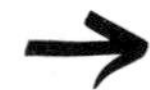

- Leave Ms. Jones' chart open and continue to the next exercise.

Exercise 2

Writing Activity—Disability Insurance Word Bank

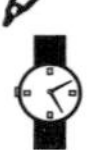

15 minutes

Let's assume that Janet Jones' illness is not work-related. She is unable to work and has no income. She is finding it impossible to maintain her home and provide for her family. Disability insurance will replace a portion of earned income while she is unable to perform her job. It is the responsibility of the health insurance professional to assist the physician in the timely filing of disability forms and assist the patient in applying for disability benefits.

1. Match each disability-related term with its definition.

	Definition	**Term**
_____	A program that provides monthly cash payments to low-income, elderly, blind, and/or disabled individuals	a. ADA
		b. Long-term disability
_____	An insurance program that protects workers from loss of income as a result of disability and provides cash benefits to disabled workers younger than 65	c. Short-term disability
		d. SSDI
		e. SSI
_____	Insurance that helps to replace income for 5 years or until the individual turns 65	f. Ticket to Work
_____	Legislation to protect the civil rights of individuals with disabilities	

_____ A program created to help individuals who receive social security benefits find and keep employment

_____ Insurance that provides an income for the early part of a disability, usually from 2 weeks to 2 years

2. Disability insurance benefits do not provide payment for medical services to the physician. Considering this, explain why it is important for the health insurance specialist to be familiar with the terms defined in question 1.

Exercise 3

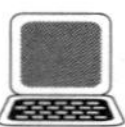

Online Activity—Completing a Workers' Compensation Claim

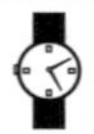

20 minutes

- You will need to access Janet Jones' medical records to complete this exercise. (*Note:* If you have exited the program, sign in again to Mountain View Clinic, select Janet Jones as your patient, and go to the Billing and Coding area. Review Ms. Jones' chart and Encounter Form as needed.)

1. Using the appropriate forms in Janet Jones' medical chart, along with her Encounter Form and the claims completion guidelines from Table B-4 in the Appendix of your textbook, complete the claim form on the next page.

HEALTH INSURANCE CLAIM FORM

APPROVED BY NATIONAL UNIFOR MCLAIM COMMITTEE (NUCC) 02/12

PICA | PICA

CARRIER

1. MEDICARE (Medicare#) ☐ MEDICAID (Medicaid#) ☐ TRICARE (ID#DoD#) ☐ CHAMPVA (Member ID#) ☐ GROUP HEALTH PLAN (ID#) ☐ FECA BLK LUNG (ID#) ☐ OTHER (ID#) ☐		1a. INSURED'S I.D. NUMBER (For Program in Item 1)
2. PATIENT'S NAME (Last Name, First Name, Middle Initial)	3. PATIENT'S BIRTH DATE MM DD YY SEX M ☐ F ☐	4. INSURED'S NAME (Last Name, First Name, Middle Initial)
5. PATIENT'S ADDRESS (No., Street)	6. PATIENT RELATIONSHIP TO INSURED Self ☐ Spouse ☐ Child ☐ Other ☐	7. INSURED'S ADDRESS (No., Street)
CITY / STATE	8. RESERVED FOR NUCC USE	CITY / STATE
ZIP CODE / TELEPHONE (Include Area Code) ( )		ZIP CODE / TELEPHONE (Include Area Code) ( )
9. OTHER INSURED'S NAME (Last Name, First Name, Middle Initial)	10. IS PATIENT'S CONDITION RELATED TO:	11. INSURED'S POLICY GROUP OR FECA NUMBER
a. OTHER INSURED'S POLICY OR GROUP NUMBER	a. EMPLOYMENT? (Current or Previous) ☐ YES ☐ NO	a. INSURED'S DATE OF BIRTH MM DD YY SEX M ☐ F ☐
b. RESERVED FOR NUCC USE	b. AUTO ACCIDENT? ☐ YES ☐ NO PLACE (State)	b. OTHER CLAIM ID (Designated by NUCC)
c. RESERVED FOR NUCC USE	c. OTHER ACCIDENT? ☐ YES ☐ NO	c. INSURANCE PLAN NAME OR PROGRAM NAME
d. INSURANCE PLAN NAME OR PROGRAM NAME	10d. CLAIM CODES (Designated by NUCC)	d. IS THERE ANOTHER HEALTH BENEFIT PLAN? ☐ YES ☐ NO *If yes,* complete items 9, 9a, and 9d.

READ BACK OF FORM BEFORE COMPLETING & SIGNING THIS FORM.

12. PATIENT'S OR AUTHORIZED PERSON'S SIGNATUREI authorize the release of any medical or other information necessary to process this claim. I also request payment of government benefits either to myself or to the party who accepts assignment below.

SIGNED ______ DATE ______

13. INSURED'S OR AUTHORIZED PERSON'S SIGNATURE I authorize payment of medical benefits to the undersigned physician or supplier for services described below.

SIGNED ______

PATIENT AND INSURED INFORMATION

14. DATE OF CURRENT: ILLNESS, INJURY, or PREGNANCY(LMP) MM DD YY QUAL.	15. OTHER DATE QUAL. MM DD YY	16. DATES PATIENT UNABLE TO WORK IN CURRENT OCCUPATION FROM MM DD YY TO MM DD YY
17. NAME OF REFERRING PROVIDER OR OTHER SOURCE	17a. / 17b. NPI	18. HOSPITALIZATION DATES RELATED TO CURRENT SERVICES FROM MM DD YY TO MM DD YY
19. ADDITIONAL CLAIM INFORMATION (Designated by NUCC)		20. OUTSIDE LAB? ☐ YES ☐ NO $ CHARGES
21. DIAGNOSIS OR NATURE OF ILLNESS OR INJURY Relate A-L to service line below (24E) ICD Ind. A. B. C. D. E. F. G. H. I. J. K. L.		22. RESUBMISSION CODE ORIGINAL REF. NO.
		23. PRIOR AUTHORIZATION NUMBER

	24. A. DATE(S) OF SERVICE From MM DD YY To MM DD YY	B. PLACE OF SERVICE	C. EMG	D. PROCEDURES, SERVICES, OR SUPPLIES (Explain Unusual Circumstances) CPT/HCPCS MODIFIER	E. DIAGNOSIS POINTER	F. $ CHARGES	G. DAYS OR UNITS	H. EPSDT Family Plan	I. ID. QUAL.	J. RENDERING PROVIDER ID. #
1									NPI	
2									NPI	
3									NPI	
4									NPI	
5									NPI	
6									NPI	

25. FEDERAL TAX I.D. NUMBER SSN EIN ☐ ☐	26. PATIENT'S ACCOUNT NO.	27. ACCEPT ASSIGNMENT? (For govt. claims, see back) ☐ YES ☐ NO	28. TOTAL CHARGE $	29. AMOUNT PAID $	30. Rsvd for NUCC Use $
31. SIGNATURE OF PHYSICIAN OR SUPPLIER INCLUDING DEGREES OR CREDENTIALS (I certify that the statements on the reverse apply to this bill and are made a part thereof.) SIGNED DATE	32. SERVICE FACILITY LOCATION INFORMATION a. NPI b.		33. BILLING PROVIDER INFO & PH # ( ) a. NPI b.		

PHYSICIAN OR SUPPLIER INFORMATION

NUCC Instruction Manual available at: www.nucc.org *PLEASE PRINT OR TYPE* OMB APPROVAL PENDING

→
- Click **Close Chart** to return to the Billing and Coding area.
- Click the exit arrow at the lower right corner of the screen to go to the Summary Menu.
- On the Summary Menu, click **Return to Map** to continue to the next lesson or click **Exit the Program**.

LESSON 14

Diagnostic Coding

Reading Assignment: Chapter 12—Diagnostic Coding

Patients: Jean Deere, Jose Imero, Kevin McKinzie

Learning Objective:

- Identify guidelines available in the ICD-9-CM manual to assist in accurate diagnosis coding.
- Demonstrate an understanding of the ICD-9-CM coding process by accurately coding patients' diagnoses to the greatest degree of specificity.
- Complete the CMS-1500 claim forms using appropriate ICD-9-CM and CPT codes.
- Identify the ICD-10-CM coding process
- Identify specified characteristics of ICD-10-CM codes.

Overview:

This lesson addresses diagnostic coding, using the most recent edition of the ICD-9-CM coding manual. You will learn to locate coding guideline and convention resources, apply coding conventions, and interpret coding guidelines. You will perform exercises designed to provide students with practice in abstracting diagnoses from patient records and coding these diagnoses to the highest degree of specificity. You will complete claim forms and choose appropriate diagnosis codes. You will also be introduced to ICD-10-CM coding process and guidelines and identify specified characteristics of ICD-10-CM codes.

Exercise 1

Writing Activity—Identifying the ICD-9-CM Coding Process and Guidelines

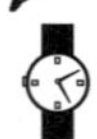

30 minutes

1. Locate the instructional steps for using Physician's Volumes 1 & 2 of the ICD-9-CM manual and outline the essential steps of diagnostic coding by completing the statements below.

   a. Locate the diagnosis in the patient's ________________________.

   b. Determine the ________________________ of the stated diagnosis.

   c. Find the main term in the ________________________________.

d. Read and apply any ____________________________ or ____________________________.

e. Cross-reference the code found to the ____.

f. Read and be guided by the ________________________ and ________________________.

g. Read through the entire category and code to the highest level of ____________________.

2. Use your textbook to answer the following questions regarding the coding process.

a. Using the alphabetic index, begin the coding process by locating the

____________________________ in the patient's medical record.

b. Identify the ____________________________ term in the diagnostic statement and locate it in the index.

c. Note any ____________________________ or ____________________________ modifiers.

d. Scan the main term for ________________________ or ________________________ notes.

e. Select the most appropriate code and verify the selected code by cross-reference to the

____________________________.

3. Use your textbook to answer the following questions regarding the ICD-10-CM coding process.

a. ICD-10-CM codes are from three to ________ characters in length.

b. Each ICD-10-CM code begins with a(n) ____________________________ character.

c. ___________ is used as a placeholder in a ICD-10-CM code.

d. The seventh character may be a ______________________ or a ______________________.

4. Indicate whether the following statement is true or false.

__________ Seventh characters are used in all chapters.

5. Never code directly from the ____________________________.

Locate the Official Coding Guidelines in the ICD-9-CM manual to answer the following questions.

6. The Official Coding Guidelines state that the instruction ____________________________ following a main term in the index means that another main term may also be referenced and may provide additional entries that might be useful.

7. The Official Coding Guidelines state that diagnosis codes are to be used at their

____________________________ number of digits available.

8. Codes for ____________________________ and ____________________________, as opposed to diagnoses, are acceptable for reporting purposes when a related definitive diagnosis has not been established.

9. The selection of the appropriate E code is guided by the ______________________ to ______________________.

10. An E code can never be listed ______________________.

11. Use the full range of E codes to completely describe the cause, the intent, and the ______________________ of ______________________.

12. When coding outpatient services, do not code diagnoses documented as "probable," "suspected," "questionable," or "______________________."

13. When coding outpatient services, code all documented conditions that coexist at the time of the encounter and require or affect patient care, ______________________, or ______________________.

Exercise 2

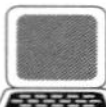

Online Activity—Applying the ICD-9-CM Coding Process and Guidelines

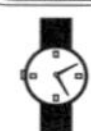

20 minutes

- Sign in to Mountain View Clinic.
- From the patient list, select **Jean Deere**.

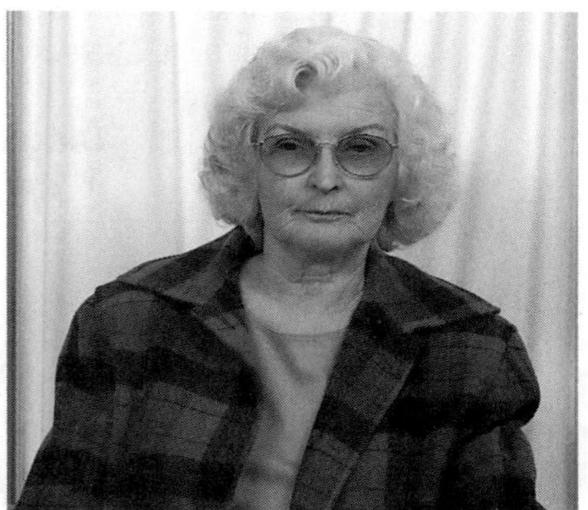

- On the office map, highlight and click on **Exam Room** to enter the Exam Room.

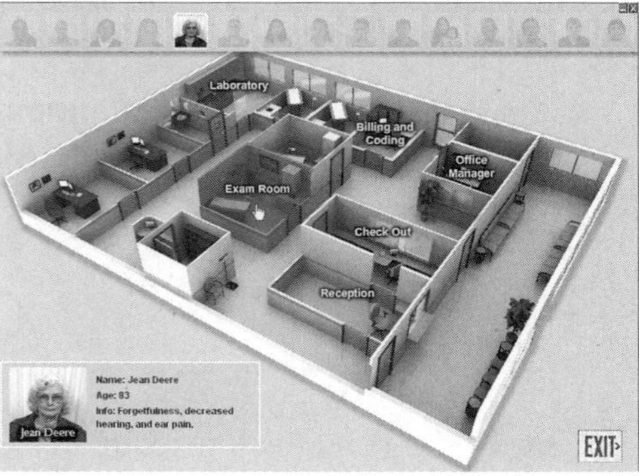

- Under the View heading, click on **Exam Notes** to read the documentation regarding Ms. Deere's visit.

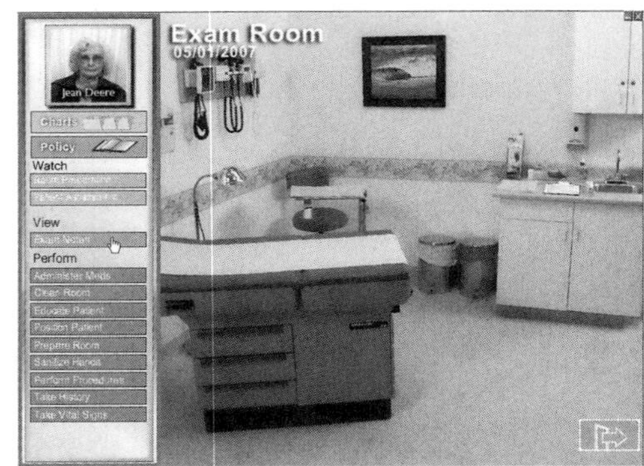

1. In the Impression portion of the Exam Notes for Jean Deere, the physician states that the patient has a "mild to moderate memory loss." Below, work through the process for selecting the appropriate ICD-9-CM code for this condition.

Main Term	Diagnosis Code Indicated in the Alphabetic Index	Diagnosis Code Confirmed by Tabular List

2. In the Impression portion of the Exam Notes for Jean Deere, the physician states that the patient has "impaired hearing." Below, work through the process for selecting the appropriate ICD-9-CM code for this condition.

Main Term	Diagnosis Code Indicated in the Alphabetic Index	Diagnosis Code Confirmed by Tabular List

3. In the Impression portion of the Exam Notes for Jean Deere, the physician states that the patient has "ear pain." Below, work through the process for selecting the appropriate ICD-9-CM code for this condition.

Main Term	Diagnosis Code Indicated in the Alphabetic Index	Diagnosis Code Confirmed by Tabular List

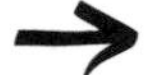

- Click **Finish** to return to the Exam Room.
- Click the exit arrow at the lower right corner of the screen to go to the Summary Menu.
- On the Summary Menu, click **Return to Map** and continue to the next exercise.

Exercise 3

Writing Activity—Applying Accurate Codes to the Diagnoses Listed on the Encounter Form

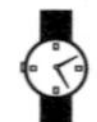

20 minutes

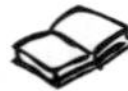

1. The staff members at Mountain View Clinic have decided to update their Encounter Form with the diagnoses most frequently reported by their practice. Using the most recent edition of the ICD-9-CM manual and the coding steps presented in the textbook, insert the correct diagnosis codes for each of the conditions listed on the form below.

______ Abscess	______ Bursitis	______ Fracture	______ Pneumonia
______ Abrasion-Sup.Injury	______ CAD	______ Gastritis	______ Pregnancy
______ Acne	______ Chest Pain	______ Gastroenteritis	______ Rectal Bleed
______ Alcohol Abuse	______ CHF	______ Gout	______ Sinusitis
______ Allergic Reaction	______ Conjunctivitis	______ Headache	______ STD ________
______ Amenorrhea	______ COPD	______ Hematuria	______ Tendonitis
______ Anemia	______ Contraception	______ Hemorrhoids	______ UTI
______ Anxiety	______ Cough	______ HIV	______ URI
______ Annual GYN exam	______ CVA	______ Hypertension	______ Vaginitis
______ Annual PE	______ Depression	______ Hypothyroidism	______ Well Baby/Child
______ Arrhythmia	______ Dermatitis	______ IBS	______ Weight Loss
______ Arthritis	______ Diabetes*	______ Low Back Pain	______ Otitis Media
______ ASHD	______ Diarrhea	______ Lymphadenopathy	______
______ Asthma	______ Dysmenorrheal	______ Nausea/Vomiting	______
______ Backache	______ Ear Impaction	______ Obesity	______
______ Breast Mass	______ Fatigue	______ Osteoporosis	______
______ Bronchitis	______ Fever	______ Pharyngitis	______

2. Based on the ICD-10-CM manual, the following diagnoses on the Encounter Form will be changed; consequently, these diagnoses will no longer be useful for reporting codes on the Encounter Form. Explain why each of these diagnoses will be changed.

   a. Diabetes:

   b. Fracture:

Exercise 4

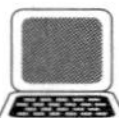

Online Activity—Diagnostic Coding for Jose Imero

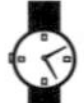

30 minutes

- From the patient list, select **Jose Imero**.

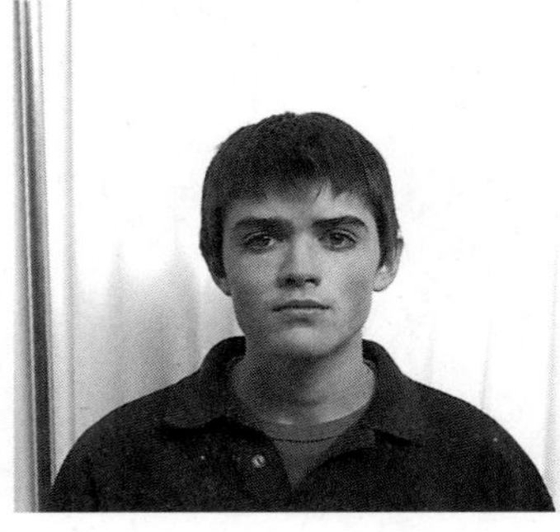

- On the office map, highlight and click on **Exam Room** to enter the Exam Room.

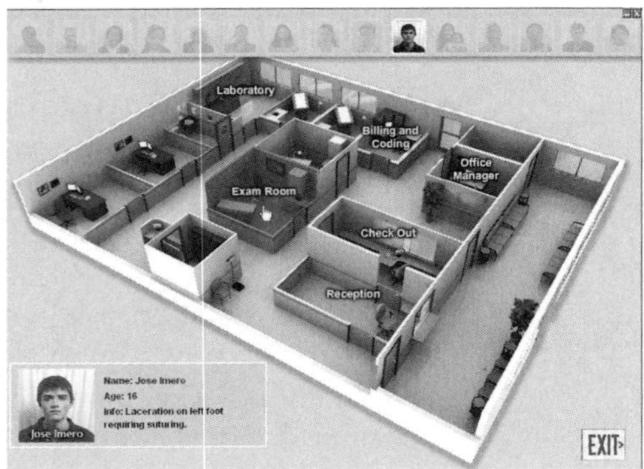

- Under the View heading, click on **Exam Notes** to read the documentation regarding Jose's visit.

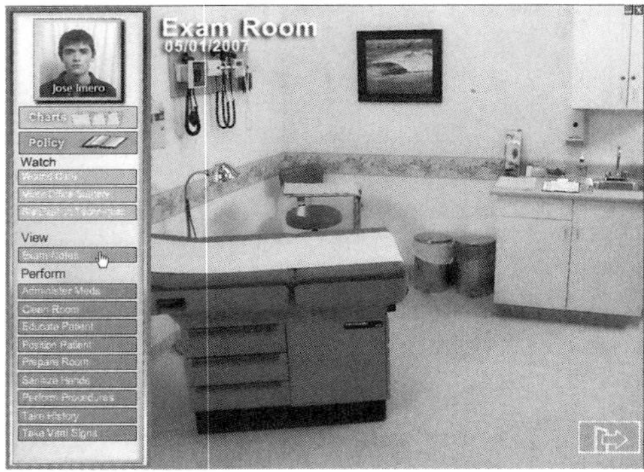

1. Based on the Exam Notes, identify why the patient is being seen today.

2. Below, work through the look-up processes identified for selecting the appropriate diagnosis code for the condition identified in question 1.

Main Term	Diagnosis Code Indicated in the Alphabetic Index	Diagnosis Code Confirmed by Tabular List

3. When you located the main term in the ICD-9-CM, what instructional note did you have to follow?

4. In addition to reporting the appropriate diagnosis code for this condition, the health insurance specialist is required to report an E code. Review the Official Coding Guidelines from the ICD-9-CM manual and using the E code index, record the appropriate code below to describe how the injury occurred.

Main Term	Diagnosis Code Indicated in the Alphabetic Index	Diagnosis Code Confirmed by Tabular List

5. The Official Coding Guidelines state that the place of occurrence should also be recorded (if it is identified) by reporting an additional E code. Using the E code index, identify the appropriate code below to describe where the injury occurred.

Main Term	Diagnosis Code Indicated in the Alphabetic Index	Diagnosis Code Confirmed by Tabular List

6. If you were using ICD-10-CM to code Jose Imero's chart, what would the extension A indicate?

7. What information would be included in an ICD-10-CM code about Jose's fracture that is not included in the ICD-9-CM code?

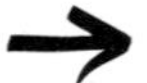

- Click **Finish** to return to the Exam Room.
- Click the exit arrow at the lower right corner of the screen to go to the Summary Menu.
- On the Summary Menu, click **Return to Map** and continue to the next exercise.

Exercise 5

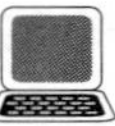

Online Activity—Completing a Claim Form

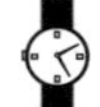

20 minutes

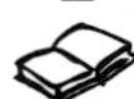

1. Jose Imero has Blue Cross/Blue Shield insurance coverage. Using the source documents in his chart and the guidelines for completion of a BC/BS claim (see Chapter 6 in your textbook), complete blocks 1 through 33 of the CMS-1500 claim form on the next page for Jose Imero. Use the ICD-9-CM codes that you identified in Exercise 2. Procedure codes to be used are as follows: 99212-25, 90703, 90471, 99070, 12004.

HEALTH INSURANCE CLAIM FORM

APPROVED BY NATIONAL UNIFOR MCLAIM COMMITTEE (NUCC) 02/12

PICA | PICA

CARRIER

1. MEDICARE (Medicare#) MEDICAID (Medicaid#) TRICARE (ID#DoD#) CHAMPVA (Member ID#) GROUP HEALTH PLAN (ID#) FECA BLK LUNG (ID#) OTHER (ID#)

1a. INSURED'S I.D. NUMBER (For Program in Item 1)

2. PATIENT'S NAME (Last Name, First Name, Middle Initial)

3. PATIENT'S BIRTH DATE MM | DD | YY SEX M F

4. INSURED'S NAME (Last Name, First Name, Middle Initial)

5. PATIENT'S ADDRESS (No., Street)

6. PATIENT RELATIONSHIP TO INSURED Self Spouse Child Other

7. INSURED'S ADDRESS (No., Street)

CITY STATE

8. RESERVED FOR NUCC USE

CITY STATE

ZIP CODE TELEPHONE (Include Area Code) ( )

ZIP CODE TELEPHONE (Include Area Code) ( )

9. OTHER INSURED'S NAME (Last Name, First Name, Middle Initial)

10. IS PATIENT'S CONDITION RELATED TO:

11. INSURED'S POLICY GROUP OR FECA NUMBER

a. OTHER INSURED'S POLICY OR GROUP NUMBER

a. EMPLOYMENT? (Current or Previous) YES NO

a. INSURED'S DATE OF BIRTH MM | DD | YY SEX M F

b. RESERVED FOR NUCC USE

b. AUTO ACCIDENT? PLACE (State) YES NO

b. OTHER CLAIM ID (Designated by NUCC)

c. RESERVED FOR NUCC USE

c. OTHER ACCIDENT? YES NO

c. INSURANCE PLAN NAME OR PROGRAM NAME

d. INSURANCE PLAN NAME OR PROGRAM NAME

10d. CLAIM CODES (Designated by NUCC)

d. IS THERE ANOTHER HEALTH BENEFIT PLAN? YES NO *If yes,* complete items 9, 9a, and 9d.

READ BACK OF FORM BEFORE COMPLETING & SIGNING THIS FORM.

12. PATIENT'S OR AUTHORIZED PERSON'S SIGNATURE I authorize the release of any medical or other information necessary to process this claim. I also request payment of government benefits either to myself or to the party who accepts assignment below.

SIGNED ______ DATE ______

13. INSURED'S OR AUTHORIZED PERSON'S SIGNATURE I authorize payment of medical benefits to the undersigned physician or supplier for services described below.

SIGNED ______

PATIENT AND INSURED INFORMATION

14. DATE OF CURRENT: ILLNESS, INJURY, or PREGNANCY(LMP) MM | DD | YY QUAL.

15. OTHER DATE QUAL. MM | DD | YY

16. DATES PATIENT UNABLE TO WORK IN CURRENT OCCUPATION FROM MM | DD | YY TO MM | DD | YY

17. NAME OF REFERRING PROVIDER OR OTHER SOURCE

17a. 17b. NPI

18. HOSPITALIZATION DATES RELATED TO CURRENT SERVICES FROM MM | DD | YY TO MM | DD | YY

19. ADDITIONAL CLAIM INFORMATION (Designated by NUCC)

20. OUTSIDE LAB? YES NO $ CHARGES

21. DIAGNOSIS OR NATURE OF ILLNESS OR INJURY Relate A-L to service line below (24E) ICD Ind.

A. ______ B. ______ C. ______ D. ______
E. ______ F. ______ G. ______ H. ______
I. ______ J. ______ K. ______ L. ______

22. RESUBMISSION CODE ORIGINAL REF. NO.

23. PRIOR AUTHORIZATION NUMBER

	24. A. DATE(S) OF SERVICE From MM DD YY To MM DD YY	B. PLACE OF SERVICE	C. EMG	D. PROCEDURES, SERVICES, OR SUPPLIES (Explain Unusual Circumstances) CPT/HCPCS MODIFIER	E. DIAGNOSIS POINTER	F. $ CHARGES	G. DAYS OR UNITS	H. EPSDT Family Plan	I. ID. QUAL.	J. RENDERING PROVIDER ID. #
1									NPI	
2									NPI	
3									NPI	
4									NPI	
5									NPI	
6									NPI	

PHYSICIAN OR SUPPLIER INFORMATION

25. FEDERAL TAX I.D. NUMBER SSN EIN

26. PATIENT'S ACCOUNT NO.

27. ACCEPT ASSIGNMENT? (For govt. claims, see back) YES NO

28. TOTAL CHARGE $

29. AMOUNT PAID $

30. Rsvd for NUCC Use $

31. SIGNATURE OF PHYSICIAN OR SUPPLIER INCLUDING DEGREES OR CREDENTIALS (I certify that the statements on the reverse apply to this bill and are made a part thereof.)

SIGNED DATE

32. SERVICE FACILITY LOCATION INFORMATION

a. NPI b.

33. BILLING PROVIDER INFO & PH # ( )

a. NPI b.

NUCC Instruction Manual available at: www.nucc.org *PLEASE PRINT OR TYPE* OMB APPROVAL PENDING

Exercise 6

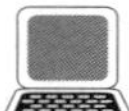

Online Activity—Diagnostic Coding for Kevin McKinzie

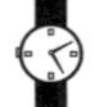

40 minutes

- From the patient list, select **Kevin McKinzie**.

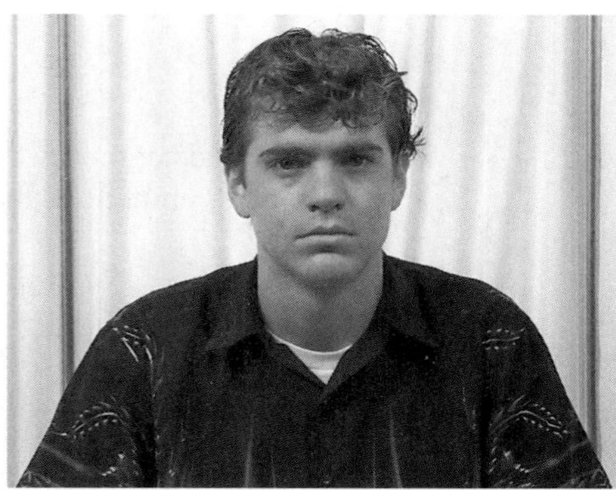

- On the office map, highlight and click on **Exam Room** to enter the Exam Room.

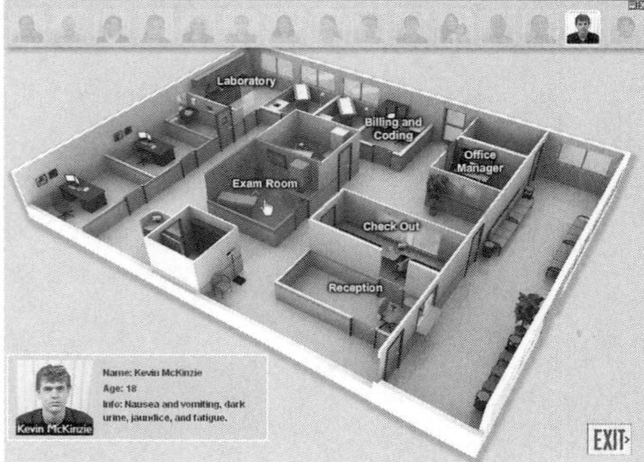

- Under the Watch heading, click on **Patient Interview** to view the video.

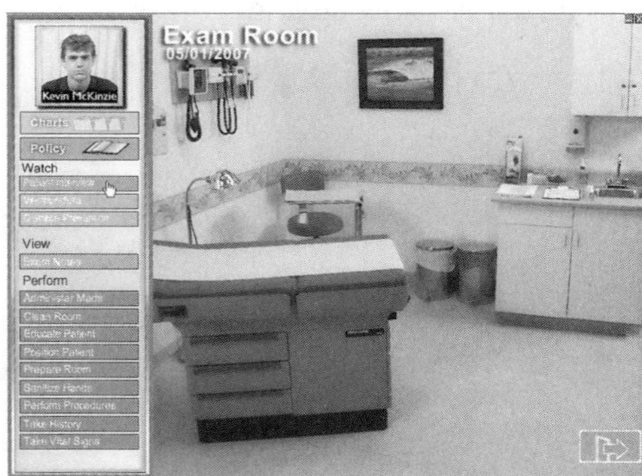

- After viewing the video, click **Close** to return to the Exam Room.
- Under the View heading, click on **Exam Notes** to read the documentation regarding Kevin McKinzie's visit.

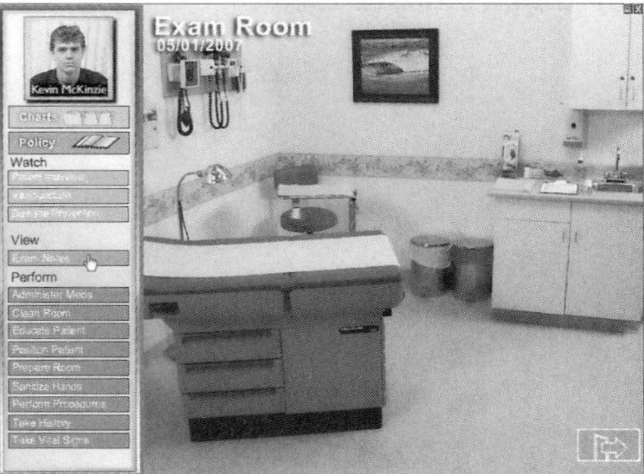

1. During the patient interview, what symptoms does the patient claim to have?

2. In the second sentence of the Exam Notes for this patient, what symptoms does the physician document as the reason for the patient's visit today?

3. In the Exam Notes for this patient, what health problems does the physician document in the Impression section?

4. One entry in the Impression section of the Exam Notes is worded "R/O hepatitis, mono." What is the rule about coding an entry like this?

5. When should an ICD-9-CM code be assigned to impressions documented as symptoms or worded as "rule out"?

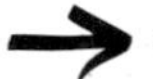

- Click **Finish** to return to the Exam Room.
- Click the exit arrow at the lower right corner of the screen to go to the Summary Menu.
- On the Summary Menu, click **Return to Map**.
- On the office map, highlight and click on **Billing and Coding** to enter the Billing and Coding area.

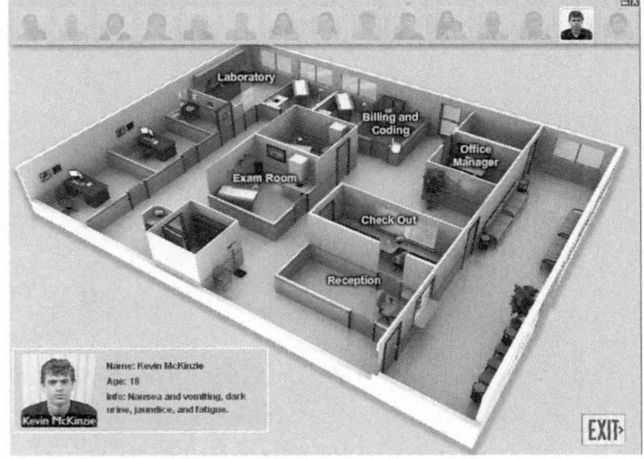

- Under the View heading, click on **Encounter Form** to examine the diagnoses indicated for this patient.

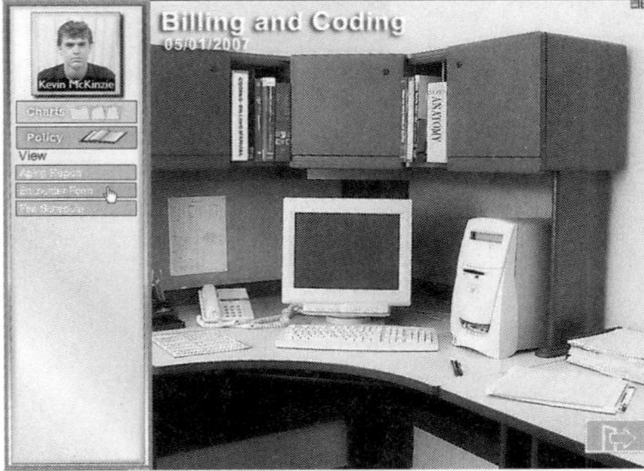

6. Indicate whether each of the following statements is true or false.

   a. __________ The diagnoses indicated on Kevin McKinzie's Encounter Form are the same as those documented in the Impression section of the Exam Notes.

   b. __________ The biller/coder should report the conditions/diagnoses documented in the patient's medical chart in block 21 of the CMS-1500, as opposed to those noted on the Encounter Form.

7. When the diagnoses listed on the Encounter Form are different from those documented in the medical record, the biller/coder should:
   a. report only the diagnosis codes noted on the Encounter Form.
   b. report only the diagnosis codes documented in the medical record.
   c. report both the diagnosis codes documented in the record and on the Encounter Form.
   d. report the discrepancy to the physician and ask for clarification regarding what specific diagnoses to code and report.
   e. insert an "addendum" to the medical record, adding the missing diagnoses codes from the Encounter Form.

8. Based on the supporting documentation, indicate which conditions should be reported on Kevin McKinzie's CMS-1500 claim form. Select all that apply.

_____ Dark urine

_____ Low-grade fever

_____ Asthma, well controlled

_____ Nausea w/vomiting

_____ Severe fatigue

_____ Weight loss

_____ Stomach pains

_____ GI symptoms

_____ Jaundice

_____ Yellow eyes

_____ R/O hepatitis/mono

_____ Seizure disorder

9. Of the conditions you did *not* select in question 8, choose four and explain below why these conditions would not be reported.

10. Indicate the appropriate ICD-9-CM code for each condition listed below.

Condition	ICD-9-CM Code
Asthma, well controlled	
Dark urine	
Fatigue	
Jaundice	
Low-grade fever	
Nausea/vomiting	
Seizure disorder	
Stomach pains	
Weight loss	

11. Let's assume that Kevin McKinzie is being seen in the office for his asthma. Using ICD-10-CM, what are the various stages of asthma that can be coded?

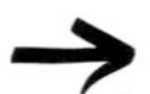

- Click **Finish** to close the Encounter Form and return to the Billing and Coding area.

Exercise 7

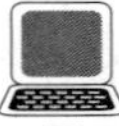

Online Activity—Completing a Claim Form

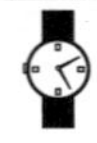

20 minutes

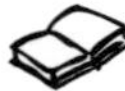

1. Kevin McKinzie has Small Business Owners Group insurance coverage. Using the source documents in his chart and the guidelines for completion of a CMS-1500 claim form (see Chapter 5 in your textbook), complete blocks 1 through 33 of the CMS-1500 claim form on the following page. Report the appropriate ICD-9-CM codes identified in the exercises above. Here are the procedure codes needed to complete this claim: 99205, 99000, 82270, 81000, 36415 86308.

HEALTH INSURANCE CLAIM FORM

APPROVED BY NATIONAL UNIFOR MCLAIM COMMITTEE (NUCC) 02/12

PICA — PICA — CARRIER

1. MEDICARE (Medicare#) MEDICAID (Medicaid#) TRICARE (ID#DoD#) CHAMPVA (Member ID#) GROUP HEALTH PLAN (ID#) FECA BLK LUNG (ID#) OTHER (ID#)

1a. INSURED'S I.D. NUMBER (For Program in Item 1)

2. PATIENT'S NAME (Last Name, First Name, Middle Initial)

3. PATIENT'S BIRTH DATE MM DD YY SEX M F

4. INSURED'S NAME (Last Name, First Name, Middle Initial)

5. PATIENT'S ADDRESS (No., Street)

6. PATIENT RELATIONSHIP TO INSURED Self Spouse Child Other

7. INSURED'S ADDRESS (No., Street)

CITY STATE

8. RESERVED FOR NUCC USE

CITY STATE

ZIP CODE TELEPHONE (Include Area Code) ( )

ZIP CODE TELEPHONE (Include Area Code) ( )

9. OTHER INSURED'S NAME (Last Name, First Name, Middle Initial)

10. IS PATIENT'S CONDITION RELATED TO:

11. INSURED'S POLICY GROUP OR FECA NUMBER

a. OTHER INSURED'S POLICY OR GROUP NUMBER

a. EMPLOYMENT? (Current or Previous) YES NO

a. INSURED'S DATE OF BIRTH MM DD YY SEX M F

b. RESERVED FOR NUCC USE

b. AUTO ACCIDENT? YES NO PLACE (State)

b. OTHER CLAIM ID (Designated by NUCC)

c. RESERVED FOR NUCC USE

c. OTHER ACCIDENT? YES NO

c. INSURANCE PLAN NAME OR PROGRAM NAME

d. INSURANCE PLAN NAME OR PROGRAM NAME

10d. CLAIM CODES (Designated by NUCC)

d. IS THERE ANOTHER HEALTH BENEFIT PLAN? YES NO *If yes,* complete items 9, 9a, and 9d.

READ BACK OF FORM BEFORE COMPLETING & SIGNING THIS FORM.

12. PATIENT'S OR AUTHORIZED PERSON'S SIGNATUREI authorize the release of any medical or other information necessary to process this claim. I also request payment of government benefits either to myself or to the party who accepts assignment below.

SIGNED ____ DATE ____

13. INSURED'S OR AUTHORIZED PERSON'S SIGNATURE I authorize payment of medical benefits to the undersigned physician or supplier for services described below.

SIGNED ____

PATIENT AND INSURED INFORMATION

14. DATE OF CURRENT: ILLNESS, INJURY, or PREGNANCY(LMP) MM DD YY QUAL.

15. OTHER DATE QUAL. MM DD YY

16. DATES PATIENT UNABLE TO WORK IN CURRENT OCCUPATION FROM MM DD YY TO MM DD YY

17. NAME OF REFERRING PROVIDER OR OTHER SOURCE

17a.

17b. NPI

18. HOSPITALIZATION DATES RELATED TO CURRENT SERVICES FROM MM DD YY TO MM DD YY

19. ADDITIONAL CLAIM INFORMATION (Designated by NUCC)

20. OUTSIDE LAB? YES NO $ CHARGES

21. DIAGNOSIS OR NATURE OF ILLNESS OR INJURY Relate A-L to service line below (24E) ICD Ind.

A. B. C. D.

E. F. G. H.

I. J. K. L.

22. RESUBMISSION CODE ORIGINAL REF. NO.

23. PRIOR AUTHORIZATION NUMBER

	24. A. DATE(S) OF SERVICE From MM DD YY To MM DD YY	B. PLACE OF SERVICE	C. EMG	D. PROCEDURES, SERVICES, OR SUPPLIES (Explain Unusual Circumstances) CPT/HCPCS MODIFIER	E. DIAGNOSIS POINTER	F. $ CHARGES	G. DAYS OR UNITS	H. EPSDT Family Plan	I. ID. QUAL.	J. RENDERING PROVIDER ID. #
1									NPI	
2									NPI	
3									NPI	
4									NPI	
5									NPI	
6									NPI	

25. FEDERAL TAX I.D. NUMBER SSN EIN

26. PATIENT'S ACCOUNT NO.

27. ACCEPT ASSIGNMENT? (For govt. claims, see back) YES NO

28. TOTAL CHARGE $

29. AMOUNT PAID $

30. Rsvd for NUCC Use $

31. SIGNATURE OF PHYSICIAN OR SUPPLIER INCLUDING DEGREES OR CREDENTIALS (I certify that the statements on the reverse apply to this bill and are made a part thereof.)

SIGNED DATE

32. SERVICE FACILITY LOCATION INFORMATION

a. NPI b.

33. BILLING PROVIDER INFO & PH # ( )

a. NPI b.

PHYSICIAN OR SUPPLIER INFORMATION

NUCC Instruction Manual available at: www.nucc.org *PLEASE PRINT OR TYPE* OMB APPROVAL PENDING

- Click the exit arrow at the lower right corner of the screen to go to the Summary Menu.
- On the Summary Menu, click **Return to Map** to continue to the next lesson or click **Exit the Program**.

LESSON 15

Procedural Coding (E&M and HCPCS)

Reading Assignment: Chapter 13—Procedural, Evaluation and Management, and HCPCS Coding

Patients: Jean Deere, Wilson Metcalf, Teresa Hernandez, John R. Simmons

Resources Needed: Current-Year CPT-4 Coding Manual

Learning Objectives:

- Identify guidelines available in the CPT manual to assist in accurate procedural coding.
- Assign correct CPT codes to services/procedures provided to selected patients.
- Complete CMS-1500 claim forms using appropriate ICD-9-CM and CPT codes.

Overview:

This lesson addresses the basics of CPT coding, using the most recent edition of the CPT-4 and HCPCS manuals. You will learn where to locate coding guideline and conventions and how to apply them. Next, you will complete exercises designed to give you practice in abstracting procedural information from patient records and coding these procedures accurately. Finally, you will complete claim forms, using appropriate procedural codes.

Exercise 1

Writing Activity—Identifying the CPT Coding Process and Guidelines

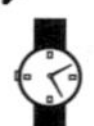

60 minutes

Before attempting to code a procedure, the health insurance professional must become familiar with the contents and structure of the CPT manual, as well as the process for selecting the appropriate code. Guidelines are placed throughout the CPT coding manual that will further assist the health insurance professional in accurately reporting procedure codes. These guidelines should be referenced at all times.

1. Using your textbook, outline the essential steps of procedural coding by completing the statements below.

   a. Identify the ____________________, ____________________, or ____________________ to be coded.

   b. Determine the ____________________ term.

   c. Locate the main term in the ____________________ and note the ____________________ or ____________________.

   d. Cross-reference the single code, multiple codes, or code range numerically in the ____________________ section of the manual.

   e. Read and follow any notes, special instructions, or ____________________ associated with the code.

   f. Determine and ____________________ the appropriate code.

Using the Introduction of your CPT manual, complete the following statements.

2. Any service or procedure reported with a CPT code must be adequately ____________________ in the medical record.

3. If no specific CPT code exists that identifies the services performed, then report the service using the appropriate ____________________ procedure code.

4. Instructions, typically included as ____________________ notes with selected codes, indicate that a code should not be reported with another code or codes.

5. ____________________ are always performed in addition to the primary service or procedure and must never be reported as stand-alone codes.

6. A ____________________ provides the means to report or indicate that a performed service or procedure has been altered by some specific circumstance but not changed in its definition or code.

7. A service that is rarely provided, unusual, variable, or new may require a ____________________.

8. The CPT manual features an expandable alphabetic index that includes listings by ____________________ and ____________________.

9. Using the index in your CPT manual, find and record the appropriate CPT codes for the following services listed on Mountain View Clinic's Encounter Form.

Service	CPT Code
New patient office visit, level IV	
Established patient office visit, level V	
New patient preventive care for child (1-4 years of age)	
New patient preventive care for patient 65+ years old	
Established patient preventive care for patient younger than 1 year	
Established patient preventive care for patient 18-39 years of age	

10. Using the index in your CPT manual, find and record the appropriate CPT codes for the following procedures listed on Mountain View Clinic's Encounter Form.

Procedure	CPT Code
Anoscopy	
Comprehensive audiometry	
Avulsion/nail	
ECG, tracing only	
Automated visual acuity screening	
Spirometry	
DT (under 7 years of age)	
DTAP (under 7 years of age; IM)	
DTP	
MMR	
OPV	

Exercise 2

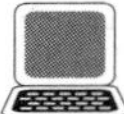

Online Activity—CPT Coding Assignment 1

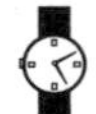

30 minutes

- Sign in to Mountain View Clinic.
- From the patient list, select **Jean Deere**.

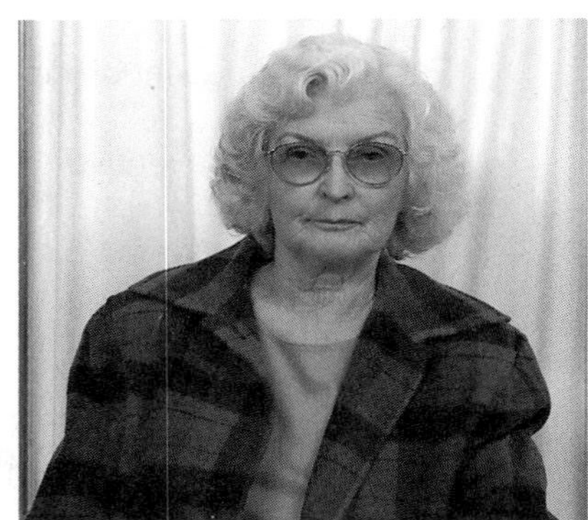

- On the office map, highlight and click on **Billing and Coding** to enter the Billing and Coding area.

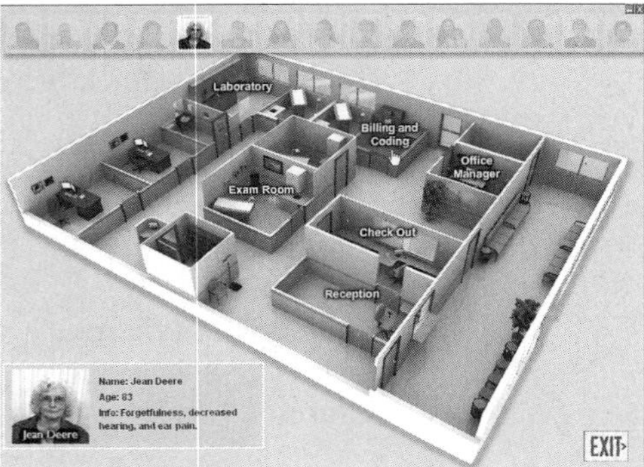

- Under the View heading, click on **Encounter Form**.

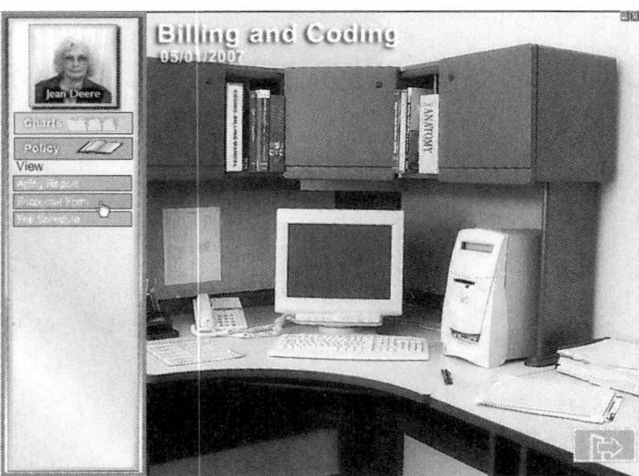

1. Ms. Deere is an established patient, and her office visit is a level IV visit. What is the correct E&M code for this visit level?

2. The procedures/services provided to Ms. Deere today include (1) ear lavage; (2) UA, dipstick; and (3) pulse oximetry. Using the most recent CPT-4 coding manual, provide the correct CPT codes for these three services/procedures.

3. Suppose Dr. Meyers admits Ms. Deere to the hospital. What is the E&M code for Dr. Meyers' admission and initial hospital care for requiring a moderate complexity of medical decision making?

4. If Dr. Meyers admitted Ms. Deere to the hospital on the same date that he saw her in the office, which E&M service would he report?

5. What code would be used for Dr. Meyers' subsequent hospital visits (moderate complexity) to Ms. Deere?

6. How many of the key components (history, examination, and medical decision making) must the physician meet or exceed in his documentation to support the code reported in question 5?

7. Assume that during Ms. Deere's hospital stay, tests indicate a heart problem, prompting Dr. Meyers to call in a cardiologist, Dr. Hudson. Dr. Hudson's inpatient consultation includes a comprehensive history, a comprehensive evaluation, and medical decision making of moderate complexity. What is the correct E&M code for Dr. Hudson's consultation?

8. If the consulting physician, Dr. Hudson, sees Ms. Deere a second time during her inpatient stay, what range of CPT codes would Dr. Hudson report?

9. Dr. Meyers spends 20 minutes with Ms. Deere on the last day of her hospitalization, which includes her discharge. The correct code would be ____________________.

10. If Ms. Deere had been admitted and discharged on the same date by Dr. Meyers, what range of CPT codes would be reported by the physician?

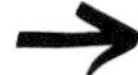

- Click **Finish** to close the Encounter Form and return to the Billing and Coding area.
- Click the exit arrow at the lower right corner of the screen to go to the Summary Menu.
- On the Summary Menu, click **Return to Map** to continue to the next exercise.

Exercise 3

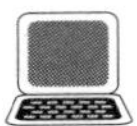

Online Activity—CPT Coding Assignment 2

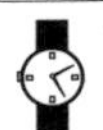

30 minutes

- From the patient list, select **Wilson Metcalf**.

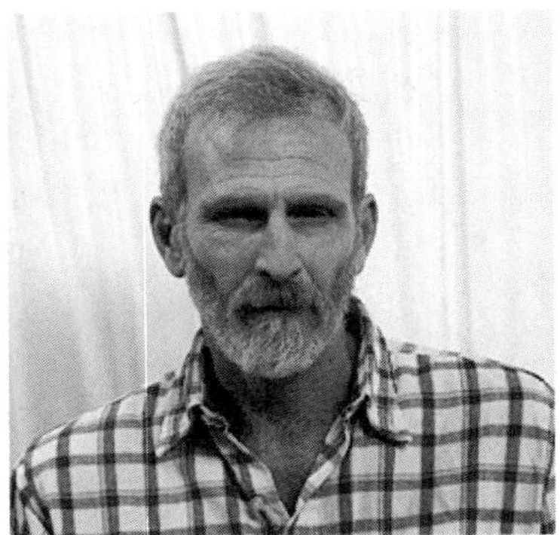

- On the office map, highlight and click on **Billing and Coding** to enter the Billing and Coding area.

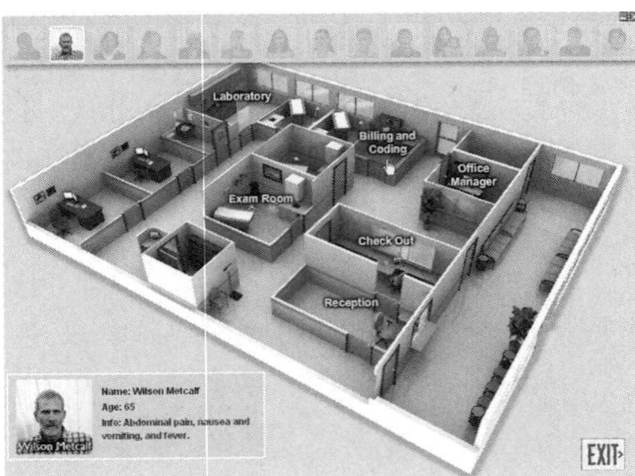

- Click on **Charts** to open Mr. Metcalf's medical record.

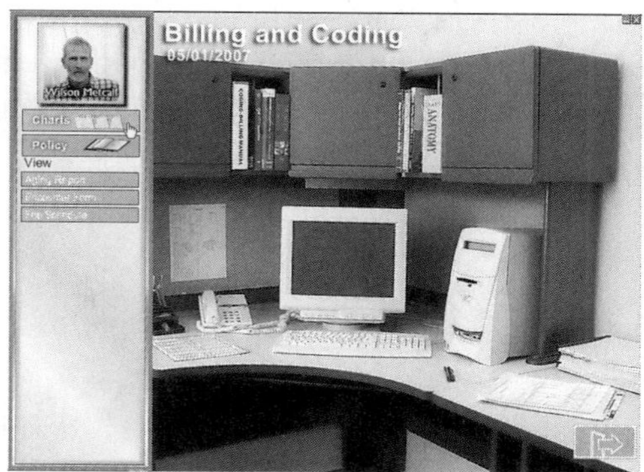

- Click on the **Patient Medical Information** tab and select **1-Progress Notes** from the drop-down menu.

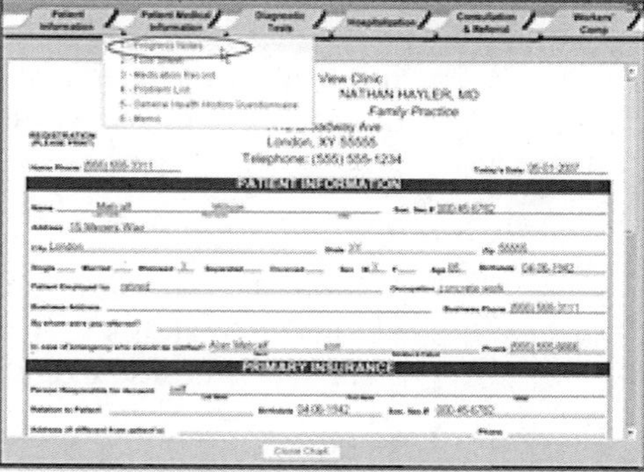

1. Were any laboratory tests completed for Mr. Metcalf on 5/1/2007? If so, list and code each test.

2. Besides the examination, were any procedures performed on 5/1/2007? If so, list and code each.

3. We know that Mr. Metcalf was subsequently admitted to the hospital. Let's look at a hypothetical scenario for his hospital stay. Assume that he had the following procedures performed in an attempt to acquire a definitive diagnosis: (1) flexible esophagoscopy (2) flexible colonoscopy, proximal to splenic flexure, with removal of two polyps; and (3) needle biopsy of the liver. From blood tests performed by the ED physician, it was determined that Mr. Metcalf was severely anemic. As a result, he was given a blood transfusion. Using the most recent CPT-4 manual, code these four procedures.

4. The use of modifiers in CPT coding can indicate that a service or procedure has been altered by some specific circumstance, but without changing its definition or code. Let's assume that documentation states that the liver biopsy took considerably more time than is typically required. Identify which modifier would be used in this example.

5. On the last day of his hospitalization, Mr. Metcalf underwent a needle biopsy of the prostate. The correct CPT code for this procedure is ____________________.

6. If it was documented that ultrasonic imaging guidance was used to perform the needle biopsy of the prostate described above, the CPT code reported for this procedure would be ____________________.

7. Wilson Metcalf was discharged from the hospital on day 4. The physician documents that he spent a total of 45 minutes documenting the medical record and then discussing test results, prognoses, and medication requirements with the patient and his son. The correct CPT code for hospital discharge is ____________________.

8. On the date of discharge, the attending physician called in a podiatrist to treat an area of cellulitis on Mr. Metcalf's left foot. What range of codes would the podiatrist use to report these concurrent care services?

→ • Click **Close Chart** when finished to return to the Billing and Coding area.
- Click the exit arrow at the lower right corner of the screen to go to the Summary Menu.
- On the Summary Menu, click **Return to Map** to continue to the next exercise.

Exercise 4

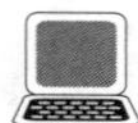

Online Activity—CPT Coding Assignment 3

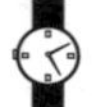

30 minutes

- From the patient list, select **Teresa Hernandez**.

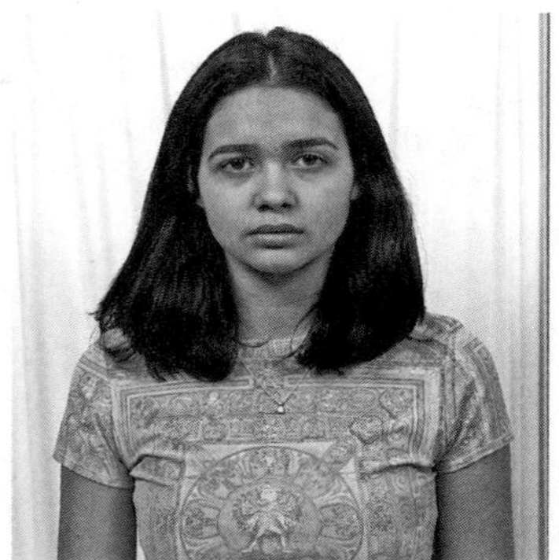

- On the office map, highlight and click on **Billing and Coding** to enter the Billing and Coding area.

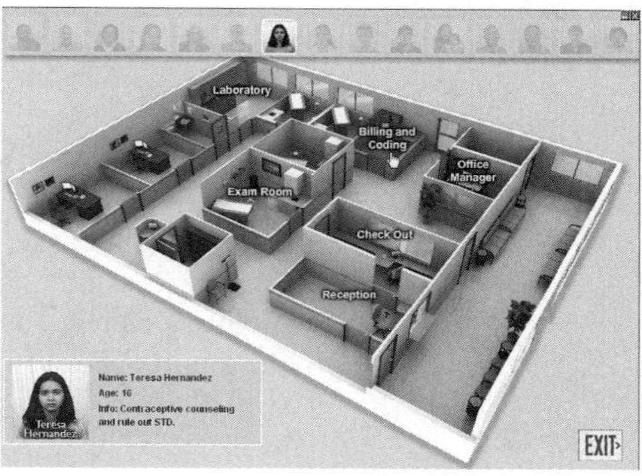

- Click on **Charts** to open Teresa's medical record.

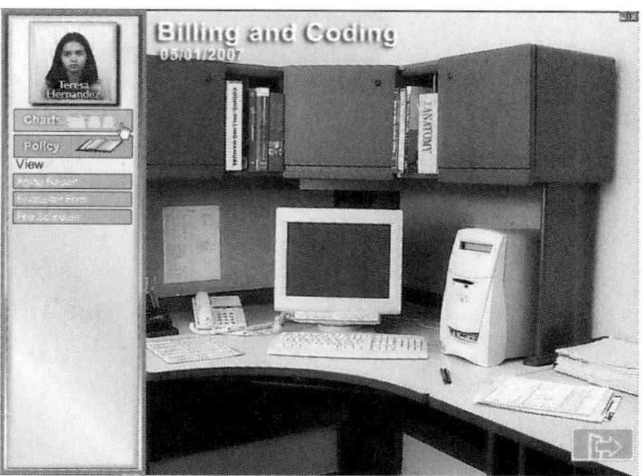

- Click on the **Patient Medical Information** and select **1-Progress Notes** from the drop-down menu. Review the Progress Notes for 5/1/2007.

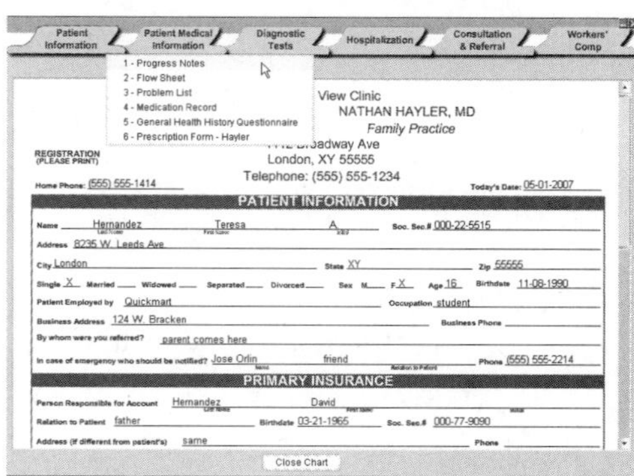

- When finished, click **Close Chart** to return to the Billing and Coding area.
- Under the View heading, click on **Encounter Form**.

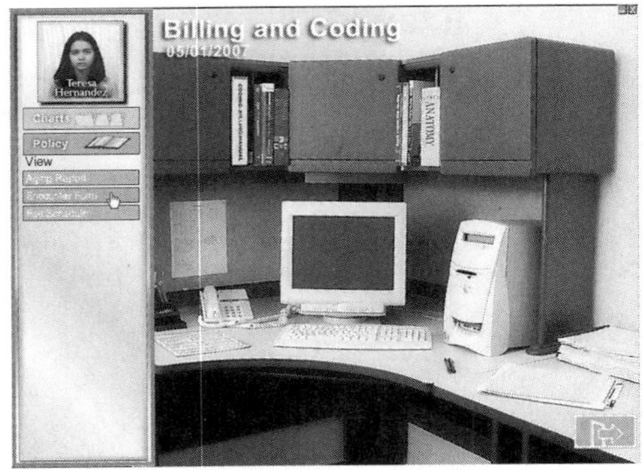

1. List and code all procedures/services that were performed on this date.

2. Let's assume that because of Teresa's multiple concurrent problems, her visit (including examination, assessment, and counseling with her and her parents) took much longer than usual. The physician spent a total of 90 minutes face to face with the patient. Is there a method to report this additional time?

3. If it is determined that Teresa has an STD and the physician decides to treat her with an antibiotic injection, what type of code will be used to report the medication being administered?

4. Teresa will return in 3 weeks for a Pap test. The CPT code used for this test will be

   ____________________.

5. Teresa was given a prescription for a "seasonal oral contraceptive pack." What CPT code will be reported for this service?

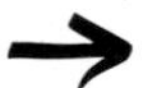

- Click **Finish** to close the Encounter Form and return to the Billing and Coding area.

Exercise 5

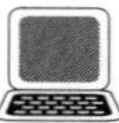

Online Activity—Completing a Claim Form

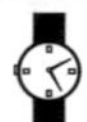

40 minutes

- From the Billing and Coding area, click on **Charts**. (*Note:* If you have exited the program, sign in again to Mountain View Clinic, select Teresa Hernandez as your patient, go to the Billing and Coding area, and open her chart.)
- Review Teresa's chart as needed to complete question 1.

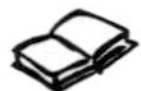

1. Teresa Hernandez has Mutual Health insurance coverage. Using the source documents in her chart and the guidelines for completion of a CMS-1500 claim form (see Chapter 5 in your textbook), complete blocks 1 through 33 of the CMS-1500 claim form on the next page. Report the appropriate ICD-9-CM and CPT codes, excluding the code for the handling fee. The diagnoses are (1) V25.01, starting oral contraceptives, and (2) V69.2, high-risk sexual behavior.

HEALTH INSURANCE CLAIM FORM

APPROVED BY NATIONAL UNIFOR MCLAIM COMMITTEE (NUCC) 02/12

PICA — PICA — CARRIER

1. MEDICARE (Medicare#) MEDICAID (Medicaid#) TRICARE (ID#DoD#) CHAMPVA (Member ID#) GROUP HEALTH PLAN (ID#) FECA BLK LUNG (ID#) OTHER (ID#)
1a. INSURED'S I.D. NUMBER (For Program in Item 1)

2. PATIENT'S NAME (Last Name, First Name, Middle Initial)
3. PATIENT'S BIRTH DATE MM DD YY SEX M F
4. INSURED'S NAME (Last Name, First Name, Middle Initial)

5. PATIENT'S ADDRESS (No., Street)
6. PATIENT RELATIONSHIP TO INSURED Self Spouse Child Other
7. INSURED'S ADDRESS (No., Street)

CITY STATE
8. RESERVED FOR NUCC USE
CITY STATE

ZIP CODE TELEPHONE (Include Area Code) ( )
ZIP CODE TELEPHONE (Include Area Code) ( )

9. OTHER INSURED'S NAME (Last Name, First Name, Middle Initial)
10. IS PATIENT'S CONDITION RELATED TO:
11. INSURED'S POLICY GROUP OR FECA NUMBER

a. OTHER INSURED'S POLICY OR GROUP NUMBER
a. EMPLOYMENT? (Current or Previous) YES NO
a. INSURED'S DATE OF BIRTH MM DD YY SEX M F

b. RESERVED FOR NUCC USE
b. AUTO ACCIDENT? YES NO PLACE (State)
b. OTHER CLAIM ID (Designated by NUCC)

c. RESERVED FOR NUCC USE
c. OTHER ACCIDENT? YES NO
c. INSURANCE PLAN NAME OR PROGRAM NAME

d. INSURANCE PLAN NAME OR PROGRAM NAME
10d. CLAIM CODES (Designated by NUCC)
d. IS THERE ANOTHER HEALTH BENEFIT PLAN? YES NO *If yes,* complete items 9, 9a, and 9d.

READ BACK OF FORM BEFORE COMPLETING & SIGNING THIS FORM.

12. PATIENT'S OR AUTHORIZED PERSON'S SIGNATUREI authorize the release of any medical or other information necessary to process this claim. I also request payment of government benefits either to myself or to the party who accepts assignment below.

SIGNED ____ DATE ____

13. INSURED'S OR AUTHORIZED PERSON'S SIGNATURE I authorize payment of medical benefits to the undersigned physician or supplier for services described below.

SIGNED ____

PATIENT AND INSURED INFORMATION

14. DATE OF CURRENT: ILLNESS, INJURY, or PREGNANCY(LMP) MM DD YY QUAL.
15. OTHER DATE QUAL. MM DD YY
16. DATES PATIENT UNABLE TO WORK IN CURRENT OCCUPATION FROM MM DD YY TO MM DD YY

17. NAME OF REFERRING PROVIDER OR OTHER SOURCE
17a.
17b. NPI
18. HOSPITALIZATION DATES RELATED TO CURRENT SERVICES FROM MM DD YY TO MM DD YY

19. ADDITIONAL CLAIM INFORMATION (Designated by NUCC)
20. OUTSIDE LAB? YES NO $ CHARGES

21. DIAGNOSIS OR NATURE OF ILLNESS OR INJURY Relate A-L to service line below (24E) ICD Ind.
A. B. C. D.
E. F. G. H.
I. J K. L.
22. RESUBMISSION CODE ORIGINAL REF. NO.
23. PRIOR AUTHORIZATION NUMBER

24. A. DATE(S) OF SERVICE From MM DD YY To MM DD YY	B. PLACE OF SERVICE	C. EMG	D. PROCEDURES, SERVICES, OR SUPPLIES (Explain Unusual Circumstances) CPT/HCPCS MODIFIER	E. DIAGNOSIS POINTER	F. $ CHARGES	G. DAYS OR UNITS	H. EPSDT Family Plan	I. ID. QUAL.	J. RENDERING PROVIDER ID. #
1								NPI	
2								NPI	
3								NPI	
4								NPI	
5								NPI	
6								NPI	

25. FEDERAL TAX I.D. NUMBER SSN EIN
26. PATIENT'S ACCOUNT NO.
27. ACCEPT ASSIGNMENT? (For govt. claims, see back) YES NO
28. TOTAL CHARGE $
29. AMOUNT PAID $
30. Rsvd for NUCC Use $

31. SIGNATURE OF PHYSICIAN OR SUPPLIER INCLUDING DEGREES OR CREDENTIALS (I certify that the statements on the reverse apply to this bill and are made a part thereof.)

SIGNED DATE

32. SERVICE FACILITY LOCATION INFORMATION
a. NPI b.

33. BILLING PROVIDER INFO & PH # ( )
a. NPI b.

PHYSICIAN OR SUPPLIER INFORMATION

NUCC Instruction Manual available at: www.nucc.org *PLEASE PRINT OR TYPE* OMB APPROVAL PENDING

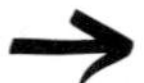

- Click **Close Chart** when finished to return to the Billing and Coding area.
- Click the exit arrow at the lower right corner of the screen to go to the Summary Menu.
- On the Summary Menu, click **Return to Map**.
- From the patient list, select **John R. Simmons**.
- On the office map, highlight and click on **Billing and Coding** to enter the Billing and Coding area.
- Click on **Charts** to open Dr. Simmons' medical records.
- Review Dr. Simmons' chart as needed to complete question 2.

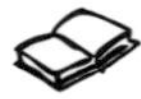

2. John R. Simmons has Teacher's Health Insurance coverage. Using the source documents in Dr. Simmons' chart and the guidelines for completion of a CMS-1500 claim form (see Chapter 5 in your textbook), complete blocks 1 through 33 of the CMS-1500 claim form on the next page. Report the appropriate ICD-9-CM and CPT codes.

HEALTH INSURANCE CLAIM FORM

APPROVED BY NATIONAL UNIFOR MCLAIM COMMITTEE (NUCC) 02/12

PICA　　　　PICA

CARRIER

1. MEDICARE (Medicare#) MEDICAID (Medicaid#) TRICARE (ID#DoD#) CHAMPVA (Member ID#) GROUP HEALTH PLAN (ID#) FECA BLK LUNG (ID#) OTHER (ID#)

1a. INSURED'S I.D. NUMBER (For Program in Item 1)

2. PATIENT'S NAME (Last Name, First Name, Middle Initial)

3. PATIENT'S BIRTH DATE MM DD YY SEX M F

4. INSURED'S NAME (Last Name, First Name, Middle Initial)

5. PATIENT'S ADDRESS (No., Street)

6. PATIENT RELATIONSHIP TO INSURED Self Spouse Child Other

7. INSURED'S ADDRESS (No., Street)

CITY STATE

8. RESERVED FOR NUCC USE

CITY STATE

ZIP CODE TELEPHONE (Include Area Code) ( )

ZIP CODE TELEPHONE (Include Area Code) ( )

9. OTHER INSURED'S NAME (Last Name, First Name, Middle Initial)

10. IS PATIENT'S CONDITION RELATED TO:

11. INSURED'S POLICY GROUP OR FECA NUMBER

a. OTHER INSURED'S POLICY OR GROUP NUMBER

a. EMPLOYMENT? (Current or Previous) YES NO

a. INSURED'S DATE OF BIRTH MM DD YY SEX M F

b. RESERVED FOR NUCC USE

b. AUTO ACCIDENT? YES NO PLACE (State)

b. OTHER CLAIM ID (Designated by NUCC)

c. RESERVED FOR NUCC USE

c. OTHER ACCIDENT? YES NO

c. INSURANCE PLAN NAME OR PROGRAM NAME

d. INSURANCE PLAN NAME OR PROGRAM NAME

10d. CLAIM CODES (Designated by NUCC)

d. IS THERE ANOTHER HEALTH BENEFIT PLAN? YES NO *If yes*, complete items 9, 9a, and 9d.

READ BACK OF FORM BEFORE COMPLETING & SIGNING THIS FORM.

12. PATIENT'S OR AUTHORIZED PERSON'S SIGNATUREI authorize the release of any medical or other information necessary to process this claim. I also request payment of government benefits either to myself or to the party who accepts assignment below.

SIGNED ______ DATE ______

13. INSURED'S OR AUTHORIZED PERSON'S SIGNATURE I authorize payment of medical benefits to the undersigned physician or supplier for services described below.

SIGNED ______

PATIENT AND INSURED INFORMATION

14. DATE OF CURRENT: ILLNESS, INJURY, or PREGNANCY(LMP) MM DD YY QUAL.

15. OTHER DATE QUAL. MM DD YY

16. DATES PATIENT UNABLE TO WORK IN CURRENT OCCUPATION FROM MM DD YY TO MM DD YY

17. NAME OF REFERRING PROVIDER OR OTHER SOURCE

17a.

17b. NPI

18. HOSPITALIZATION DATES RELATED TO CURRENT SERVICES FROM MM DD YY TO MM DD YY

19. ADDITIONAL CLAIM INFORMATION (Designated by NUCC)

20. OUTSIDE LAB? YES NO $ CHARGES

21. DIAGNOSIS OR NATURE OF ILLNESS OR INJURY Relate A-L to service line below (24E) ICD Ind.

A. ____ B. ____ C. ____ D. ____

E. ____ F. ____ G. ____ H. ____

I. ____ J. ____ K. ____ L. ____

22. RESUBMISSION CODE ORIGINAL REF. NO.

23. PRIOR AUTHORIZATION NUMBER

	24. A. DATE(S) OF SERVICE From MM DD YY To MM DD YY	B. PLACE OF SERVICE	C. EMG	D. PROCEDURES, SERVICES, OR SUPPLIES (Explain Unusual Circumstances) CPT/HCPCS MODIFIER	E. DIAGNOSIS POINTER	F. $ CHARGES	G. DAYS OR UNITS	H. EPSDT Family Plan	I. ID QUAL.	J. RENDERING PROVIDER ID. #
1									NPI	
2									NPI	
3									NPI	
4									NPI	
5									NPI	
6									NPI	

PHYSICIAN OR SUPPLIER INFORMATION

25. FEDERAL TAX I.D. NUMBER SSN EIN

26. PATIENT'S ACCOUNT NO.

27. ACCEPT ASSIGNMENT? (For govt. claims, see back) YES NO

28. TOTAL CHARGE $

29. AMOUNT PAID $

30. Rsvd for NUCC Use $

31. SIGNATURE OF PHYSICIAN OR SUPPLIER INCLUDING DEGREES OR CREDENTIALS (I certify that the statements on the reverse apply to this bill and are made a part thereof.)

SIGNED DATE

32. SERVICE FACILITY LOCATION INFORMATION

a. NPI b.

33. BILLING PROVIDER INFO & PH # ( )

a. NPI b.

NUCC Instruction Manual available at: www.nucc.org　　*PLEASE PRINT OR TYPE*　　OMB APPROVAL PENDING

- Click **Close Chart** when finished to return to the Billing and Coding area.
- Click the exit arrow at the lower right corner of the screen to go to the Summary Menu.
- On the Summary Menu, click **Return to Map** to continue to the next lesson or click **Exit the Program**.

LESSON 16

The Claims Process

Reading Assignment: Chapter 14—The Patient

Patients: Rhea Davison, Shaunti Begay, Jean Deere

Learning Objectives:

- Identify methods to meet and exceed self-pay patient expectations.
- Identify the self-pay patient and establish appropriate billing and collection procedures for them.
- Understand the importance of keeping patients informed of billing policies and procedures.
- Provide billing and collection tips and techniques.
- Identify laws affecting credit and collection.
- Understand general accounting principles related to all patient transactions.

Overview:

This lesson addresses patient management, including billing policies and practices. Learning opportunities include recognizing acceptable methods for minimizing appointment delays, keeping patients informed, following the procedure for legally terminating the patient-physician relationship, and understanding acceptable collection procedures.

You will view Rhea Davison's check-in video to determine whether the patient's expectations were met and explore methods in exceeding self-pay patient expectations. Next, you will view Shaunti Begay's check-in and check-out videos to identify acceptable collection procedures. You will also view Jean Deere's check-in and check-out videos to identify specific issues related to aging patients and identify methods for meeting their expectations. Finally, you will complete exercises related to the recording of patient transactions.

Exercise 1

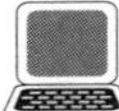

Online Activity—Meeting the Self-Pay Patient's Expectations

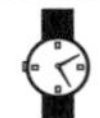

45 minutes

- Sign in to Mountain View Clinic.
- From the patient list, select **Rhea Davison**.

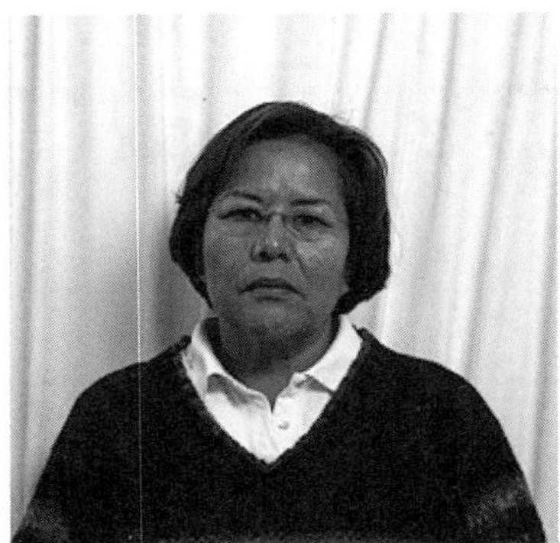

- On the office map, highlight and click on **Reception** to enter the Reception area.

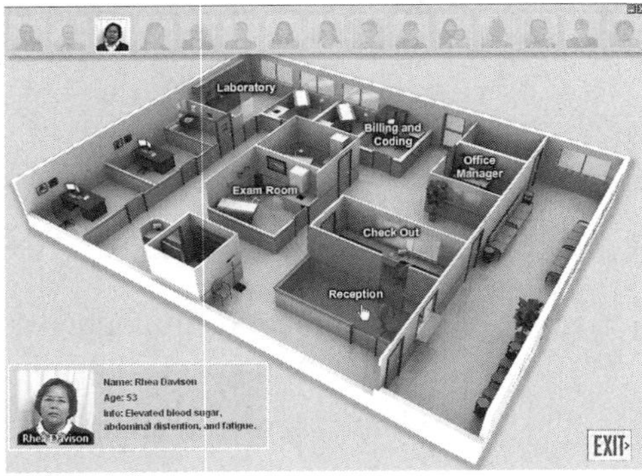

- Under the Watch heading, click on **Patient Check-In** to view the video.

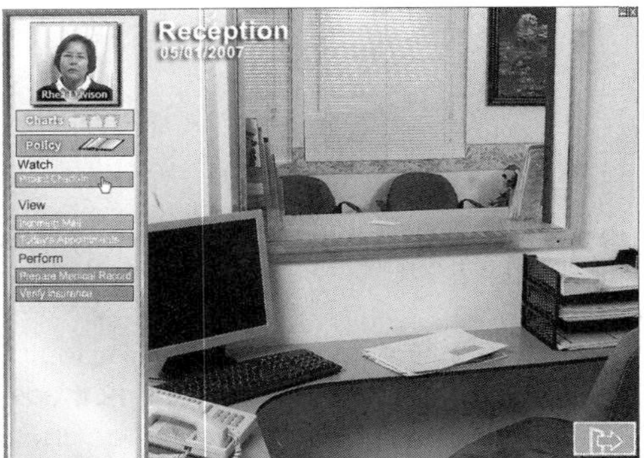

1. The initial part of the check-in process for an established patient such as Ms. Davison is to verify the patient's insurance coverage as identified on the Patient Information Form. Ms. Davison's insurance coverage is confirmed as "self-pay," which means:
   a. Ms. Davison has deliberately tried to avoid paying her bill.
   b. Ms. Davison's insurance will pay her directly and she will then pay the provider.
   c. Ms. Davison has exceeded her health insurance benefits.
   d. Ms. Davison has inadequate health insurance coverage or no insurance at all.

2. During Rhea Davison's check-in process, she is told that Kristin is "certified." Kristin's certification seems to affect Ms. Davison's judgment in a positive way about the quality of care she will receive from the office and seems to put her mind at ease. This concept is referred to as having:
   a. peace of mind.
   b. a surrogate.
   c. reassurance.
   d. tangible services.

3. During the check-in process, Kristin advises Ms. Davison of several policies at Mountain View Clinic. Which of the following policies/procedures are addressed in the check-in video? Select all that apply.

   _____ Late arrival policy—if the patient is 15 minutes late or more, the clinic will reschedule the appointment.

   _____ Late arrival policy—there is a $25 charge for a late arrival.

   _____ Privacy policy—the entire clinic staff adheres to HIPAA confidentiality standards for all patients coming to the clinic.

   _____ Payment at time of service policy—all charges for services provided are expected to be paid in full at the time of service.

- At the end of the video, click **Close** to return to the Reception area.
- Click on **Policy** to open the office Policy Manual and review as needed to answer the next questions.

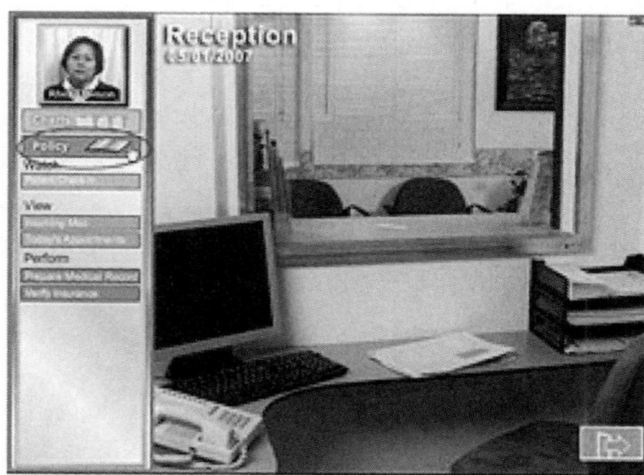

4. In the Mountain View Clinic Policy Manual, the section titled "Telephone Policy" states that patients should be reminded that any payment due is expected:
   a. before the scheduled appointment.
   b. at the time the service is rendered.
   c. within 30 days after the service is provided.
   d. within 60 days after the service is provided.

5. In Mountain View Clinic's Policy Manual, the "Patient Insurance Policy" states that if a patient does not have insurance coverage, he or she should be advised of the charges when the appointment is made and provided with a detailed statement of all charges after services have been provided. A detailed statement of charges could be provided to the patient with a copy of the:
   a. Assignment of Benefits Form.
   b. Patient Information Form.
   c. Encounter Form.
   d. Progress Note.

6. According to the "Billing Schedule" outlined in the Mountain View Clinic Policy Manual, Ms. Davison can expect to receive a statement of her outstanding balance:
   a. every day.
   b. every week.
   c. every 30 days.
   d. every 60 days.

7. If Ms. Davison does not make any payment on her account within 120 days from the date of service, Mountain View Clinic's policy is to:
   a. make a telephone call to Ms. Davison requesting payment within 7 to 10 days.
   b. turn the account over to a collection agency.
   c. write off the balance of the bill as uncollectible debt.
   d. file a small claims suit for the delinquent account.

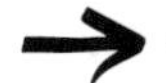

- Click **Close Manual** to return to the Reception area.
- Click the exit arrow to go to the Summary Menu.
- On the Summary Menu, click **Return to Map**.
- On the office map, highlight and click on **Check Out** to enter the Check Out area.

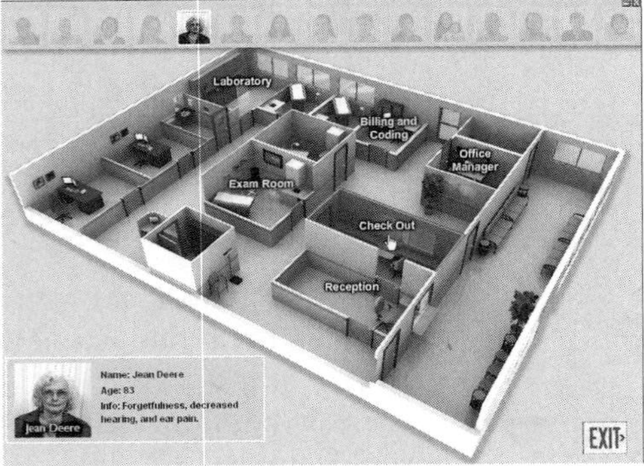

- Under the Watch heading, click on **Patient Check-Out** to view the video.
- At the end of the video, click **Close** to return to the Check Out area.

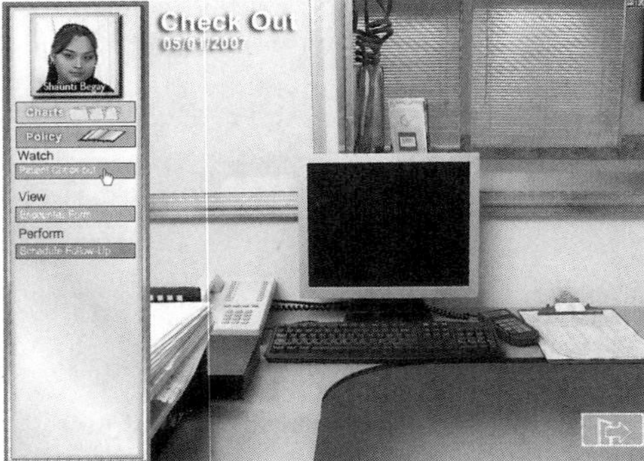

8. Based on the conversation with Ms. Davison at check-out, it appears that credit arrangements and a payment plan have been established. It is important for the health insurance professional to keep in mind that an installment payment plan of more than four payments comes under the federal Truth in Lending Act of 1968, which requires that the business disclose:
   a. any monthly finance charges.
   b. the date when payments are due.
   c. the amount of any late-payment charges.
   d. all of the above.

9. If Ms. Davison stops making payments on her bill, the physicians at Mountain View Clinic can terminate their patient-provider relationship as long as the termination is carried out within the confines of the law. Which of the following actions must be taken in order to do this legally and avoid any accusation of "abandonment"? Select all that apply.

_____ The patient must be sent a letter stating that he or she can no longer be treated by the clinic.

_____ The letter must be sent by certified mail with a return receipt to prove the patient received the communication.

_____ The clinic must write off any outstanding balance.

_____ The clinic must allow a specified time for the patient to find an alternative caregiver.

_____ The clinic must inform the new care provider of the reason for patient-provider termination.

_____ The letter sent to the patient must state the reason why the clinic or physician is terminating the patient-provider relationship.

10. Based on the check-in and check-out videos, do you think the staff at Mountain View Clinic met (or exceeded) Ms. Davison's expectations as a self-pay patient?

- Click the exit arrow to leave the Check Out area and return to the map.
- On the map, click on **Billing and Coding**.
- In the Billing and Coding area, access Ms. Davison's **Encounter Form** and the office's **Fee Schedule**.

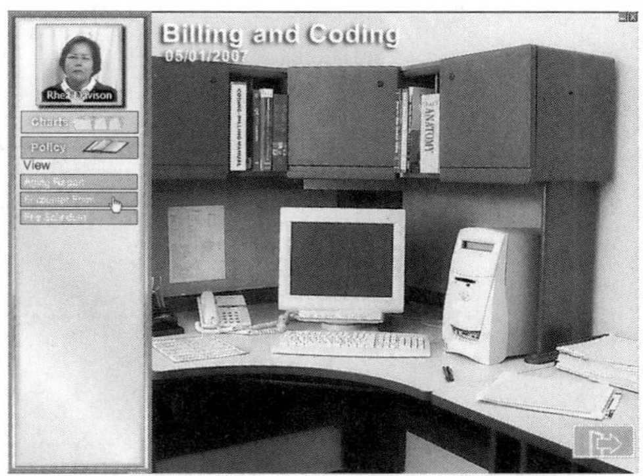

11. Using the information on Ms. Davison's Encounter Form, complete the following ledger card. Include all charges and payments for her visit to Mountain View Clinic on this date.

Mountain View Clinic
Patient Ledger

DATE:
Patient ID:
Patient Name:
Insurance Type:

Date	Professional Service	Fee ($)	Payment ($)	Adj. ($)	Prev. Bal. ($)	New Balance ($)
	Totals					

- Click the exit arrow at the lower right corner of the screen to go to the Summary Menu.
- On the Summary Menu, click **Return to Map** to continue to the next exercise.

Exercise 2

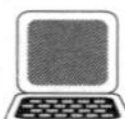

Online Activity—Performing Acceptable Collection Procedures

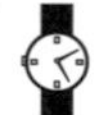

30 minutes

- From the patient list, select **Shaunti Begay**. (*Note:* If you have exited the program, sign in again to Mountain View Clinic and select Shaunti Begay as your patient.)

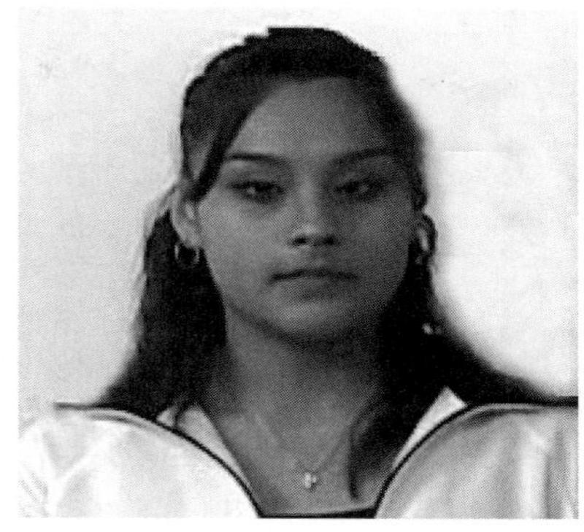

- On the office map, highlight and click on **Reception** to enter the Reception area.

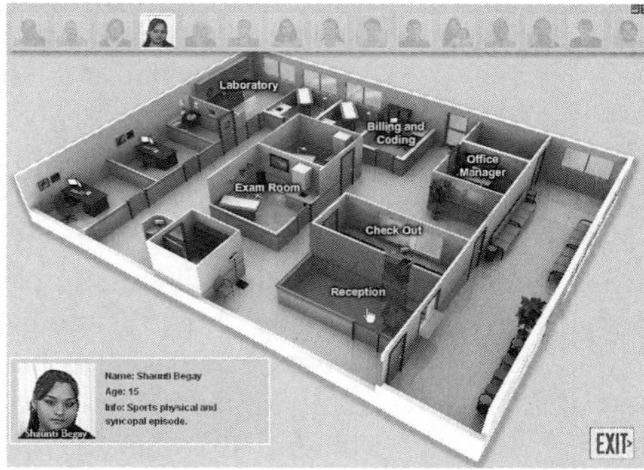

- Under the Watch heading, click on **Patient Check-In** to view the video.

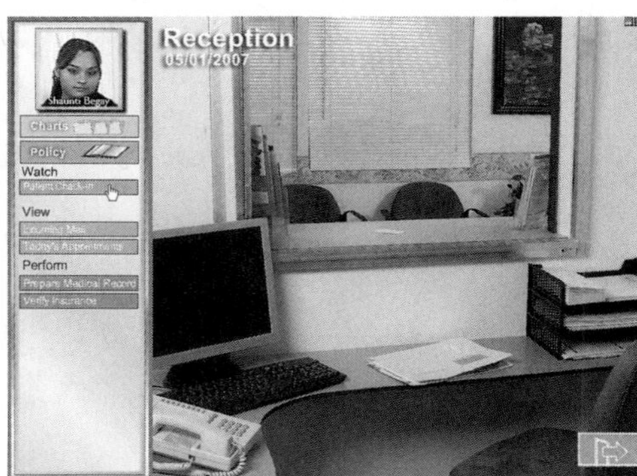

- At the end of the video, click **Close** to return to the Reception area.
- Click the exit arrow at the lower right corner of the screen to go to the Summary Menu.
- On the Summary Menu, click **Return to Map**.
- On the office map, highlight and click on **Check Out** to enter the Check Out area.

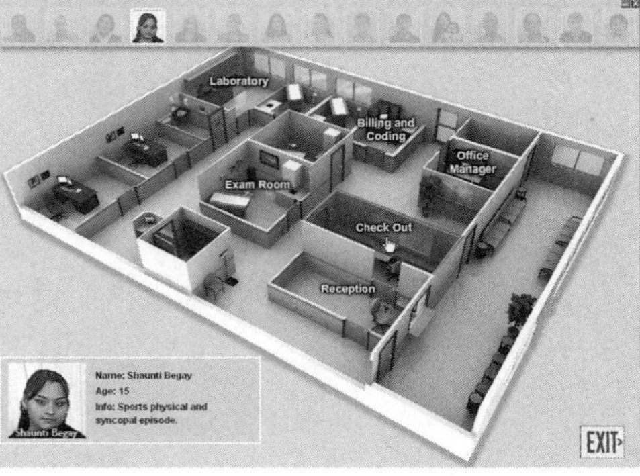

- Under the Watch heading, click on **Patient Check-Out** to view the video.
- At the end of the video, click the **X** in the upper right corner to return to the Check Out area.

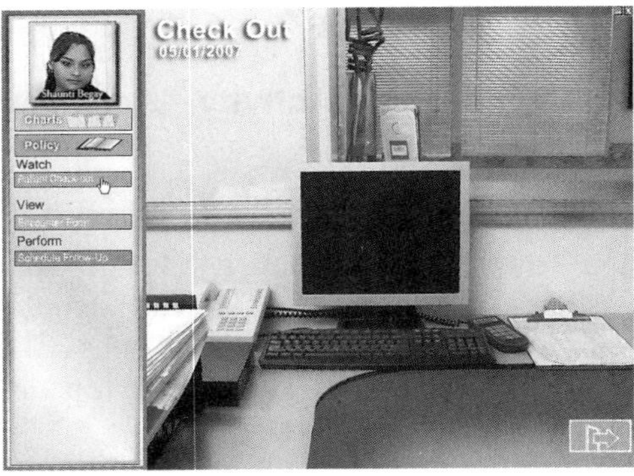

1. What mistake was made by Mountain View Clinic when the appointment for Shaunti Begay was scheduled related to payment of the services she received?
   a. The staff member did not ask what type of insurance the patient had.
   b. The staff member did not did not confirm whether the practice participated with Shaunti's insurance.
   c. The staff member did not call Shaunti's insurance to confirm her benefits.
   d. No mistake was made by the clinic; the patient's mother did not know the name of her insurance carrier at the time.

2. Based on what occurred in the video, think about ways to improve the staff's handling of the initial interaction with Shaunti's mother when she called to schedule her daughter's appointment. What actions by the staff would have been advisable to address the cost of Shaunti's health care up front and help to meet the Begay's expectations?
   a. Provide Shaunti's mother with an approximate cost of what the initial fee would be
   b. Advise Shaunti's mother that payment would be expected at time of service
   c. Explain insurance "participation" and how it would affect payment of services; then ask Shaunti's mother to call back to schedule the appointment once she has the name of her insurance carrier
   d. Do all of the above

3. The clinic has asked you to establish a policy for increasing financial success. Which of the following are appropriate for inclusion in this policy? Select all that apply.

   _____ Discussing payment policies when a patient telephones for an appointment

   _____ Sending statements promptly

   _____ Establishing an action plan for bills over 30 days old

   _____ Sending a statement to the patient's place of employment

   _____ Calling or sending a letter to the patient/debtor if payment has not been received within 60 days

   _____ Calling the patient early in the morning before he or she leaves for work to make sure you are successful in reaching the patient at home

   _____ Insisting that all copayments are paid at the time services are provided

4. Let's assume that 3 months have passed and Mr. Begay has not made further payment on this account. Name four methods the clinic staff could use to collect this outstanding account.

5. In which of the following ways would the Fair Debt Collection Practices Act affect the efforts of the clinic staff to collect this outstanding balance from Mr. Begay? Select all that apply.

_____ Unless the court or the debtor consents, collection calls may not be made at any time that is unusual or inconvenient to the consumer—that is, before 8 a.m. or after 9 p.m.

_____ Clinic staff members may not call Mr. Begay if he informs them that he has hired an attorney.

_____ If Ms. Begay informs the staff that she is ill, collection calls may not be made.

_____ If there is a change of address, collection calls may not be made.

_____ If Mr. Begay's employer prohibits phone calls to him at work, no calls can be made to him there.

6. After the clinic has made numerous attempts to collect the outstanding balance from Mr. Begay, it is determined that a small claims suit should be launched. Identify the steps involved in small claims litigation. Select all that apply.

_____ Acquire correct forms and instructions for completing them.

_____ Enter all necessary information on the forms.

_____ Attach any applicable documentation that provides amount and proof of debt.

_____ Send a copy of the completed forms to the patient/debtor.

_____ Return completed forms (and copies) to the court office.

_____ Provide patient/debtor with the filing fee.

_____ Appear in court on the required date to substantiate the case.

_____ Ask the sheriff's office to collect the total amount from the debtor.

7. Based on the check-in and check-out videos, do you think the staff at Mountain View Clinic met (or exceeded) the expectations of Shaunti Begay and her parents?

- Click the exit arrow to leave the Check Out area and return to the map.
- On the map, click on **Billing and Coding**.
- In the Billing and Coding area, access Shaunti Begay's **Encounter Form** and the office's **Fee Schedule** as needed to complete the following question.

8. Using the information on Shaunti Begay's Encounter Form, complete the following ledger card. Include all charges and payments for her visit to Mountain View Clinic on this date.

Mountain View Clinic
Patient Ledger

DATE:
Patient ID:
Patient Name:
Insurance Type:

Date	Professional Service	Fee ($)	Payment ($)	Adj. ($)	Prev. Bal. ($)	New Balance ($)
	Totals					

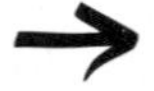

- Click the exit arrow at the lower right corner of the screen to go to the Summary Menu.
- On the Summary Menu, click **Return to Map** to continue to the next exercise.

Exercise 3

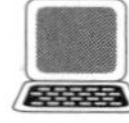

Online Activity—Meeting the Expectations of the Aging Population

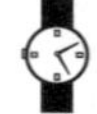

30 minutes

- From the patient list, select **Jean Deere**. (*Note:* If you have exited the program, sign in again to Mountain View Clinic and select Jean Deere as your patient.)

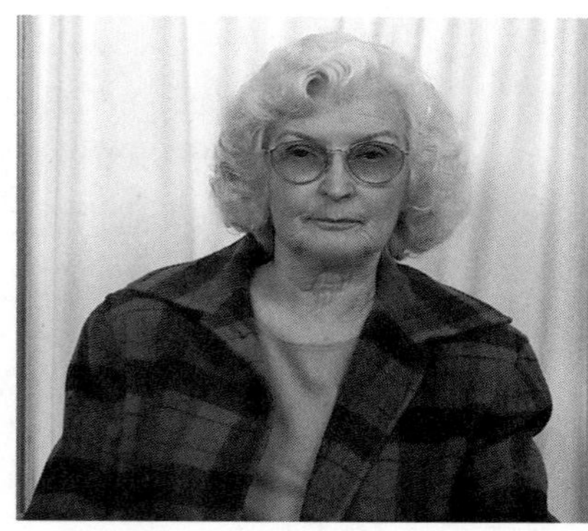

- On the office map, highlight and click on **Reception** to enter the Reception area.

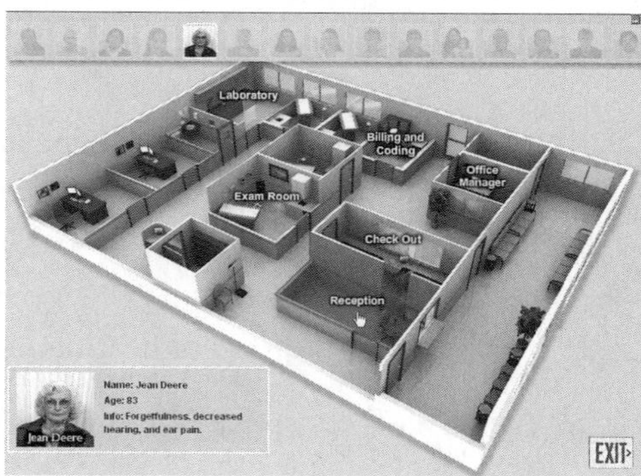

- Under the Watch heading, click on **Patient Check-In** to view the video.

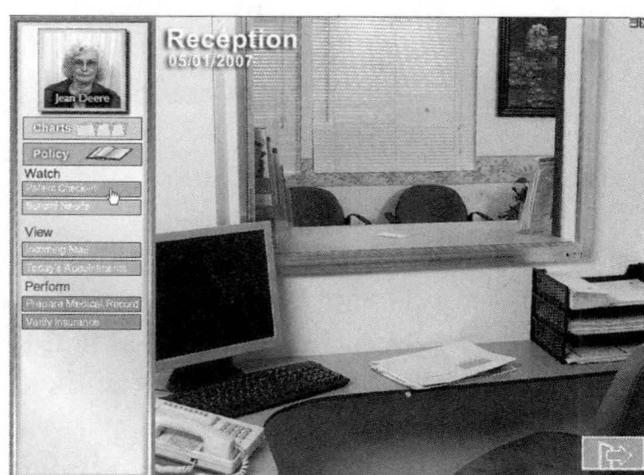

- At the end of the video, click **Close** to return to the Reception area.
- Click the exit arrow at the lower right corner of the screen to go to the Summary Menu.
- On the Summary Menu, click **Return to Map**.
- On the office map, highlight and click on **Check Out** to enter the Check Out area.

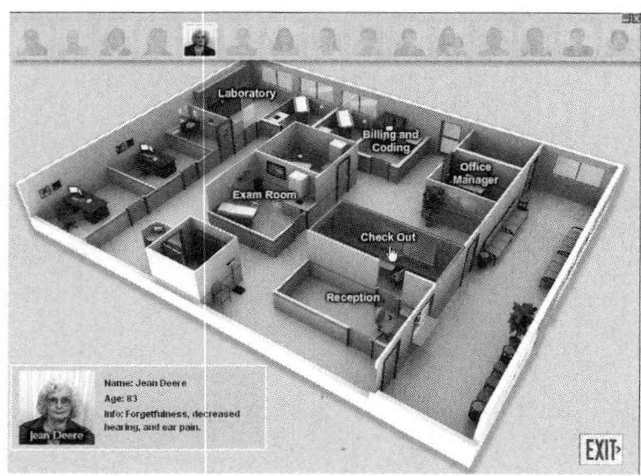

- Under the Watch heading, click on **Patient Check-Out** to view the video.
- At the end of the video, click **Close** to return to the Check Out area.

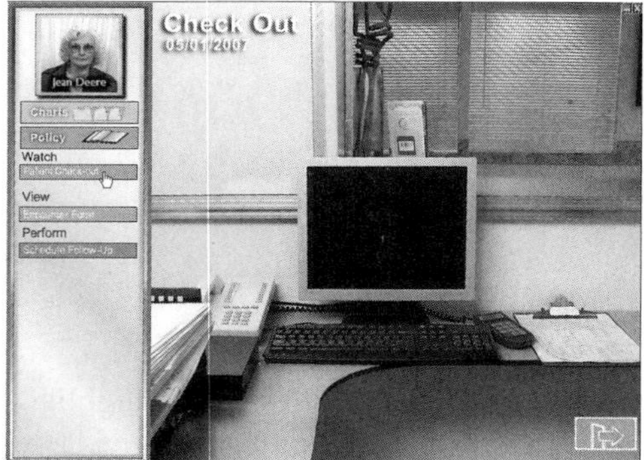

1. When dealing with older adult patients, the health insurance professional will need particular skills that may be quite different from those needed to deal with younger patients. Identify all of Jean Deere's special needs that the health insurance professional must take into consideration.

 _____ Hard of hearing

 _____ Poor vision

 _____ Moves slowly with a walker

 _____ Poor memory

 _____ Irritable

2. According to Jean Deere's Patient Information Form, she has Medicare coverage and Oasis Health Supplement. Therefore the health insurance professional should keep the patient informed of professional fees by stating:
 a. not to worry about them, she has insurance coverage.
 b. that the practice will bill Medicare and Oasis Health Supplement for the services and will advise the patient if there is any balance.
 c. that she is responsible for the balance, regardless of the type of insurance she has.
 d. that all balances are due at the time of service; if payment is made by the insurance, the practice will refund the money to her.

3. Upon submission of Jean Deere's claim to Oasis Health Supplement for the balance after Medicare, the health insurance professional is notified that the patient has terminated her coverage with Oasis Health Supplement and they have denied the claim. What is the next step the health insurance professional should take?
   a. Bill the patient for the balance.
   b. Write off the balance.
   c. Request an appeal of the claim.

4. Before Ms. Deere received any services on this visit, was she made aware that any balances due to Mountain View Clinic would be her responsibility?
   a. Yes
   b. No

5. Let's assume that amount of Ms. Deere's patient responsibility is quite large once it is discovered that she no longer has Oasis Health Supplement coverage to pick up the balance after Medicare. The practice decides that because of her age, they do not want to extend credit to her. What law would prevent them from denying her credit based on her age?
   a. Truth in Lending Act
   b. Fair Credit Billing Act
   c. Equal Credit Opportunity Act
   d. Fair Debt Collection Practices Act.

6. Based on the check-in and check-out videos, do you think the staff at Mountain View Clinic met (or exceeded) the expectations of Jean Deere?

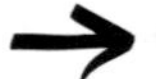

- Click the exit arrow to leave the Check Out area and return to the map.
- On the map, click on **Billing and Coding**.
- In the Billing and Coding area, access Jean Deere's **Encounter Form** and the office's **Fee Schedule** as needed to complete the next question.

7. Using the information on Jean Deere's Encounter Form, complete the following ledger card. Include all charges and payments for her visit to Mountain View Clinic on this date.

Mountain View Clinic
Patient Ledger

DATE:
Patient ID:
Patient Name:
Insurance Type:

Date	Professional Service	Fee ($)	Payment ($)	Adj. ($)	Prev. Bal. ($)	New Balance ($)
	Totals					

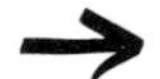

- Click the exit arrow at the lower right corner of the screen to go to the Summary Menu.
- On the Summary Menu, click **Return to Map**.

Exercise 4

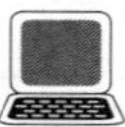

Online Activity—Recording Daily Patient Transactions

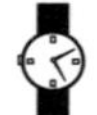

30 minutes

This exercise is a group activity to be performed with the assistance of your instructor.

1. Using the information you recorded on the patient ledger cards for Rhea Davison, Shaunti Begay, and Jean Deere earlier in this lesson, complete the day sheet on the next page by recording each patient's transactions, including any previous balances, charges, payments, and current balances for the day.

Mountain View Clinic
Daysheet

Date	Professional Service	Fee	Payment	Adjustment	New Balance	Old Balance	Patient's Name	Distribution: Dr. Hayler	Distribution: Dr. Meyer
	TOTALS						TOTALS		

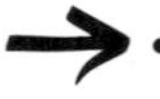

- Return to the Office Map and select Jean Deere as your patient.
- Highlight and click on **Reception** to enter the Reception area.

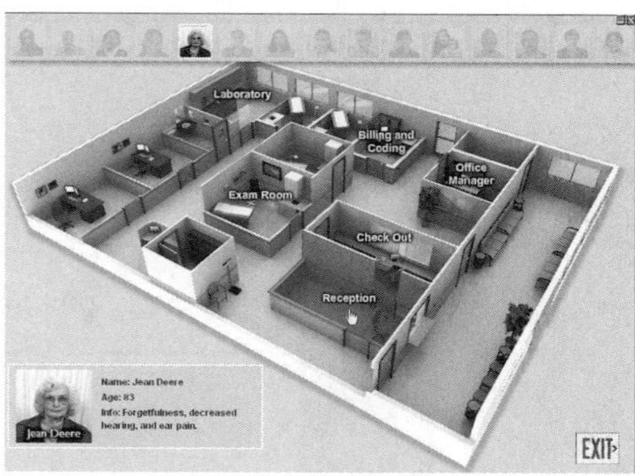

- Under the View heading, click on **Incoming Mail** to view the mail received by the clinic.

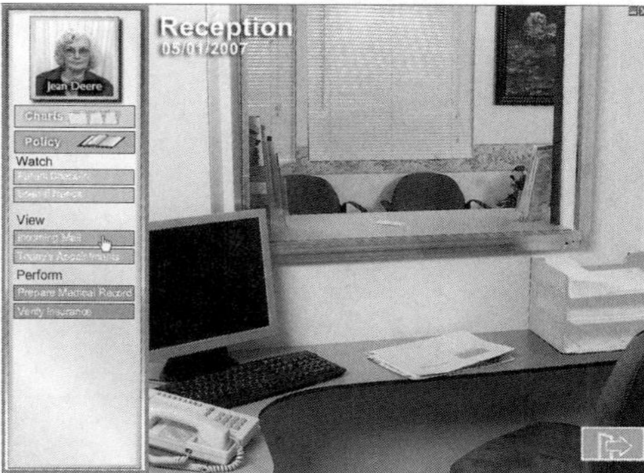

- Click the numbers or arrows at the top of the page to examine and read each piece of mail.

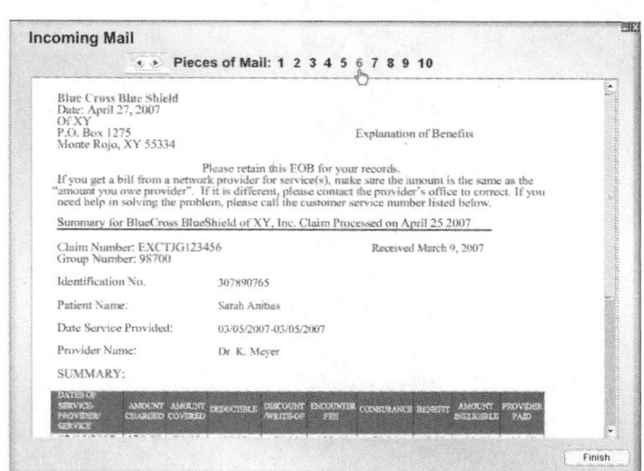

2. On the next page, post to the day sheet any payments that were received in the incoming mail.

Mountain View Clinic
Daysheet

Date	Professional Service	Fee	Payment	Adjustment	New Balance	Old Balance	Patient's Name	Distribution	
								Dr. Hayler	Dr. Meyer
	TOTALS						TOTALS		

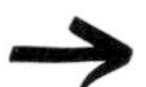

- Click **Finish** to return to the Reception area.
- Click the exit arrow at the lower right corner of the screen to go to the Summary Menu.
- On the Summary Menu, click **Return to Map** to continue to the next lesson or click **Exit the Program**.

LESSON 17

Successful Claims Processing

Reading Assignment: Chapter 15—Keys to Successful Claims Management

Patients: Wilson Metcalf, Renee Anderson, Louise Parlet

Learning Objectives:

- Identify the steps of the claims process.
- Track a claim.
- Post charges and payments to patient ledger cards.
- Successfully process claim denials and appeals.
- Complete blocks 9 through 9d of the CMS-1500 form for secondary claims.

Overview:

This lesson covers the claims process and the keys to successful claims processing. You will identify the various levels of the Medicare appeals process. You will post payments to patient ledger cards and process claims for patients with secondary insurance coverage. You will also practice calculating payments based on percentages of reimbursement.

Exercise 1

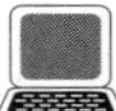

Online Activity—Keys to Successful Claims Processing

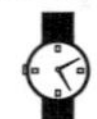

60 minutes

1. Using your textbook, identify the six keys to successful claims submission.

- Sign in to Mountain View Clinic.
- From the patient list, select **Wilson Metcalf**.

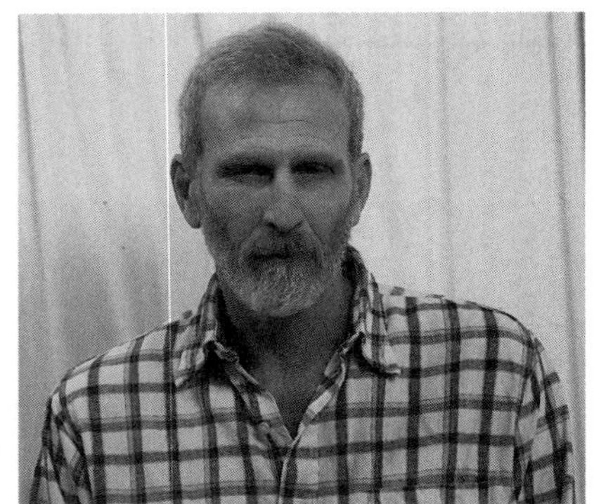

- On the office map, highlight and click on **Billing and Coding** to enter the Billing and Coding area.

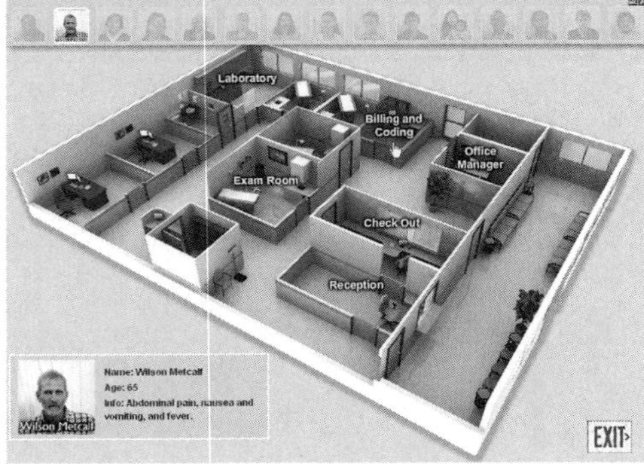

- Click on **Charts** to open Mr. Metcalf's medical record.

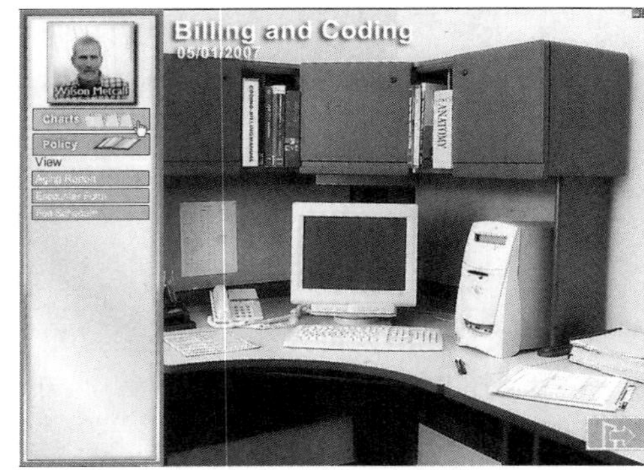

- Review the Patient Information Form (the chart automatically displays this form when first opened).
- Now click on the **Patient Information** tab and select **3-Insurance Cards** from the drop-down menu to review Mr. Metcalf's current insurance cards.

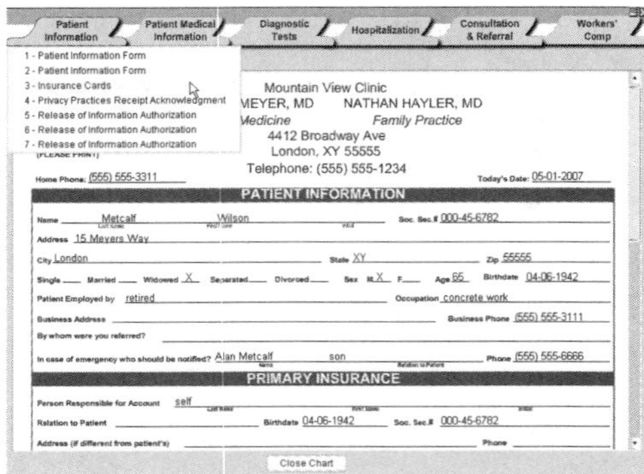

Mountain View Clinic
MEYER, MD NATHAN HAYLER, MD
Medicine Family Practice
4412 Broadway Ave
London, XY 55555
Telephone: (555) 555-1234

Home Phone: (555) 555-3311 Today's Date: 05-01-2007

PATIENT INFORMATION

Name Metcalf Wilson Soc. Sec.# 000-45-6782
Address 15 Meyers Way
City London State XY Zip 55555
Single ___ Married ___ Widowed X Separated ___ Divorced ___ Sex M X F ___ Age 65 Birthdate 04-06-1942
Patient Employed by retired Occupation concrete work
Business Address ___ Business Phone (555) 555-3111
By whom were you referred? ___
In case of emergency who should be notified? Alan Metcalf son Phone (555) 555-6666

PRIMARY INSURANCE

Person Responsible for Account self
Relation to Patient ___ Birthdate 04-06-1942 Soc. Sec.# 000-45-6782
Address (if different from patient's) ___ Phone ___

2. One of the keys to successful claims processing is obtaining the necessary preauthorization or precertification. In reviewing Mr. Metcalf's patient information for the visit on 5/1/2007, note that he is now eligible for Medicare. What is Medicare's rule regarding preauthorization?
   a. Medicare does not require prior authorization for medically necessary services.
   b. Medicare requires preauthorization for office visits only.
   c. Medicare requires preauthorization for all services.
   d. Medicare should be contacted to determine whether prior authorization is required.

3. Indicate whether each of the following statements is true or false.

   a. _________ Because Mr. Metcalf is an established patient with Mountain View Clinic, it is not necessary to verify his insurance information at check-in.

   b. _________ When completing the claim form, the health insurance professional should record the diagnosis code that the provider checked on Mr. Metcalf's Encounter Form without question.

   c. _________ Upon completion of the CMS-1500 claim form for Mr. Metcalf, the health insurance professional should review the completed claim form to ensure that the physician has signed it.

   d. _________ If Medicare receives a clean claim for the service provided to Mr. Metcalf, the claim will be paid in a timely manner.

4. Listed in the right column below are common phrases used to describe various steps of the claims process. Match each phrase with the specific step it refers to.

	Specific Step of the Claims Process	**Common Descriptive Phrase**
_____	Claim is received, dated, and processed through an OCR scanner.	a. Tracking claims
		b. Claims adjudication
_____	The insurance/billing specialist determines how much of the claim was paid, what the patient is responsible for, and/or why some charges were not allowed.	c. Claim arrival at the insurance office
		d. Posting payment
_____	In the provider's office, claims are documented on a columnar form for a follow-up process.	e. Interpreting the EOB
_____	The insurer sends payment and remittance advice to the provider.	f. Receiving payment
_____	Data are entered into the payer's computer system, and proceeds are determined.	
_____	The insurance/billing specialist notes the amount paid by the insurer on the patient's ledger card.	

5. Mr. Metcalf's charge for today's encounter is $45. Assuming he has satisfied his annual deductible and that Medicare's allowable fee for these services is $30, what amount will Medicare pay?

6. How much must Mr. Metcalf pay out-of-pocket for this encounter?

7. Mountain View Clinic is a Medicare PAR provider; therefore what will the amount of the contractual adjustment be?

8. Complete the ledger card below for Mr. Metcalf, posting today's charge, Mr. Metcalf's co-insurance, and Medicare's payment. Also show how the remaining balance, if any, is handled.

Mountain View Clinic
Patient Ledger

DATE:
Patient ID:
Patient Name:
Insurance Type:

Date	Professional Service	Fee ($)	Payment ($)	Adj. ($)	Prev. Bal. ($)	New Balance ($)
	Totals					

9. Let's assume that Medicare has denied this claim for Mr. Metcalf. The health insurance professional at Mountain View Clinic believes this claim has been wrongly denied. What are the five different levels of the Medicare appeals process that the health insurance professional should be familiar with?

10. The health insurance professional must request the Medicare appeal for Mr. Metcalf's claim within __________ days from the date of the original determination for Part A and B appeals.

11. What is the health insurance professional required to do in order to avoid Mr. Metcalf's request for an appeal being denied as a duplicate claim?

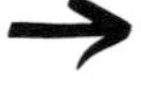

- Click **Close Chart** when finished to return to the Billing and Coding area.
- Click the exit arrow at the lower right corner of the screen to go to the Summary Menu.
- On the Summary Menu, click **Return to Map** and continue to the next exercise.

Exercise 2

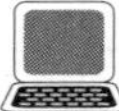

Online Activity—Following the Claim Process

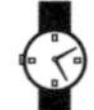

30 minutes

- From the patient list, select **Renee Anderson**. (*Note:* If you have exited the program, sign in again to Mountain View Clinic and select Renee Anderson as your patient.)

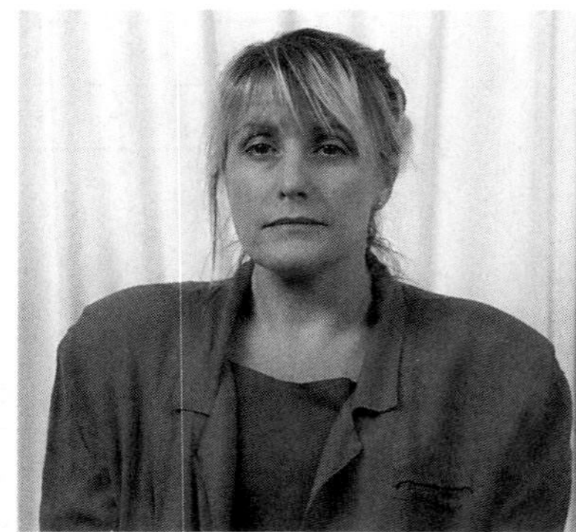

- On the office map, highlight and click on **Billing and Coding** to enter the Billing and Coding area.

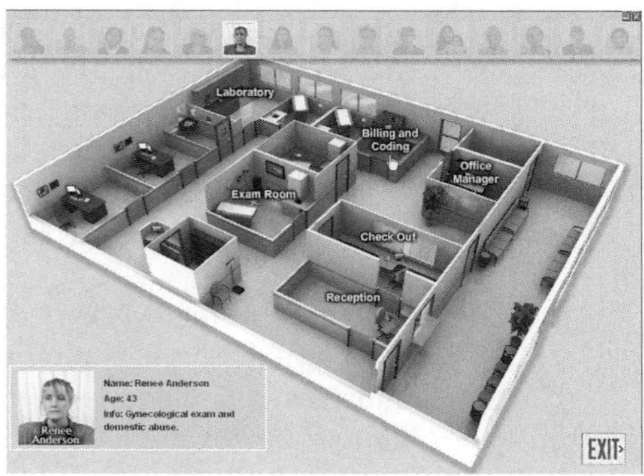

- Click on **Charts** to open Ms. Anderson's medical record.

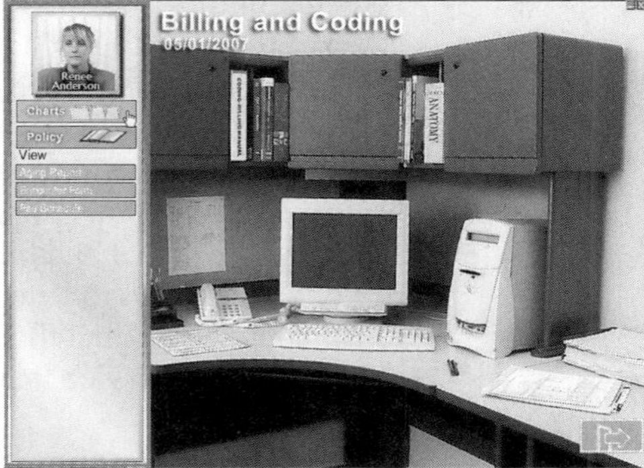

1. Renee Anderson's Patient Information Form states that she has coverage under Blue Cross/Blue Shield. After BC/BS receives the claim from Mountain View Clinic, it will be dated, scanned through an optical character recognition (OCR) device, and undergo a decision-making process by the carrier referred to as:
   a. review.
   b. processing.
   c. adjudication.
   d. appeals.

2. Within what time frame can a response regarding payment on a claim be expected in "real-time adjudication"?
   a. Before the patient leaves the office
   b. Within 2 hours
   c. Within 2 days
   d. Within 2 weeks

3. When preparing Ms. Anderson's claim form, the health insurance professional ensures successful OCR scanning by using:
   a. preprinted black and white CMS-1500 claim forms.
   b. dashes for hyphenated names.
   c. capital letters for all alphabet characters.
   d. red ink to make corrections on claim forms.

4. Assume that Ms. Anderson's claim is returned by Blue Cross/Blue Shield, stating that an error has been made and a correct claim should be prepared and submitted. The health insurance professional should:
   a. correct only the error and resubmit the claim.
   b. correct the error and mark "not duplicate claim" on the claim.
   c. correct the error and mark "for review" on the claim.
   d. correct the error and mark "appeal" on the claim.

5. The health insurance professional should have a mechanism in place to track Ms. Anderson's claim if it is not processed timely by Blue Cross/Blue Shield:
   a. within a week from claim submission.
   b. within 3 weeks from claim submission.
   c. within 4-6 weeks from claim submission.
   d. within 2-3 months from claim submission.

6. In the event that Ms. Anderson's claim is not processed promptly and an inquiry to Blue Cross/Blue Shield is required to determine the status of the unpaid claim, what would be the most efficient and most effective method for the health insurance professional to handle the follow-up?
   a. Contacting the carrier by phone
   b. Resubmitting the claim
   c. Faxing a follow-up claim to the carrier
   d. Copying a system-generated report of unpaid claims and sending it to the carrier

7. In the event that Ms. Anderson's claim is processed and the explanation of benefits (EOB) has denied the claim, the health insurance professional should:
   a. record the denial and bill the patient.
   b. review the EOB to determine why the claim was denied and confirm its legitimacy.
   c. immediately appeal the claim.
   d. write off the service that is denied.

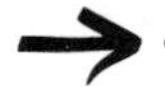

- When finished, click **Close Chart** to return to the Billing and Coding area.
- Under the View heading, click on **Encounter Form** to review the charges for Ms. Anderson's visit.
- You will also need to refer to the **Fee Schedule** as you complete the next question.

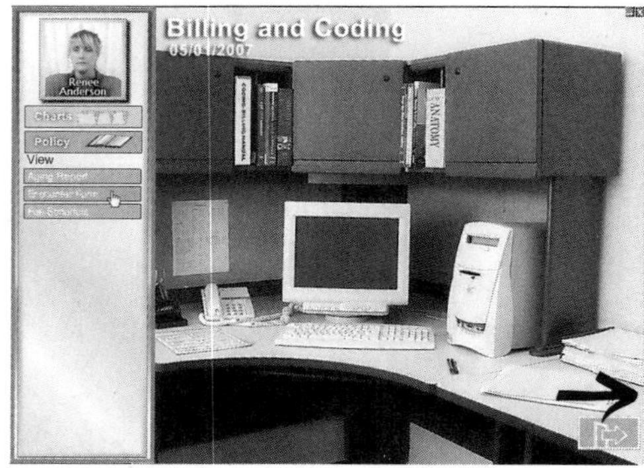

8. The total charge for Renee Anderson's encounter today was $275.00. BC/BS will pay 90% of the remaining charges, and this was filed as a "real time adjudication" claim. On the ledger card below, post today's charges for Ms. Anderson, along with her copayment and the BC/BS payment. Total the columns.

Mountain View Clinic
Patient Ledger

DATE:
Patient ID:
Patient Name:
Insurance Type:

Date	Professional Service	Fee ($)	Payment ($)	Adj. ($)	Prev. Bal. ($)	New Balance ($)
	Totals					

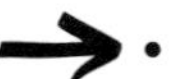

- Click **Finish** to close the Encounter Form and return to the Billing and Coding area.
- Click the exit arrow at the lower right corner of the screen to go to the Summary Menu.
- On the Summary Menu, click **Return to Map** and continue to the next exercise.

Exercise 3

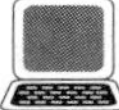

Online Activity—Processing Denials, Appeals, and Secondary Claim Filing

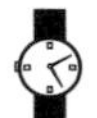

30 minutes

- From the patient list, select **Louise Parlet**. (*Note:* If you have exited the program, sign in again to Mountain View Clinic and select Louise Parlet as your patient.)

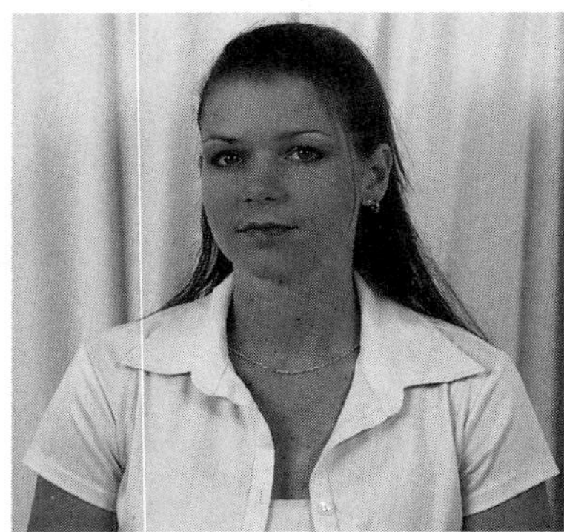

- On the office map, highlight and click on **Billing and Coding** to enter the Billing and Coding area.

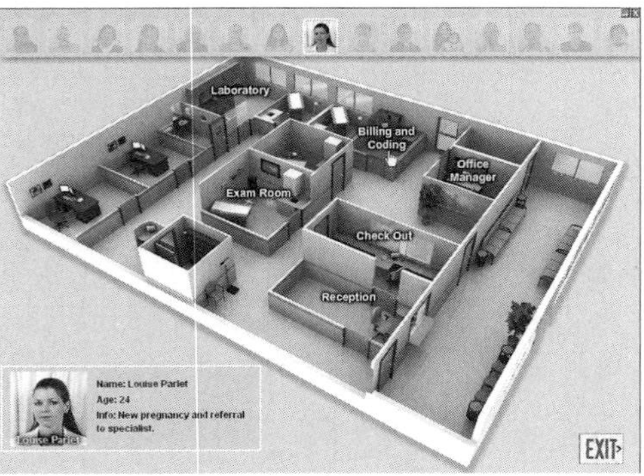

- Click on **Charts** to open Ms. Parlet's medical record.

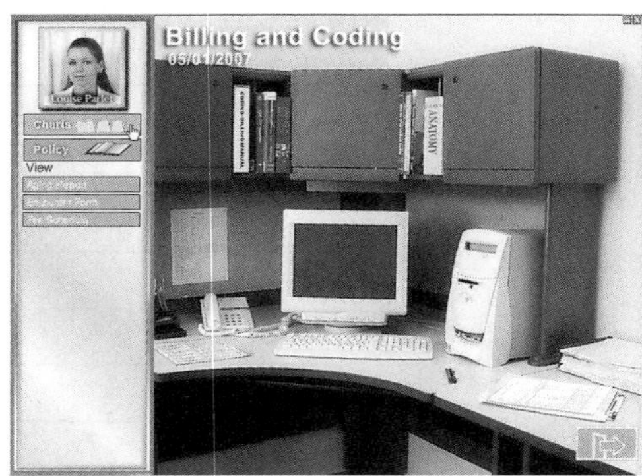

1. Note that Ms. Parlet is covered under two insurance policies, Teachers' Health Group and BC/BS. Fill in the form below with the correct secondary insurance information.

1. MEDICARE ☐ (Medicare#) MEDICAID ☐ (Medicaid#) TRICARE ☐ (ID#DoD#) CHAMPVA ☐ (Member ID#) GROUP HEALTH PLAN ☐ (ID#) FECA BLK LUNG ☐ (ID#) OTHER ☐ (ID#)		1a. INSURED'S I.D. NUMBER (For Program in Item 1)
2. PATIENT'S NAME (Last Name, First Name, Middle Initial)	3. PATIENT'S BIRTH DATE MM DD YY SEX M ☐ F ☐	4. INSURED'S NAME (Last Name, First Name, Middle Initial)
5. PATIENT'S ADDRESS (No., Street)	6. PATIENT RELATIONSHIP TO INSURED Self ☐ Spouse ☐ Child ☐ Other ☐	7. INSURED'S ADDRESS (No., Street)
CITY STATE	8. RESERVED FOR NUCC USE	CITY STATE
ZIP CODE TELEPHONE (Include Area Code) ( )		ZIP CODE TELEPHONE (Include Area Code) ( )
9. OTHER INSURED'S NAME (Last Name, First Name, Middle Initial)	10. IS PATIENT'S CONDITION RELATED TO:	11. INSURED'S POLICY GROUP OR FECA NUMBER
a. OTHER INSURED'S POLICY OR GROUP NUMBER	a. EMPLOYMENT? (Current or Previous) ☐ YES ☐ NO	a. INSURED'S DATE OF BIRTH MM DD YY SEX M ☐ F ☐
b. RESERVED FOR NUCC USE	b. AUTO ACCIDENT? ☐ YES ☐ NO PLACE (State)	b. OTHER CLAIM ID (Designated by NUCC)
c. RESERVED FOR NUCC USE	c. OTHER ACCIDENT? ☐ YES ☐ NO	c. INSURANCE PLAN NAME OR PROGRAM NAME
d. INSURANCE PLAN NAME OR PROGRAM NAME	10d. CLAIM CODES (Designated by NUCC)	d. IS THERE ANOTHER HEALTH BENEFIT PLAN? ☐ YES ☐ NO *If yes*, complete items 9, 9a, and 9d.
READ BACK OF FORM BEFORE COMPLETING & SIGNING THIS FORM. 12. PATIENT'S OR AUTHORIZED PERSON'S SIGNATURE I authorize the release of any medical or other information necessary to process this claim. I also request payment of government benefits either to myself or to the party who accepts assignment below. SIGNED ______	DATE ______	13. INSURED'S OR AUTHORIZED PERSON'S SIGNATURE I authorize payment of medical benefits to the undersigned physician or supplier for services described below. SIGNED ______

2. Let's assume that upon receipt of the EOB for Ms. Parlet's claim (as completed above), the health insurance professional determines that the insurance company has downcoded the claim. This means:
   a. the insurance carrier has denied the claim based on the diagnosis submitted.
   b. the insurance carrier does not recognize the CPT code submitted.
   c. the insurance carrier has assigned a substitute code (one that the carrier believes fits the service performed) at a lower level than reported.
   d. the insurance carrier has requested additional information from the provider.

3. In the event of downcoding by the insurance carrier, the health insurance professional should:
   a. write off the unpaid balance by the insurance carrier.
   b. bill the patient for any unpaid balance by the insurance carrier.
   c. change coding techniques based on the carrier's interpretation of them.
   d. contact the claims adjuster and ask the reason for downcoding.

4. Assume that the EOB for Ms. Parlet's claim indicates that the venipuncture performed (36415) is inclusive in the lab and visit codes reported. This is referred to as:
   a. downcoding.
   b. bundled or integral to the main procedure.
   c. considered to be "medically unnecessary."
   d. a noncovered service.

5. Which resource would the health insurance professional use to determine whether Ms. Parlet's services denied as "inclusive" are appropriate, reasonable, or valid?
   a. Federal Register
   b. Medicare Fee Schedule
   c. Relative Value Unit
   d. National Correct Coding Initiative

6. In the event that the EOB for Ms. Parlet's claim indicates that the claim is denied because the claim was not filed within the time limit set by the insurance carrier, the health insurance professional should immediately:
   a. appeal the claim.
   b. bill the patient.
   c. write off the service.
   d. examine the practice's contract with the insurance carrier to confirm timely filing guidelines and determine whether there any allowances for late filing of claims that may be relevant.

7. If Ms. Parlet's claim must be appealed with the insurance carrier, which of the following is *not* a basic rule for appealing the claim?
   a. Include a copy of the EOB.
   b. Provide additional documentation to support the appeal.
   c. Provide a cover letter.
   d. Contact the state insurance's commissioner.

→ • When finished, click **Close Chart** to return to the Billing and Coding area.
- Click the exit arrow at the lower right corner of the screen to go to the Summary Menu.
- On the Summary Menu, click **Exit the Program**.